Depression

Guest Editor

DAVID L. MINTZ, MD

PSYCHIATRIC CLINICS OF NORTH AMERICA

www.psych.theclinics.com

March 2012 • Volume 35 • Number 1

SAUNDERS an imprint of ELSEVIER, Inc.

W.B. SAUNDERS COMPANY
A Division of Elsevier Inc.

1600 John F. Kennedy Boulevard • Suite 1800 • Philadelphia, PA 19103-2899

http://www.theclinics.com

PSYCHIATRIC CLINICS OF NORTH AMERICA Volume 35, Number 1
March 2012 ISSN 0193-953X, ISBN-13: 978-1-4557-3925-7

Editor: Joanne Husovski
Developmental Editor: Donald Mumford

Psychiatric Clinics of North America (ISSN 0193-953X) is published quarterly by Elsevier Inc., 360 Park Avenue South, New York, NY 10010-1710. Months of issue are March, June, September, and December. Business and Editorial Offices: 1600 John F. Kennedy Blvd., Suite 1800, Philadelphia, PA 19103-2899. Periodicals postage paid at New York, NY and additional mailing offices. Subscription prices are $286.00 per year (US individuals), $504.00 per year (US institutions), $141.00 per year (US students/residents), $347.00 per year (Canadian individuals), $627.00 per year (Canadian Institutions), $431.00 per year (foreign individuals), $627.00 per year (foreign institutions), and $210.00 per year (international & Canadian students/residents). Foreign air speed delivery is included in all *Clinics'* subscription prices. All prices are subject to change without notice. **POSTMASTER:** Send address changes to *Psychiatric Clinics of North America,* Elsevier Health Sciences Division, Subscription Customer Service, 3251 Riverport Lane, Maryland Heights, MO 63043. Customer Service: 1-800-654-2452 (US). From outside the United States, call 1-314-447-8871. Fax: 1-314-447-8029. E-mail: journalscustomerservice-usa@elsevier.com (for print support) and journalsonlinesupport-usa@elsevier.com (for online support).

Reprints. For copies of 100 or more, of articles in this publication, please contact the Commercial Reprints Department, Elsevier Inc., 360 Park Avenue South, New York, New York 10010-1710. Tel.: (212) 633-3813, Fax: (212) 462-1935, E-mail: reprints@elsevier.com.

Psychiatric Clinics of North America is covered in *MEDLINE/PubMed (Index Medicus), Current Contents/Social and Behavioral Sciences, Social Science Citation Index, Embase/Excerpta Medica,* and PsycINFO.

Printed and bound by CPI Group (UK) Ltd, Croydon, CR0 4YY
Transferred to Digital Print 2012

Contributors

GUEST EDITOR

DAVID L. MINTZ, MD
Director of Psychiatric Education, The Austen Riggs Center, Stockbridge, Massachusetts

AUTHORS

SIDNEY J. BLATT, PhD
Departments of Psychiatry and Psychology, Yale University, New Haven, Connecticut

J. MICHAEL BOSTWICK, MD
Professor of Psychiatry, Department of Psychiatry and Psychology, Mayo Clinic College of Medicine, Rochester, Minnesota

FREDRIC N. BUSCH, MD
Clinical Associate Professor of Psychiatry, Weill Cornell Medical College; Faculty, Columbia University Center for Psychoanalytic Training and Research, New York, New York

DANIEL CARLAT, MD
Associate Clinical Professor, Department of Psychiatry, Tufts University School of Medicine, Boston, Massachusetts

YULIA E. CHENTSOVA-DUTTON, PhD
Assistant Professor, Department of Psychology, Georgetown University, Washington, DC

MARY LYNN DELL, MD, DMin
Associate Professor of Psychiatry, Pediatrics, and Bioethics, Case Western Reserve University School of Medicine; Director, Child and Adolescent Psychiatry Consultation Liaison Service, Rainbow Babies and Children's Hospital/University Hospitals Case Medical Center, Cleveland, Ohio

JAMES M. ELLISON, MD, MPH, DFAPA
Associate Professor of Psychiatry, Harvard Medical School, Boston; Clinical Director, Geriatric Psychiatry Program, McLean Hospital, Belmont, Massachusetts

GIOVANNI A. FAVA, MD
Professor of Clinical Psychology, Department of Psychology, University of Bologna, Bologna, Italy; Clinical Professor of Psychiatry, Department of Psychiatry, State University of New York, Buffalo, New York

DAVID F. FLYNN, MD
Staff Psychiatrist, The Austen Riggs Center, Stockbridge, Massachusetts

S. NASSIR GHAEMI, MD
Director, Mood Disorders Program, Tufts Medical Center; Professor of Psychiatry, Tufts University School of Medicine, Boston, Massachusetts

DAVID G. HARPER, PhD
Assistant Professor of Psychology, Department of Psychiatry, Harvard Medical School, Boston; Associate Psychologist, McLean Hospital, Belmont, Massachusetts

GABOR I. KEITNER, MD
Professor, Department of Psychiatry and Human Behavior, The Warren Alpert Medical School of Brown University; Associate Psychiatrist-in-Chief, Department of Psychiatry, Rhode Island Hospital and The Miriam Hospital, Providence, Rhode Island

RONALD C. KESSLER, PhD
Professor, Department of Health Care Policy, Harvard Medical School, Boston, Massachusetts

HELEN H. KYOMEN, MD, MS, DFAPA
Clinical Instructor in Psychiatry, Harvard Medical School; Associate Psychiatrist, McLean Hospital, Belmont; Director of Education and Research for Geriatric Psychiatry, North Shore Medical Center, Salem, Massachusetts

PATRICK LUYTEN, PhD
Department of Psychology, University of Leuven, Leuven, Belgium; Research Department of Clinical, Educational and Health Psychology, University College, London, United Kingdom

ABIGAIL K. MANSFIELD, PhD
Assistant Professor of Psychiatry, Department of Psychiatry and Human Behavior, The Warren Alpert Medical School of Brown University; Psychologist, Department of Psychiatry, Rhode Island Hospital, Providence, Rhode Island

DAVID L. MINTZ, MD
Director of Psychiatric Education, The Austen Riggs Center, Stockbridge, Massachusetts

CHARLES B. NEMEROFF, MD, PhD
Leonard M. Miller Professor and Chairman, and Director, Center on Aging, Department of Psychiatry and Behavioral Sciences, Leonard M. Miller School of Medicine, University of Miami, Miami, Florida

SANDRA RACKLEY, MD
Assistant Professor of Psychiatry and Pediatrics, The George Washington University School of Medicine; Director, Psychiatry Consultation-Liaison and Emergency Department Services, Children's National Medical Center, Washington, DC

ANDREW G. RYDER, PhD
Associate Professor, Department of Psychology, Concordia University; Affiliated Researcher, Culture and Mental Health Research Unit, Sir Mortimer B. Davis—Jewish General Hospital, Montreal, Quebec, Canada

LARRY S. SANDBERG, MD
Clinical Assistant Professor of Psychiatry, Weill Cornell Medical College; Faculty, Columbia University Center for Psychoanalytic Training and Research, New York, New York

RADU V. SAVEANU, MD
Professor and Vice Chairman for Educational Affairs, Director, Psychiatric Residency Training Program, Department of Psychiatry and Behavioral Sciences, Leonard M. Miller School of Medicine, University of Miami, Miami, Florida

NADA L. STOTLAND, MD, MPH
Professor of Psychiatry, Rush Medical College, Chicago, Illinois

DONNA M. SUDAK, MD
Professor of Psychiatry, Director of Psychotherapy Training, Department of Psychiatry, Drexel University College of Medicine, Philadelphia, Pennsylvania

ELENA TOMBA, PhD
Assistant Professor of Clinical Psychology, Department of Psychology, University of Bologna, Bologna, Italy

DERICK E. VERGNE, MD
Clinical Assistant Professor of Psychiatry, Mood Disorders Program, Tufts Medical Center, Tufts University School of Medicine, Boston, Massachusetts

PAUL A. VÖHRINGER, MD
Assistant Professor of Psychiatry, Hospital Clinico, Facultad de Medicina, Universidad de Chile, Santiago, Chile; Research Fellow, Mood Disorders Program, Tufts Medical Center, Tufts University School of Medicine, Boston, Massachusetts

Contents

> Data are reviewed on the societal costs of major depressive disorder (MDD). Early-onset MDD predicts difficulties in subsequent role transitions, including low educational attainment, high risk of teen childbearing, marital disruption, and unstable employment. MDD is also associated with elevated risk of onset, persistence, and severity of a chronic physical disorders as well as with increased early mortality. Although effectiveness trials show that expanded MDD treatment can reverse many of these adverse effects, only a minority of people with MDD receives treatment and the quality of treatment is unacceptably low among the majority of those in treatment.

> Chinese depressed patients emphasize somatic symptoms; this represents one sustained line of evidence-based inquiry about how culture shapes depression. Some explanations highlight cultural variations in experience and expression of symptoms; others emphasize language use and social positioning. We propose an alternative to this dichotomy, starting from a model of culture, mind, and brain as 3 deeply interconnected levels of one system. We can then propose ways in which the social world shapes depressive symptom presentation, including the personal experience of these symptoms. Such a view has potential impact on how mental health professionals think about, study, and treat depression.

> In the past, persistent or chronic symptoms of depression have often been labeled depressive personality. Full recovery from depression is a relatively new concept and therapeutic goal and is difficult to define; however, pursuit is underway for new treatment options for full recovery. These options include more standardized and aggressive treatment with antidepressants; matching patients to specific medications at the outset of treatment using pharmacogenetics, electroencephalography, or other tools; cognitive interventions; treatment of cooccurring disorders including substance abuse; better doctor-patient relationships

and active involvement of patients in selecting and carrying out treatment modalities; and combining of psychopharmacologic and psychotherapeutic treatments.

Efficacy of currently available antidepressants and psychotherapy for treatment of depression is unacceptably low. Development of new treatments is dependent on a comprehensive understanding of genetic and environmental contributions to depression. The authors review new discoveries regarding brain alterations in depression including gene-environment interactions. They demonstrate how molecular neurobiology and structural and functional brain imaging techniques have helped to inform understanding of brain activities. They focus on the association between adverse life events including childhood maltreatment, genetic variations, and the risk for developing major depression, and they discuss how gene-environment interactions and epigenetic modifications may inform treatment choices and modalities.

In this conceptual review, the authors critique the unitary concept of "major depressive disorder" (MDD) and identify four major subtypes: neurotic, mixed, melancholic, and pure depression. The biopsychosocial model is critiqued as leading to an extreme eclecticism which has led to a simplistic acceptance of the unitary view of MDD with little scientific solidity. An alternative to biopsychosocial eclecticism, based on medical humanism, is proposed. The authors advocate a return to careful psychopathology as the basis of all nosology.

Treatment indications that derive from randomized controlled trials and meta-analyses refer to the average patient and often clash with the variety of clinical situations. Clinical judgment should mediate the choice of the main evidence-based treatment ingredients in depression (pharmacotherapy and psychotherapy). For the treatment of the acute episode of unipolar depression, pharmacotherapy appears to be the most viable strategy for most of the patients. For preventing recurrence of depression, the sequential use of pharmacotherapy and psychotherapy, when available, may be the treatment of choice in many cases, though long-term drug treatment or intermittent pharmacotherapy may be applied to other cases.

Cognitive Behavioral Therapy for Depression

Donna M. Sudak

Cognitive–behavioral therapy (CBT) is a valuable treatment for mild, moderate, and severe forms of major depression. It is equally effective and more durable than medication alone, and the combination of medication and CBT may increase the response rate and extend durability when CBT is employed after pharmacotherapy is successful. Behavioral activation, specific CBT strategies for suicidal and hopeless patients, and cognitive restructuring are key components of treatment.

Psychodynamic Treatment of Depression

Patrick Luyten and Sidney J. Blatt

This article reviews the theoretical assumptions of psychodynamic treatments of depression, as well as evidence supporting the efficacy of these interventions. Brief psychoanalytic therapy (BPT) is more effective than control conditions and as effective as other active psychotherapeutic treatments or pharmacotherapy in depression, with effects tending to be maintained in the longer term. The combination of BPT and medication is superior to medication alone. Longer-term psychoanalytic treatment (LTPT) is efficacious for patients suffering from chronic depression and co-morbid personality problems. Together, these findings warrant the inclusion of psychoanalytic therapy as a first-line treatment in depression in adults, children and adolescents.

Evidence-Based Somatic Treatment of Depression in Adults

Daniel Carlat

This article reviews recent studies and controversies about the effectiveness of antidepressant medications for depression. It is divided into three broad topics: (1) the heated controversy regarding how one should interpret "efficacy studies" of antidepressants, that is, the standard placebo-controlled double-blind studies used by drug companies to gain Food and Drug Administration approval; (2) "effectiveness studies," open-label studies enrolling types of patients who are excluded from efficacy studies, focusing on one enormous study in particular—the STAR-D trial; and (3) the evidence base that can guide clinicians in the choice of antidepressants for particular patients.

How (Not What) to Prescribe: Nonpharmacologic Aspects of Psychopharmacology

David L. Mintz and David F. Flynn

From an evidence-based perspective, it has become apparent that pharmacologic treatment of depression has so far fallen short of its promise. One source of disappointing outcomes may be the dearth of attention to psychosocial aspects of the prescribing process. Evidence suggests that how the doctor prescribes may be even more potent than what the doctor prescribes. Providing medications while neglecting effective prescribing behaviors means patients are likely to receive less than optimally effective treatment. This article reviews the psychological and interpersonal mechanisms that can help or hinder pharmacologic treatment outcomes and offers recommendations for enhancing the process of prescribing.

Although multiple medications and some forms of psychotherapy have demonstrated efficacy for major depression, many patients have persistent symptoms and experience relapse. Combination treatment has been employed by clinicians who believe that it provides the maximal potential for sustained remission and increased treatment adherence. Research suggests that although many patients may respond to a single approach, combined treatment should be strongly considered for patients with chronic depression (other than dysthymia), a history of trauma, or accompanying personality disorders. Further studies are essential to better determine the best treatments or combination of treatments for particular depressive disorders.

Whether because of the critical shortage and geographical distribution patterns of child and adolescent psychiatrists, third-party payer constrictions, patient preferences, or the fact that many primary care physicians diagnose and treat depression as a regular part of their medical practices, psychotropic medication prescriptions for youth often are written by clinicians who have not completed child and adolescent psychiatry fellowships. This article reviews information helpful for those prescribing antidepressant medications for pediatric depression, including descriptions of other mental health disciplines partnering in the care of depressed youth; current psychotherapeutic modalities commonly used in treatment; and ethical and regulatory issues inherent to prescribing antidepressant medications for this patient population.

The increasing numbers of older adults who are surviving to more advanced ages and the greater recognition of late-life depression's prevalence emphasize how important it is to detect and treat this disorder. Evidence-based psychotherapeutic, pharmacologic, and neurotherapeutic treatment interventions offer many treatment alternatives, allowing substantial individualization of treatment approach. Demonstration of the effectiveness of depression treatment in primary care suggests the feasibility of increasing our patients' access to care. Growing appreciation of the pathophysiology of depression and its interrelationships with cognitive impairment may increase our ability to limit or delay certain aspects of cognitive impairment through more aggressive treatment of depression.

RELATED INTEREST ARTICLE

Social Science & Medicine, September 1996 (Vol. 43, No. 6, Pages 967-974)
**Age differences among Japanese on the center for epidemiologic studies
depression scale: An ethnocultural perspective on somatization**
Noboru Iwata and Robert E. Roberts

THE CLINICS ARE NOW AVAILABLE ONLINE!

Access your subscription at:
www.theclinics.com

Preface

Integrative Approaches to Depression and Its Treatment

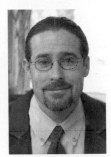

David L. Mintz, MD
Guest Editor

Thomas Kuhn, the noted philosopher of science, tells us that there is a predictable movement of scientific development.[1] During periods of normal science, our understanding grows, and models of understanding become more precise. However, with increasing rigor, it becomes easier to appreciate the limits of any particular explanatory model. The eventual result is what he coined a "paradigm shift." I am hopeful that there is a psychiatric paradigm shift in the making, which seems to be emerging around our treatment of depression.

The last two decades have seen a period of unprecedented scientific development in psychiatry. While overall human knowledge doubles approximately every 33 years, and medical knowledge at least every 19 years,[2] it is immediately obvious that the growth in the neurosciences far outstrips that rate. With increasingly precise tools from the biological sciences, such as genetic testing and neuroimaging, we are unlocking not only the secrets of the brain but also of the mind. The current generation of psychiatrists prescribe medications that have been intelligently designed rather than serendipitously discovered. Against the backdrop of such optimistic growth in the neurosciences (as well as certain economic pressures), the old paradigm, psychoanalysis, was declared dead in the mainstream media and in mainstream psychiatry. The 1990s were, by Presidential proclamation, the "Decade of the Brain."

Now we are in an era of evidence-based practice. The quality of evidence that we have is often better, and the consumers of that evidence are more sophisticated. One consequence of the focus on evidence is the growing recognition that mainstream approaches to depression have fallen far short of our optimism for those treatments. Analysis of our entire research corpus on antidepressant treatment suggests that, while our treatments are effective, in general they hold only a slight edge over placebo for the average patient.

Psychiatr Clin N Am 35 (2012) xiii–xvi
doi:10.1016/j.psc.2012.01.002
0193-953X/12/$ – see front matter © 2012 Elsevier Inc. All rights reserved.

psych.theclinics.com

Just as psychoanalysis was once declared dead, major media outlets such as *Newsweek*,[3] *The Wall Street Journal*,[4] *New Yorker Magazine*,[5] *Salon.com*,[6] and *The New York Times*[7] have all recently run features that question the utility of psychopharmacology and challenge psychiatric overreliance on antidepressant medications. Increasingly, we are hearing these concerns in our clinics and consulting rooms.

In the two most recent volumes of the *Psychiatric Clinics of North America* to address the topic of depression, the content was dominated by a biological focus that reflected the optimism of the times. The current issue differs in this way. While the bulk of these articles still largely hinge on "biological" approaches (except those specifically addressing the psychotherapies), the articles here share an understanding that depression and its treatment should not be reductionistically conceptualized. The paradigm shift that is heralded is not back to a psychological model, but toward a greater integration of bio- and psycho- and social.

In this volume, Ronald Kessler takes an epidemiologic view on depression. He explores not only the personal costs of depression and the economic toll of its treatment but also the significant social costs of depression. In this sense, depression is not simply an illness located in the biology of one person but is a social problem. Similarly, by cross-cultural comparison, Ryder and Chentsova-Dutton explore the ways that depression is not simply a brain disease, but that its symptoms and presentation are profoundly shaped by psychological and cultural factors.

Against the backdrop of our growing awareness that full recovery eludes far too many of our patients, Nada Stotland considers the recovery concept, broadening it beyond a simple symptom-focused conceptualization, and considers psychosocial impediments to recovery, including social and economic factors that interfere with access to adequate care. Daniel Carlat also takes a sober look at the state of antidepressant outcome research, exploring the controversies surrounding both efficacy and effectiveness studies, offering guidance both about how to understand the research and about how to select antidepressant medications based on the available evidence.

Saveanu and Nemeroff examine cutting edge understandings of the biology of depression, including the role of neurotransmitters, neuroanatomy, and neuroendocrine factors. However, in a breathtaking synthesis of the evidence, they show how old dichotomies such as nature-nurture break down. Early life experiences such as trauma and neglect affect not only the mind, but also the brain, producing marked changes in the expression of genes that are linked to depression. Conversely, "psychological" treatments such as psychotherapy are shown, for example, to promote up-regulation of serotonin receptors, questioning historical distinctions between psychological and biological treatments.

Although taking issue with the constraints of the biopsychosocial model, Drs Ghaemi, Vöhringer, and Vergne argue effectively against a "one size fits all" approach to depression. Depression, in their view, is a heterogeneous construct, with some presentations shaped more by character and others shaped more by biology. It is only by paying attention to phenomenological data, the patient's experience, that we can know best what we are treating and how to treat it. In a similar vein, Tomba and Fava look at the topic of treatment selection. Given significant limitations in our current clinical taxonomies, they argue for the importance of using "clinical judgment" in treatment selection. Focusing on the particular impact of treatment sequencing, they suggest that the manner in which treatments are provided have significant effects on outcome. Mintz and Flynn take this point further. Exploring the extensive but oft-neglected evidence base regarding effective prescribing behaviors for depression, they argue specifically that how we prescribe may be more potent than what we prescribe.

Evidence-based psychotherapies seem increasingly relevant in light of the limitations of purely pharmacologic approaches. Donna Sudak explores the place of cognitive behavioral therapy in depression treatment, arguably the most highly supported of any treatment for depression. Luyten and Blatt look at the burgeoning evidence base in support of psychodynamic treatment for depression and place it among the ranks of evidence-based psychotherapies, giving guidance in thinking about which patients might be most likely to benefit from psychodynamic treatment. Recognizing that many patients may be failed by unimodal treatments (either psychotherapy or pharmacotherapy alone), Busch and Sandberg consider the evidence for integrating biological and psychological treatments in order to enhance outcomes, arguing that many patients require a bio-psycho-social approach.

Looking at depression in special populations (the medically ill, the elderly, and children and adolescents), Rackley and Bostwick, Ellison, Kyomen, and Harper, and Dell, respectively, all present perspectives that consider pharmacologic treatments against the backdrop of broader psychosocial considerations such as the locus of care, existential and ethical concerns, and the meanings, to patients, of treatment.

This issue is rounded out by Dr Keitner and Mansfield-Marcaccio's examination of treatment-resistant depression. For a great many of those patients, they conclude, we must get beyond a simple biomedical (or even psychotherapeutic) model and empower patients as active agents in recovery through disease management approaches that have proven effective in other medical disciplines.

I am grateful to the authors who have put such time, consideration, and wisdom into these articles. It is my hope that the articles here, and the underlying call for more integrated and biopsychosocial ways of thinking about depression treatment, will contribute usefully to our field and to our patients. While psychiatry may not necessarily need therapy,[4] it does need something more than it currently has at its disposal.[8] In my view, it is by embracing the psychological and social aspects of our intellectual inheritance and integrating them thoughtfully with cutting-edge neurobiological understandings that psychiatry will be able most potently to address the needs of those who struggle with depression.

David L. Mintz, MD
The Austen Riggs Center
25 Main Street, PO Box 962
Stockbridge, MA 01262, USA

E-mail address:
david.mintz@austenriggs.net

REFERENCES

1. Kuhn T. The structure of scientific revolutions. Chicago: University of Chicago Press; 1962.
2. Heathfield H, Louw G. New challenges for clinical informatics: knowledge management tools. Health Informat J 1999;5:67–73.
3. Begley S. The depressing news about antidepressants. Newsweek Magazine. February 10, 2010:34–41.
4. Shorter E. Why psychiatry needs therapy. Wall Street Journal. February 27, 2010. Available at: http://online.wsj.com/article/SB10001424052748704188104575508370 0227601116.html. Accessed December 19, 2011.

5. Menand L. Head case: can psychiatry be a science? The New Yorker. March 1, 2010. Available at: http://www.newyorker.com/arts/critics/atlarge/2010/03/01/100301crat_atlarge_menand. Accessed December 19, 2011.

6. Bayard L. My antidepressant gets harder to swallow. Salon.com. April 5, 2010. Available at: http://www.salon.com/2010/04/05/is_my_lexapro_working/. Accessed December 19, 2011.

7. Carlat D. Mind over meds. The New York Times. April 19, 2010. Available at: http://www.nytimes.com/2010/04/25/magazine/25Memoir-t.html?pagewanted=all. Accessed December 19, 2011.

8. Plakun EM. Treatment resistance and psychodynamic psychiatry: concepts psychiatry needs from psychoanalysis. Psychodynam Psychiatry 2012, in press.

The Costs of Depression

Ronald C. Kessler, PhD

KEYWORDS

- Absenteeism • Costs of illness • Disability • Illness burden
- Impairment • Major depressive disorder

Major depression is a commonly occurring, seriously impairing, and often recurrent mental disorder.[1,2] The World Health Organization (WHO) ranks major depressive disorder (MDD) as the fourth leading cause of disability worldwide[3] and projects that by 2020 it will be the second leading cause owing to currently unexplained increasing prevalence in recent cohorts.[4] Although data on the prevalence and costs of MDD do not exist for most countries, psychiatric epidemiologic surveys of the general population, students, and primary care patients have been carried out in many developed countries as well as in an increasing number of developing countries. The results of these surveys are reviewed in this chapter. The paper begins with an overview of information on the descriptive epidemiology of major depression (prevalence, age of onset, course, comorbidity) and then focuses primarily on data documenting the individual and societal costs of depression.

Before turning to the review, it is noteworthy that a number of the largest epidemiologic surveys of major depression focused on major depressive episodes (MDE) rather than MDD. The difference between the two is that MDE includes depressive episodes that occur as part of bipolar disorder, whereas MDD excludes bipolar depression. Because the vast majority of lifetime MDE is MDD, the difference between the two is not of great importance when examining lifetime disorders. However, because bipolar depression is considerably more persistent than non-bipolar depression,[5] the proportion of MDE cases owing to bipolar depression increases as the time frame of assessment decreases, making it important to distinguish MDE from MDD in examining current prevalence and correlates. We consequently focus in the current report on MDD, but report data on MDE when they are the only data available for some major studies.

BASIC DESCRIPTIVE EPIDEMIOLOGY
Prevalence

Weissman and colleagues[6] published the first cross-national data on the prevalence of MDD, using the same methods as, the landmark US Epidemiologic Catchment

Disclosure: See last page of article.
Department of Health Care Policy, Harvard Medical School, 180 Longwood Avenue, Boston, MA 02115, USA
E-mail address: ncs@hcp.med.harvard.edu

Psychiatr Clin N Am 35 (2012) 1–14
doi:10.1016/j.psc.2011.11.005
0193-953X/12/$ – see front matter © 2012 Elsevier Inc. All rights reserved.

Area Study.[7] Lifetime prevalence estimates in these surveys were in the range of 1.5% to 19.0%, with a midpoint of 9.4% and generally higher rates in higher income than lower income countries. Twelve-month prevalence estimates were in the range of 0.8% to 5.8%, with a midpoint of 3.7%. Subsequent studies[8] using a diagnostic interview developed by the WHO explicitly for cross-national comparative research found prevalence estimates of MDD that were very similar to those in the earlier US Epidemiologic Catchment Area–based surveys, again finding higher rates in higher income than lower income countries.[8] Moussavi and associates[9] more recently reported data on the 12-month prevalence of MDE (ICD-10 criteria) from the massive (n = 245,404 respondents) WHO World Health Survey, a 60-country survey designed to assess the recent prevalence and impairment of a wide range of health problems in every region of the world (http://www.who.int/healthinfo/survey/whsresults/en/index.html). Major depression was the only mental disorder included in the World Health Survey. The 12-month prevalence of major depression was 3.2% and between 9.3% and 23.0% among participants with a chronic condition. Bromet and co-workers[10] more recently reported data on the 12-month and lifetime prevalence of MDE from the 18-country WHO World Mental Health (WMH) Surveys (n = 89,037). Mean lifetime and 12-month prevalence estimates of DSM-IV MDE were 14.6% and 5.5% in high-income countries compared with 11.1% and 5.9% in low- and middle-income countries, respectively.

The wide cross-national variation in prevalence estimates and generally elevated rates in high-income countries might reflect cross-national differences in the threshold for defining clinically significant depression in diagnostic interviews. However, if that was the case, we would expect that depression detected in countries with the lowest estimated prevalence would be the most severe cases, resulting in high impairment rates, and that reports of core depressive symptoms would be more similar across countries than estimates of disorder prevalence. Neither of these expectations was borne out, however, when they were examined in the WMH data, adding indirect support to a substantive interpretation of the cross-national differences in MDE. But why do these prevalence differences exist? Differences in stress exposure, reactivity to stress, and endogenous depression unrelated to environmental provoking factors are all possibilities. On 1 level it seems counterintuitive that people in high-income countries would experience more stress than those in low- or middle-income countries. However, it has been suggested that depression is to some extent an illness of affluence.[11] A related argument is that income inequality, which is for the most part greater in high- than low- or middle-income countries, promotes a wide variety of chronic conditions that includes depression.[12] Although further analyses of existing epidemiologic data might shed some light on these perspectives, such analyses have not yet been carried out.

COURSE OF ILLNESS

Few large-scale, longitudinal, general population studies of MDD exist, but clinical studies show that a substantial proportion of people who seek treatment for major depression have a chronic–recurrent course of illness.[13,14] Subtyping is complicated by the fact that chronic depression subtypes are poorly understood.[15] The community survey finding that lifetime prevalence is 2 to 3 times that of 12-month prevalence suggests that between one third and one half of lifetime cases have recurrent episodes in a given year. However, long-term longitudinal studies also show that some people with lifetime MDD fail to report their history of depression in cross-section studies.[16,17] We would expect this recall failure to be lower in the WMH surveys because of special probes used for lifetime recall,[18] but it would nonetheless be prudent to consider the 12-month–to–lifetime prevalence ratios in the WMH surveys upper-bound estimates on persistence and WMH lifetime prevalence estimates lower-bound estimates on true lifetime prevalence because of likely recall failure in retrospective reports of lifetime prevalence.

THE COSTS OF MAJOR DEPRESSION
Life Course Role Incumbency, Timing, and Transitions

Given their typically early age of onset, mental disorders might be expected to have adverse effects on critical developmental transitions, such as educational attainment and timing of marriage. A number of epidemiologic studies have examined these effects, with a focus on 4 domains: Education, marital timing and stability, childbearing, and occupation.

Education

Several studies show early-onset mental disorders associated with termination of education.[19–26] Although disruptive behavior disorders and bipolar disorder tend to have the strongest associations in these studies, MDD also is significantly associated with a roughly 60% elevated odds of failure to complete secondary school than otherwise comparable youth in high-income countries.

Marital Timing and Stability

Several studies have examined associations of premarital mental disorders with subsequent marriage.[27–29] Early-onset mental disorders predict low probability of ever marrying, but are either positively associated[28] or unrelated[27] with early (before age 18) marriage, which is known to be associated with a number of adverse outcomes, and negatively associated with on-time and late marriage, which are known to be associated with a number of benefits (eg, financial security, social support). These associations are largely the same for men and women and across countries. MDD is among the most important of these premarital mental disorders. A separate set of studies has shown that premarital history of mental disorders predicts divorce,[30,31] again with associations quite similar for husbands and wives across all countries and MDD among the most important disorders in this regard.[27]

Teen Childbearing

We are aware of only 1 study that examined the association between child–adolescent mental disorder and subsequent teen child bearing.[32] MDD and a number of other early-onset mental disorders were significant predictors of increased teen childbearing. Disaggregation found that the overall associations were due to disorders predicting increased sexual activity but not decreased use of contraception.

Employment Status

Although depression is known to be associated with unemployment, most research on this association has emphasized the impact of job loss on depression rather than depression as a risk factor for job loss.[33] A recent analysis from the WMH surveys documented the latter association by showing that history of mental disorders as of the age of completing schooling predicted current (at the time of interview) unemployment and work disability. (Kawakami N, Abdulghani EA, Alonso J, et al. Early-life mental disorders and adult household income in the World Mental Health Surveys. Submitted for publication.) However, these associations were only significant in high-income countries, raising the possibility that MDD becomes more detrimental to work performance as the substantive complexity of work increases.

Role Performance

A considerably larger amount of research has been carried out on the associations of mental disorders with various aspects of role performance, with a special focus on marital quality, work performance, and financial success.

Marital functioning

It has long been known that marital dissatisfaction and discord are strongly related to depressive symptoms (eg, Culp and associates[34] and Wishman[35]), with an average correlation between marital dissatisfaction and depressive symptoms of approximately $r = 0.4$ across studies and very similar patterns for men and women.[36] Longitudinal studies show that the association is bidirectional,[37,38] but with a stronger time-lagged association of marital discord predicting depressive symptoms than vice versa.[39] Fewer studies have considered the effects of clinical depression on marital functioning,[40–42] but those studies consistently document significant adverse effects.

Considerable research documents that both perpetration of and victimization by physical violence in marital relationships are significantly associated with depression.[43] Although these studies have generally focused on presumed mental health consequences of relationship violence,[44–46] a growing body of research has more recently suggested that marital violence is partly a consequence of preexisting mental disorders.[47–50] Indeed, longitudinal studies consistently find that premarital history of mental disorders, including depression, predict subsequent marital violence perpetration[48,51] and victimization.[43,49,50,52] However, few of these studies adjusted for comorbidity. A recent study in the WMH surveys[53] found that the association between premarital history of MDD and subsequent marital violence disappears after controls are introduced for disruptive behavioral disorders and substance use disorders, suggesting that depression might be a risk marker rather than a causal risk factor.

Parental functioning

A number of studies have documented significant associations of both maternal[54] and paternal[55] depression with negative parenting behaviors. These associations are found throughout the age range of children, but are most pronounced for the parents of young children. Although only an incomplete understanding exists of pathways, both laboratory and naturalistic studies of parent–infant microinteractions have documented subtle ways in which parental depression leads to maladaptive interactions that impede infant affect regulation and later child development.[56]

Days out of role

Considerable research has examined days out of role associated with various physical and mental disorders in an effort to produce data on comparative disease burden for health policy planning purposes.[57,58] These studies typically find that MDD is associated with among the highest number of days out of role at the societal level of any physical or mental disorder owing to its combination of comparatively high prevalence and comparatively strong individual-level association.[59–61] In the WMH surveys, for example, 62,971 respondents across 24 countries were assessed for a wide range of common physical and mental disorders as well as for days out of role in the 30 days before interview.[62] MDD was associated with 5.1% of all days out of role, the fourth highest population-attributable risk proportion of all the disorders considered (exceeded only by headache/migraine, other chronic pain conditions, and cardiovascular disorders) and by far the largest among the mental disorder. A number of epidemiologic surveys in the United States have estimated the workplace costs of either MDE or MDD on absenteeism and low work performance (often referred to as *presenteeism*).[63–66] All these studies found that MDE and MDD significantly predict overall lost work performance. Several studies attempted to estimate the annual salary-equivalent human capital value of these losses. These estimates were in the range $30.1 billion[65] to $51.5 billion.[63]

Financial Success

One of most striking aspects of the impairment associated with MDD is that the personal earnings and household income of people with MDD are substantially lower than those of people without depression.[67–72] However, it is unclear whether depression is primarily a cause, consequence, or both in these associations owing to the possibility of reciprocal causation between income-earnings and MDD.[73] Causal effects of low income on depression have been documented in quasi-experimental studies of job loss.[33] Time series analyses have also documented aggregate associations between unemployment rates and suicide rates.[74] Previous studies of the effects of mental disorders on reductions in income have not controlled for these reciprocal effects, making the size of the adverse effects of depression on income earnings uncertain. One way to sort out this temporal order would be to take advantage of the fact that depression often starts in childhood or adolescence and use prospective epidemiologic data to study long-term associations between early-onset disorders and subsequent income earnings. Several such studies exist, all of them suggesting that depression in childhood–adolescence predicts reduced income earnings in adulthood.[75,76]

Comparative Impairments

A number of community surveys, most of them carried out in the United States, have examined the comparative effects of diverse diseases on various aspects of role functioning.[58,61,77–80] MDE was included in a number of these studies and the results typically showed that musculoskeletal disorders and MDE were associated with the highest levels of disability at the individual level among all commonly occurring disorders assessed. The most compelling study of this sort outside the United States was based on 15 national surveys carried out as part of the WMH surveys.[81] Disorder-specific disability scores were compared across people who experienced each of 10 chronic physical disorders and ten mental disorders in the year before interview. MDD and bipolar disorder were the mental disorders most often rated severely impairing in both developed and developing countries. None of the physical disorders considered had impairment levels as high as those for MDD or bipolar disorder despite the fact that the physical disorders included such severe conditions as cancer, diabetes, and heart disease. Nearly all the higher mental-than-physical ratings were statistically significant at the .05 level. Comparable results were obtained when analyses focused exclusively on sub-samples of cases in treatment and when comparisons were restricted to respondents who had both disorders in a given pair (eg, respondents who had both MDD and cancer or both MDD and heart disease).

Another set of surveys examined comparative decrements in perceived health associated with a wide range of disorders.[9,82,83] MDD was the focus of 2 such studies. The first study was part of the WHO World Health Surveys of nearly one quarter of a million respondents across 60 countries.[9] A consistent pattern was found in these surveys across countries and sociodemographic subgroups within countries for MDD to be associated with a greater decrement in perceived health than any of the 4 physical disorders compared with it (angina, arthritis, asthma, and diabetes). The second study was part of the WMH surveys, where MDD was compared with 18 other physical (eg, cancer, cardiovascular disorders, diabetes) and mental (eg, bipolar disorder, panic disorder, posttraumatic stress disorder) disorders in predicting a summary measure of perceived health.[84] MDD was among the 3 disorders associated with the highest decrements in perceived health, the other 2 being severe insomnia and neurologic disorders (epilepsy, Parkinson's disease, and multiple sclerosis).

Morbidity and Mortality

It is now well established that MDD is significantly associated with a wide variety of chronic physical disorders, including arthritis, asthma, cancer, cardiovascular disease, diabetes, hypertension, chronic respiratory disorders, and a variety of chronic pain conditions.[85–93] Although most of the data documenting these associations comes from clinical samples in the United States, similar data also exist from community epidemiologic surveys carried out throughout the world.[94,95] These associations have considerable individual and public health significance and can be thought of as representing costs of depression in at least 2 ways. First, to the extent that MDD is a causal risk factor, it leads to an increased prevalence of these physical disorders, with all their associated financial costs, impairments, and increased mortality risk. Evidence about MDD as a cause of these physical disorders is spotty, however, although we know from meta-analyses of longitudinal studies that MDD is a consistent predictor of the subsequent first onset of coronary artery disease,[96,97] stroke,[98] diabetes,[99] heart attacks,[100,101] and certain types of cancer.[102] A number of biologically plausible mechanisms have been proposed to explain the prospective associations of MDD with these disorders.[103–107] These include a variety of poor health behaviors known to be linked with MDD, such as elevated rates of smoking and drinking,[108] obesity,[109] low compliance with treatment regimens,[110,111] and a variety of biological dysregulations, such as hypothalamic–pituitary–adrenal hyperactivity and impaired immune function.[112] Based on these observations, there is good reason to believe that MDD might be a causal risk factor for at least some chronic physical disorders. Second, even if depression is more a consequence than a cause of chronic physical disorders, as it seems to be for some disorders based on stronger prospective associations of depression onset subsequent to, rather than before, onset of the physical disorder, comorbid depression is often associated with a worse course of the physical disorder.[113–115] A number of reasons could be involved here, but one of the most consistently documented is that depression is often associated with nonadherence to treatment regimens.[111,116,117]

Based on these considerations, it should not be surprising that MDD is associated with a significantly elevated risk of early death.[103,105,118] This is true partly because people with MDD have a high suicide risk,[119–121] but also because depression is associated with elevated risk of the many types of disorders noted. MDD is also associated with elevated mortality risk among people with certain kinds of disorders as part of a larger pattern of associations of MDD with disorder severity. There has been particular interest in MDD as a risk factor for cardiovascular mortality due to heart attack and stroke among people with cardiovascular disease.[122–125] Indeed, a number of interventions have been developed to detect and treat depression among people with cardiovascular disease in an effort to prolong life, although the results of these studies have so far been only modest.[126]

SUMMARY

The data reported herein show clearly that major depression is a commonly occurring and burdensome disorder. The high prevalence, early age of onset, and high persistence of MDD in the many different countries where epidemiologic surveys have been administered confirm the high worldwide importance of depression. Although evidence is not definitive that MDD plays a causal role in its associations with the many adverse outcomes reviewed here, there is clear evidence that depression has causal effects on a number of important mediators, making it difficult to assume anything other than that depression has strong causal effects on many dimensions of burden. These results have been used to argue for the likely cost -effectiveness of expanded depression treatment from a societal perspective.[127] Two separate, large-scale, randomized, workplace depression treatment effectiveness trials have been carried out in the United States to evaluate the cost effectiveness of expanded treatment from an employer perspective.[128,129] Both trials had positive returns on investment to employers. A substantial expansion of worksite depression care management programs has occurred in the United States subsequent to the publication of these trials.[130] However, the proportion of people with depression who receive treatment remains low in the United States and even lower in other parts of the world. A recent US study found that only about half of workers with MDD received treatment in the year of interview and that fewer than half of treated workers received treatment consistent with published treatment guidelines.[131] Although the treatment rate was higher for more severe cases, even some with severe MDD often failed to receive treatment.[132] The WMH surveys show that treatment rates are even lower in many other developed countries and consistently much lower in developing countries.[133] Less information is available on rates of depression treatment among patients with chronic physical disorders, but available evidence suggests that expanded treatment could be of considerable value.[134] Randomized, controlled trials are needed to expand our understanding of the effects of detection and treatment of depression among people in treatment for chronic physical disorders. In addition, controlled effectiveness trials with long-term follow-ups are needed to increase our understanding of the effects of early MDD treatment interventions on changes in life course role trajectories, role performance, and onset of secondary physical disorders.

DISCLOSURE

This report was prepared in conjunction with the author's participation in the World Health Organization World Mental Health (WMH) Survey Initiative. WMH is supported by the United States National Institute of Mental Health (R01MH070884), the John D. and Catherine T. MacArthur Foundation, the Pfizer Foundation, the US Public Health Service (R13-MH066849, R01-MH069864, and R01 DA016558), the Fogarty International Center (FIRCA R03-TW006481), the Pan American Health Organization, the Eli Lilly & Company Foundation, Ortho-McNeil Pharmaceutical, Inc., GlaxoSmithKline, Sanofi Aventis and Bristol-Myers Squibb. A complete list of WMH publications can be found at http://www.hcp.med.harvard.edu/wmh/.

Dr Kessler has been a consultant for AstraZeneca, Analysis Group, Bristol-Myers Squibb, Cerner-Galt Associates, Eli Lilly & Company, GlaxoSmithKline Inc., Health-Core Inc., Health Dialog, Integrated Benefits Institute, John Snow Inc., Kaiser Permanente, Matria Inc., Mensante, Merck & Co, Inc., Ortho-McNeil Janssen Scientific Affairs, Pfizer Inc., Primary Care Network, Research Triangle Institute, Sanofi-Aventis Groupe, Shire US Inc., SRA International, Inc., Takeda Global Research & Development, Transcept Pharmaceuticals Inc., and Wyeth-Ayerst; has served on advisory boards for Appliance Computing II, Eli Lilly & Company, Mindsite, Ortho-McNeil Janssen Scientific Affairs, Plus One Health Management and Wyeth-Ayerst; and has had research support for his epidemiologic studies from Analysis Group Inc., Bristol-Myers Squibb, Eli Lilly & Company, EPI-Q, GlaxoSmithKline, Johnson & Johnson Pharmaceuticals, Ortho-McNeil Janssen Scientific Affairs., Pfizer Inc., Sanofi-Aventis Groupe, and Shire US, Inc.

REFERENCES

1. Spijker J, Graaf R, Bijl RV, et al. Functional disability and depression in the general population. Results from the Netherlands Mental Health Survey and Incidence Study (NEMESIS). Acta Psychiatr Scand 2004;110:208–14.
2. U'stün TB, Ayuso-Mateos JL, Chatterji S, et al. Global burden of depressive disorders in the year 2000. Br J Psychiatry 2004;184:386–92.
3. Murray CJ, Lopez AD. Evidence-based health policy—lessons from the Global Burden of Disease Study. Science 1996;274:740–3.
4. Murray CJL, Lopez AD. The Global Burden of Disease: a comprehensive assessment of mortality and disability from diseases, injuries and risk factors in 1990 and projected to 2020. Harvard University Press, 1996.
5. Merikangas KR, Jin R, He JP, et al. Prevalence and correlates of bipolar spectrum disorder in the World Mental Health Survey Initiative. Arch Gen Psychiatry 2011;68: 241–51.
6. Weissman MM, Bland RC, Canino GJ, et al. Cross-national epidemiology of major depression and bipolar disorder. JAMA 1996;276:293–9.
7. Robins LN, Regier DA, editors. Psychiatric disorders in America: the Epidemiologic Catchment Area Study. New York: The Free Press; 1991.
8. Andrade L, Caraveo-Anduaga JJ, Berglund P, et al. The epidemiology of major depressive episodes: results from the International Consortium of Psychiatric Epidemiology (ICPE) Surveys. Int J Methods Psychiatr Res 2003;12:3–21.
9. Moussavi S, Chatterji S, Verdes E, et al. Depression, chronic diseases, and decrements in health: results from the World Health Surveys. Lancet 2007;370:851–8.
10. Bromet E, Andrade LH, Hwang I, et al. Cross-national epidemiology of DSM-IV major depressive episode. BMC Med 2011;9:90.
11. Koplewicz HS, Gurian A, Williams K. The era of affluence and its discontents. J Am Acad Child Adolesc Psychiatry 2009;48:1053–5.
12. Wilkinson RG, Pickett KE. Income inequality and population health: a review and explanation of the evidence. Soc Sci Med 2006;62:1768–84.
13. Hardeveld F, Spijker J, De Graaf R, et al. Prevalence and predictors of recurrence of major depressive disorder in the adult population. Acta Psychiatr Scand 2010;122: 184–91.
14. Torpey DC, Klein DN. Chronic depression: update on classification and treatment. Curr Psychiatry Rep 2008;10:458–64.
15. Benazzi F. Various forms of depression. Dialogues Clin Neurosci 2006;8:151–61.
16. Moffitt TE, Caspi A, Taylor A, et al. How common are common mental disorders? Evidence that lifetime prevalence rates are doubled by prospective versus retrospective ascertainment. Psychol Med 2010;40:899–909.
17. Patten SB, Williams JV, Lavorato DH, et al. Recall of recent and more remote depressive episodes in a prospective cohort study. Soc Psychiatry Psychiatr Epidemiol 2011. [Epub ahead of print].
18. Knäuper B, Cannell CF, Schwarz N, et al. Improving accuracy of major depression age-of-onset reports in the US National Comorbidity Survey. Int J Methods Psychiatr Res 1999;8:39–48.

19. Breslau J, Lane M, Sampson N, et al. Mental disorders and subsequent educational attainment in a US national sample. J Psychiatr Res 2008;42:708–16.
20. Breslau J, Miller E, Joanie Chung WJ, et al. Childhood and adolescent onset psychiatric disorders, substance use, and failure to graduate high school on time. J Psychiatr Res 2011;45:295–301.
21. Kessler RC, Foster CL, Saunders WB, et al. Social consequences of psychiatric disorders, I: Educational attainment. Am J Psychiatry 1995;152:1026–32.
22. Lee S, Tsang A, Breslau J, et al. Mental disorders and termination of education in high-income and low- and middle-income countries: epidemiological study. Br J Psychiatry 2009;194:411–7.
23. McLeod JD, Kaiser K. Childhood emotional and behavioral problems and educational attainment. Am Sociological Rev 2004;69:636–58.
24. Porche MV, Fortuna LR, Lin J, et al. Childhood trauma and psychiatric disorders as correlates of school dropout in a national sample of young adults. Child Dev 2011;82:982–98.
25. Vaughn MG, Wexler J, Beaver KM, et al. Psychiatric correlates of behavioral indicators of school disengagement in the United States. Psychiatr Q 2011;82:191–206.
26. Woodward LJ, Fergusson DM. Life course outcomes of young people with anxiety disorders in adolescence. J Am Acad Child Adolesc Psychiatry 2001;40:1086–93.
27. Breslau J, Miller E, Jin R, et al. A multinational study of mental disorders, marriage, and divorce. Acta Psychiatr Scand 2011;124:474–86.
28. Forthofer MS, Kessler RC, Story AL, et al. The effects of psychiatric disorders on the probability and timing of first marriage. J Health Soc Behav 1996;37:121–32.
29. Whisman MA, Tolejko N, Chatav Y. Social consequences of personality disorders: probability and timing of marriage and probability of marital disruption. J Pers Disord 2007;21:690–5.
30. Butterworth P, Rodgers B. Mental health problems and marital disruption: is it the combination of husbands and wives' mental health problems that predicts later divorce? Soc Psychiatry Psychiatr Epidemiol 2008;43:758–63.
31. Kessler RC, Walters EE, Forthofer MS. The social consequences of psychiatric disorders, III: probability of marital stability. Am J Psychiatry 1998;155:1092–6.
32. Kessler RC, Berglund PA, Foster CL, et al. Social consequences of psychiatric disorders, II: Teenage parenthood. Am J Psychiatry 1997;154:1405–11.
33. Dooley D, Fielding J, Levi L. Health and unemployment. Annu Rev Public Health 1996;17:449–65.
34. Culp LN, Beach SRH. Marriage and depressive symptoms: the role and bases of self-esteem differ by gender. Psychol Women Quart 1998;22:647–63.
35. Whisman MA. Marital dissatisfaction and psychiatric disorders: results from the National Comorbidity Survey. J Abnorm Psychol 1999;108:701–6.
36. Whisman SA. The association between depression and marital dissatisfaction. In: Beach SRH, editor. Marital and family processes in depression: a scientific foundation for clinical practice. Washington, DC: American Psychological Association; 2001. p. 3–24.
37. Mamun AA, Clavarino AM, Najman JM, et al. Maternal depression and the quality of marital relationship: a 14-year prospective study. J Womens Health (Larchmt) 2009;18:2023–31.
38. Whisman MA, Uebelacker LA. Prospective associations between marital discord and depressive symptoms in middle-aged and older adults. Psychol Aging 2009;24:184–9.
39. Proulx CM, Helms HM, Buehler C. Marital quality and personal well-being: a meta-analysis. J Marriage Fam 2007;69:576–93.

40. Coyne JC, Thompson R, Palmer SC. Marital quality, coping with conflict, marital complaints, and affection in couples with a depressed wife. J Fam Psychol 2002; 16:26–37.
41. Kronmuller KT, Backenstrass M, Victor D, et al. Quality of marital relationship and depression: results of a 10-year prospective follow-up study. J Affect Disord 2011; 128:64–71.
42. Pearson KA, Watkins ER, Kuyken W, et al. The psychosocial context of depressive rumination: ruminative brooding predicts diminished relationship satisfaction in individuals with a history of past major depression. Br J Clin Psychol 2010;49:275–80.
43. Stith SM, Smith DB, Penn CE, et al. Intimate partner physical abuse perpetration and victimization risk factors: A meta-analytic review. Aggress Viol Behav 2004;10:65–98.
44. Afifi TO, MacMillan H, Cox BJ, et al. Mental health correlates of intimate partner violence in marital relationships in a nationally representative sample of males and females. J Interpers Violence 2009;24:1398–417.
45. Kim HK, Laurent HK, Capaldi DM, et al. Men's aggression toward women: a 10-year panel study. J Marriage Fam 2008;70:1169–87.
46. Renner LM. Intimate partner violence victimization and parenting stress: assessing the mediating role of depressive symptoms. Violence Against Women 2009;15: 1380–401.
47. Kessler RC, Molnar BE, Feurer ID, et al. Patterns and mental health predictors of domestic violence in the United States: results from the National Comorbidity Survey. Int J Law Psychiatry 2001;24:487–508.
48. Lorber MF, O'Leary KD. Predictors of the persistence of male aggression in early marriage. J Fam Viol 2004;19:329–38.
49. O'Leary KD, Tintle N, Bromet EJ, et al. Descriptive epidemiology of intimate partner aggression in Ukraine. Soc Psychiatry Psychiatr Epidemiol 2008;43:619–26.
50. Riggs DS, Caulfield MB, Street AE. Risk for domestic violence: factors associated with perpetration and victimization. J Clin Psychol 2000;56:1289–316.
51. Fang X, Massetti GM, Ouyang L, et al. Attention-deficit/hyperactivity disorder, conduct disorder, and young adult intimate partner violence. Arch Gen Psychiatry 2010;67:1179–86.
52. Lehrer JA, Buka S, Gortmaker S, et al. Depressive symptomatology as a predictor of exposure to intimate partner violence among US female adolescents and young adults. Arch Pediatr Adolesc Med 2006;160:270–6.
53. Miller E, Breslau J, Petukhova M, et al. Premarital mental disorders and physical violence in marriage: cross-national study of married couples. Br J Psychiatry 2011;199:330–7.
54. Lovejoy MC, Graczyk PA, O'Hare E, et al. Maternal depression and parenting behavior: a meta-analytic review. Clin Psychol Rev 2000;20:561–92.
55. Wilson S, Durbin CE. Effects of paternal depression on fathers' parenting behaviors: a meta-analytic review. Clin Psychol Rev 2010;30:167–80.
56. Tronick E, Reck C. Infants of depressed mothers. Harv Rev Psychiatry 2009;17: 147–56.
57. Alonso J, Angermeyer MC, Bernert S, et al. Disability and quality of life impact of mental disorders in Europe: results from the European Study of the Epidemiology of Mental Disorders (ESEMeD) project. Acta Psychiatr Scand Suppl 2004:38–46.
58. Merikangas KR, Ames M, Cui L, et al. The impact of comorbidity of mental and physical conditions on role disability in the US adult household population. Arch Gen Psychiatry 2007;64:1180–8.

59. Collins JJ, Baase CM, Sharda CE, et al. The assessment of chronic health conditions on work performance, absence, and total economic impact for employers. J Occup Environ Med 2005;47:547–57.
60. Munce SE, Stansfeld SA, Blackmore ER, et al. The role of depression and chronic pain conditions in absenteeism: results from a national epidemiologic survey. J Occup Environ Med 2007;49:1206–11.
61. Wang PS, Beck A, Berglund P, et al. Chronic medical conditions and work performance in the health and work performance questionnaire calibration surveys. J Occup Environ Med 2003;45:1303–11.
62. Alonso J, Petukhova M, Vilagut G, et al. Days out of role due to common physical and mental conditions: results from the WHO World Mental Health surveys. Mol Psychiatry 2010;16(12):1234–46.
63. Greenberg PE, Kessler RC, Birnbaum HG, et al. The economic burden of depression in the United States: how did it change between 1990 and 2000? J Clin Psychiatry 2003;64:1465–75.
64. Kessler RC, Akiskal HS, Ames M, et al. Prevalence and effects of mood disorders on work performance in a nationally representative sample of U.S. workers. Am J Psychiatry 2006;163:1561–8.
65. Stewart WF, Ricci JA, Chee E, et al. Cost of lost productive work time among US workers with depression. JAMA 2003;289:3135–44.
66. Wang PS, Simon G, Kessler RC. The economic burden of depression and the cost-effectiveness of treatment. Int J Methods Psychiatr Res 2003;12:22–33.
67. Ford E, Clark C, McManus S, et al. Common mental disorders, unemployment and welfare benefits in England. Public Health 2010;124:675–81.
68. Insel TR. Assessing the economic costs of serious mental illness. Am J Psychiatry 2008;165:663–5.
69. Kessler RC, Heeringa S, Lakoma MD, et al. Individual and societal effects of mental disorders on earnings in the United States: results from the national comorbidity survey replication. Am J Psychiatry 2008;165:703–11.
70. Levinson D, Lakoma MD, Petukhova M, et al. Associations of serious mental illness with earnings: results from the WHO World Mental Health surveys. Br J Psychiatry 2010;197:114–21.
71. Marcotte DE, Wilcox-Gok V. Estimating the employment and earnings costs of mental illness: recent developments in the United States. Soc Sci Med 2001;53:21–7.
72. McMillan KA, Enns MW, Asmundson GJ, et al. The association between income and distress, mental disorders, and suicidal ideation and attempts: findings from the collaborative psychiatric epidemiology surveys. J Clin Psychiatry 2010;71:1168–75.
73. Muntaner C, Eaton WW, Miech R, et al. Socioeconomic position and major mental disorders. Epidemiol Rev 2004;26:53–62.
74. Jones L. The health consequences of economic recessions. J Health Soc Policy 1991;3:1–14.
75. Smith JP, Smith GC. Long-term economic costs of psychological problems during childhood. Soc Sci Med 2010;71:110–5.
76. Goodman A, Joyce R, Smith JP. The long shadow cast by childhood physical and mental problems on adult life. Proc Natl Acad Sci U S A 2011;108:6032–7.
77. Kessler RC, Greenberg PE, Mickelson KD, et al. The effects of chronic medical conditions on work loss and work cutback. J Occup Environ Med 2001;43:218–25.
78. Lerner D, Allaire SH, Reisine ST. Work disability resulting from chronic health conditions. J Occup Environ Med 2005;47:253–64.

79. Stewart WF, Ricci JA, Chee E, et al. Lost productive work time costs from health conditions in the United States: results from the American Productivity Audit. J Occup Environ Med 2003;45:1234–46.
80. Verbrugge LM, Patrick DL. Seven chronic conditions: their impact on US adults' activity levels and use of medical services. Am J Public Health 1995;85:173–82.
81. Ormel J, Petukhova M, Chatterji S, et al. Disability and treatment of specific mental and physical disorders across the world. Br J Psychiatry 2008;192:368–75.
82. Alonso J, Ferrer M, Gandek B, et al. Health-related quality of life associated with chronic conditions in eight countries: results from the International Quality of Life Assessment (IQOLA) Project. Qual Life Res 2004;13:283–98.
83. Manuel DG, Schultz SE, Kopec JA. Measuring the health burden of chronic disease and injury using health adjusted life expectancy and the Health Utilities Index. J Epidemiol Community Health 2002;56:843–50.
84. Alonso J, Vilagut G, Chatterji S, et al. Including information about co-morbidity in estimates of disease burden: results from the World Health Organization World Mental Health Surveys. Psychol Med 2011;41:873–86.
85. Anderson RJ, Freedland KE, Clouse RE, et al. The prevalence of comorbid depression in adults with diabetes: a meta-analysis. Diabetes Care 2001;24:1069–78.
86. Buist-Bouwman MA, de Graaf R, Vollebergh WAM, et al. Comorbidity of physical and mental disorders and the effect on work-loss days. Acta Psychiatr Scand 2005;111: 436–43.
87. Chapman DP, Perry GS, Strine TW. The vital link between chronic disease and depressive disorders. Prev Chronic Dis 2005;2:A14.
88. Derogatis LR, Morrow GR, Fetting J, et al. The prevalence of psychiatric disorders among cancer patients. JAMA 1983;249:751–7.
89. Dew MA. Psychiatric disorder in the context of physical illness. In: Dohrenwend BP, editor. Adversity, stress and psychopathology. New York: Oxford University Press; 1998.
90. McWilliams LA, Cox BJ, Enns MW. Mood and anxiety disorders associated with chronic pain: an examination in a nationally representative sample. Pain 2003;106: 127–33.
91. Nemeroff CB, Musselman DL, Evans DL. Depression and cardiac disease. Depress Anxiety 1998;8(Suppl 1):71–9.
92. Ortega AN, Feldman JM, Canino G, et al. Co-occurrence of mental and physical illness in US Latinos. Soc Psychiatry Psychiatr Epidemiol 2006;41:927–34.
93. Wells KB, Golding JM, Burnam MA. Chronic medical conditions in a sample of the general population with anxiety, affective, and substance use disorders. Am J Psychiatry 1989;146:1440–6.
94. Scott KM, Bruffaerts R, Tsang A, et al. Depression-anxiety relationships with chronic physical conditions: results from the World Mental Health Surveys. J Affect Disord 2007;103:113–20.
95. Von Korff MR, Scott KM, Gureje O. Global perspectives on mental-physical comorbidity in the WHO World Mental Health Surveys. New York: Cambridge University Press; 2009.
96. Van der Kooy K, van Hout H, Marwijk H, et al. Depression and the risk for cardiovascular diseases: systematic review and meta analysis. Int J Geriatr Psychiatry 2007;22:613–26.
97. Wulsin LR, Singal BM. Do depressive symptoms increase the risk for the onset of coronary disease? A systematic quantitative review. Psychosom Med 2003;65: 201–10.

98. Ohira T, Iso H, Satoh S, et al. Prospective study of depressive symptoms and risk of stroke among Japanese. Stroke 2001;32:903–8.
99. Carnethon MR, Kinder LS, Fair JM, et al. Symptoms of depression as a risk factor for incident diabetes: findings from the National Health and Nutrition Examination Epidemiologic Follow-up Study, 1971-1992. Am J Epidemiol 2003;158:416–23.
100. Pratt LA, Ford DE, Crum RM, et al. Depression, psychotropic medication, and risk of myocardial infarction. Prospective data from the Baltimore ECA follow-up. Circulation 1996;94:3123–9.
101. Scherrer JF, Virgo KS, Zeringue A, et al. Depression increases risk of incident myocardial infarction among Veterans Administration patients with rheumatoid arthritis. Gen Hosp Psychiatry 2009;31:353–9.
102. Gross AL, Gallo JJ, Eaton WW. Depression and cancer risk: 24 years of follow-up of the Baltimore Epidemiologic Catchment Area sample. Cancer Causes Control 2010;21:191–9.
103. Carney RM, Freedland KE, Miller GE, et al. Depression as a risk factor for cardiac mortality and morbidity: a review of potential mechanisms. J Psychosom Res 2002;53:897–902.
104. Cohen S, Rodriquez MS. Pathways linking affective disturbances and physical disorders. Health Psychol 1995;14:374–80.
105. Cuijpers P, Schoevers RA. Increased mortality in depressive disorders: a review. Curr Psychiatry Rep 2004;6:430–7.
106. Katon W, Ciechanowski P. Impact of major depression on chronic medical illness. J Psychosom Res 2002;53:859–63.
107. Stapelberg NJ, Neumann DL, Shum DH, et al. A topographical map of the causal network of mechanisms underlying the relationship between major depressive disorder and coronary heart disease. Aust N Z J Psychiatry 2011;45:351–69.
108. Davis L, Uezato A, Newell JM, et al. Major depression and comorbid substance use disorders. Curr Opin Psychiatry 2008;21:14–8.
109. Cizza G. Major depressive disorder is a risk factor for low bone mass, central obesity, and other medical conditions. Dialogues Clin Neurosci 2011;13:73–87.
110. Schlenk EA, Dunbar-Jacob J, Engberg S. Medication non-adherence among older adults: a review of strategies and interventions for improvement. J Gerontol Nurs 2004;30:33–43.
111. Ziegelstein RC, Fauerbach JA, Stevens SS, et al. Patients with depression are less likely to follow recommendations to reduce cardiac risk during recovery from a myocardial infarction. Arch Intern Med 2000;160:1818–23.
112. Kiecolt-Glaser JK, Glaser R. Depression and immune function: central pathways to morbidity and mortality. J Psychosom Res 2002;53:873–6.
113. Gillen R, Tennen H, McKee TE, et al. Depressive symptoms and history of depression predict rehabilitation efficiency in stroke patients. Arch Phys Med Rehabil 2001;82:1645–9.
114. Mancuso CA, Rincon M, McCulloch CE, et al. Self-efficacy, depressive symptoms, and patients' expectations predict outcomes in asthma. Med Care 2001;39:1326–38.
115. Peyrot M, Rubin RR. Levels and risks of depression and anxiety symptomatology among diabetic adults. Diabetes Care 1997;20:585–90.
116. Breitbart W, Rosenfeld B, Pessin H, et al. Depression, hopelessness, and desire for hastened death in terminally ill patients with cancer. JAMA 2000;284:2907–11.
117. Cluley S, Cochrane GM. Psychological disorder in asthma is associated with poor control and poor adherence to inhaled steroids. Respir Med 2001;95:37–9.
118. Wulsin LR, Vaillant GE, Wells VE. A systematic review of the mortality of depression. Psychosom Med 1999;61:6–17.

119. Bostwick JM, Pankratz VS. Affective disorders and suicide risk: a reexamination. Am J Psychiatry 2000;157:1925–32.
120. Moller HJ. Suicide, suicidality and suicide prevention in affective disorders. Acta Psychiatr Scand Suppl 2003:73–80.
121. Rihmer Z. Suicide risk in mood disorders. Curr Opin Psychiatry 2007;20:17–22.
122. Barth J, Schumacher M, Herrmann-Lingen C. Depression as a risk factor for mortality in patients with coronary heart disease: a meta-analysis. Psychosom Med 2004;66:802–13.
123. Gump BB, Matthews KA, Eberly LE, et al. Depressive symptoms and mortality in men: results from the Multiple Risk Factor Intervention Trial. Stroke 2005;36:98–102.
124. Lesperance F, Frasure-Smith N, Talajic M, et al. Five-year risk of cardiac mortality in relation to initial severity and one-year changes in depression symptoms after myocardial infarction. Circulation 2002;105:1049–53.
125. van Melle JP, de Jonge P, Spijkerman TA, et al. Prognostic association of depression following myocardial infarction with mortality and cardiovascular events: a meta-analysis. Psychosom Med 2004;66:814–22.
126. Thombs BD, de Jonge P, Coyne JC, et al. Depression screening and patient outcomes in cardiovascular care: a systematic review. JAMA 2008;300:2161–71.
127. Wang PS, Patrick A, Avorn J, et al. The costs and benefits of enhanced depression care to employers. Arch Gen Psychiatry 2006;63:1345–53.
128. Rost K, Smith JL, Dickinson M. The effect of improving primary care depression management on employee absenteeism and productivity. A randomized trial. Med Care 2004;42:1202–10.
129. Wang PS, Simon GE, Avorn J, et al. Telephone screening, outreach, and care management for depressed workers and impact on clinical and work productivity outcomes: a randomized controlled trial. JAMA 2007;298:1401–11.
130. Rost K, Marshall D, Shearer B, et al. Depression care management: can employers purchase improved outcomes? Depress Res Treat 2011;2011:942519.
131. Kessler RC, Merikangas KR, Wang PS. The prevalence and correlates of workplace depression in the national comorbidity survey replication. J Occup Environ Med 2008;50:381–90.
132. Birnbaum HG, Kessler RC, Kelley D, et al. Employer burden of mild, moderate, and severe major depressive disorder: mental health services utilization and costs, and work performance. Depress Anxiety 2010;27:78–89.
133. Wang PS, Aguilar-Gaxiola S, Alonso J, et al. Use of mental health services for anxiety, mood, and substance disorders in 17 countries in the WHO world mental health surveys. Lancet 2007;370:841–50.
134. Katon W, Lin EH, Kroenke K. The association of depression and anxiety with medical symptom burden in patients with chronic medical illness. Gen Hosp Psychiatry 2007;29:147–55.

Depression in Cultural Context: "Chinese Somatization," Revisited

Andrew G. Ryder, PhD[a,b],*, Yulia E. Chentsova-Dutton, PhD[c],*

KEYWORDS

- Chinese • Culture • Depression • Somatization

Consider 2 cases from the same urban outpatient clinic in a large North American city.

> Mrs Liu is a married woman in her early 40s, a recent immigrant who arrived 2 years ago from Mainland China. Presenting complaints are "tiredness," "bad sleep," "difficulty paying attention," and "headache." She acknowledges low mood on direct questioning, which she sees as understandable given the impact of her other symptoms. Concentration problems are attributed to the effects of fatigue and insomnia, and she denies other psychological symptoms. Indeed, she openly wonders on several occasions, "Why does everyone here want to know about thoughts and feelings and so on?" She has few friends, has difficulties improving her English, and spends most days at home while her husband works, but does not see these issues as relevant to her current symptoms. Rather, they are part of what one expects from the migration experience, although she acknowledges that she prefers to discuss life difficulties with her one close friend rather than with health professionals. She is not willing to consider psychosocial interventions, but accepts treatment with a selective serotonin reuptake inhibitor when the purpose of the medication is clearly linked to relief of fatigue.

Supported by a New Investigator Award from the Canadian Institutes of Health Research to the A.G.R.

The authors have nothing to disclose.

[a] Department of Psychology, Concordia University (PY153-2), 7141 Sherbrooke Street West, Montreal, QC H4V 2E7, Canada

[b] Culture and Mental Health Research Unit, Sir Mortimer B. Davis—Jewish General Hospital, 4333 Côte-Ste-Catherine Rd, Montreal, QC H3T 1E4, Canada

[c] Department of Psychology, Georgetown University, 306 White Gravenor Hall, 3700 O Street, NW, Washington, DC 20057, USA

* Corresponding author. Department of Psychology, Concordia University (PY153-2), 7141 Sherbrooke Street West, Montreal, QC H4V 2E7, Canada.

E-mail address: andrew.ryder@concordia.ca; yec2@georgetown.edu

Ms Chan is a single woman in her mid 30s, also a recent immigrant who arrived 5 years ago from Mainland China. Presenting complaints are "exhaustion," "difficulty getting to sleep," "no appetite," and "depressed mood." She agrees that psychosocial explanations are plausible, related to trouble finding permanent employment or a romantic partner, and admits to shame about "being weak." "I am very embarrassed that I have this problem and I make sure my family back home doesn't know anything about it." Pessimistic or even hopeless thoughts about the future are also acknowledged on direct questioning, but she does not really see these thoughts as symptoms; other psychological symptoms are denied. She is willing to consider antidepressant medication so long as it is not a permanent solution, but ends up dropping out of psychotherapy after 2 sessions. After a few months, she agrees to take part in weekly group therapy sessions emphasizing a skills approach for new immigrants, and completes the program with no sessions missed.

Both cases exemplify a pattern of clinical presentation sometimes called somatization, most closely associated with depressed patients of Chinese cultural origin, and one of the best-known findings from cultural psychiatry. To what extent does the "somatization" represented here fit with classic ideas of a real psychological problem masked by somatic symptoms? Are these somatic symptoms emphasized (and psychological symptoms deemphasized) strategically, for example, to secure health care resources or avoid psychiatric stigma? Might there instead be a sense in which an emphasis on somatic symptoms really does reflect subjective experience shaped by culture? Indeed, can we assume that the somatic symptoms presented by Chinese patients always reflect the same process?

Although it is old news that "culture matters" in depression, there is not much research on the specific ways in how it does so. Work on "Chinese somatization," beginning in the 1970s and continuing today, is an important exception. Discussion has centered on explanations for this phenomenon, and whether these somatic symptoms are best understood as a particular way of presenting depression or as a different syndrome specific to this cultural context. Proposed explanations have also differed markedly in whether they postulate deep cultural shaping of both subjective experience and outward expression of symptoms, or instead emphasize more-or-less conscious processes of strategic presentation.

In using Chinese somatization as our example of a relatively well-researched topic on culture and depression, we return to a well-trodden path. The issue and its attendant debate might be familiar to many readers. We return nonetheless, and we do so with 2 aims. First, we aspire to say something new: We present an approach to culture and mental health, apply it to Chinese somatization, and in so doing point the way toward new ways of thinking about research and clinical work. Second, we hope that several decades of theory and research on Chinese somatization, seen through our interpretive lens, might serve as a model for how researchers might study psychopathology in other cultural contexts.

We begin with a brief review of international research on depression before narrowing in on the Chinese case. Then, we turn to studies establishing Chinese somatization, followed by the literature that attempts to explain these findings. We then pause to consider an approach to the study of culture that draws on ongoing developments in cultural psychology, influenced also by anthropology and cultural psychiatry.[1] This view allows us to expand our attentional approach to Chinese somatization. We conclude by considering implications for treatment, and then expand outward again to propose some future directions for culturally grounded depression studies and interventions.

CULTURE, DEPRESSION, AND SYMPTOM PRESENTATION

International studies in psychiatric epidemiology have shown that DSM-defined major depressive disorder (MDD) can be identified in many different parts of the world, albeit with considerable variation in prevalence rates. The Cross-National Study[2] studied 10 sites and found lifetime prevalence estimates ranging from 1.5% (Taiwan) to 19% (Lebanon). A group of studies conducted by the International Consortium of Psychiatric Epidemiology[3] also covered 10 sites and found lifetime prevalence estimates ranging from 3.0% (Japan) to 16.9% (United States).

Finding cases worldwide that conform to DSM-based MDD does not mean MDD best captures depression in every cultural group, let alone that depression is the same in each group. Universal features are important and facilitate group comparisons, but tend toward the general and abstract (we make this point elsewhere for personality disorders[4]). We could decide that we are going to compare cultural contexts in terms of how people experience profound distress. We could focus on prolonged problematic responses to losses of various kinds[5] and call that set of responses "depression"—but that category would be broader than DSM-defined MDD. These responses are embodied as genetic predispositions, neurochemical events, and bodily reactions. Similarly, they are deeply embedded in, and hence profoundly shaped by, their cultural context.[1,6–10] (Chentsova-Dutton YE, Choi E, Ryder AG, et al. Cultural variation in the effects of anhedonia on well-being. Submitted for publication.) A "disembedded" symptom makes as much sense as a disembodied one.

CHINESE SOMATIZATION

Despite the "Western" emphasis on psychological experience, the DSM-IV includes a range of somatic symptoms. Given these symptoms are almost always an important part of depressive presentations, the issue may instead be one of emphasis—why do some patients have predominantly or exclusively somatic presentations while others emphasize psychological symptoms? We discuss "Chinese somatization," well aware that one could easily frame the phenomenon as "Western psychologization." "Western" contexts are also cultural contexts; variation in "somatization" and "psychologization" is inherently comparative. With this caveat in mind, we refer to and largely focus on Chinese somatization, for ease of use and in keeping with the available literature.

Evidence

One of the first systematically reported cultural group differences in mental health was a low rate of depression in Chinese contexts.[11] A mental health survey was undertaken in 12 regions of China in 1982, and replicated in seven of these regions in 1993.[12] The 1993 follow-up reported lifetime- and point-prevalence estimates of 0.08% and 0.05%, respectively, which are several hundred times higher than the rate found in 1982. The Global Burden of Disease project reported a 1-year incidence rate for unipolar depression in China of 2.3%,[13] compared with the 10.3% previously found in the United States.[14] National community surveys in Taiwan have identified similarly low depression rates compared with other countries,[2,15] although not as low as rates from the mainland.

Although some researchers asked why Chinese people were unusually protected from depression, others wondered whether reporting biases or differences in symptom presentation might play a role. Use of the Chinese diagnostic category shenjing-shuairuo (SJSR; also known as neurasthenia) might reflect either or both of these possibilities. Originally described by Beard[16] in the United States, the diagnosis was adopted first by Pavlov and then introduced to China by Russian psychiatrists after the 1949 revolution.[1,17] SJSR describes symptoms similar to MDD, but with an emphasis on the somatic—the cardinal symptom is physical and mental fatigue.

By the 1960s, as many as 80% of psychiatric outpatients in China carried SJSR diagnoses,[18,19] a figure that persisted at least until the early 1980s.[11,20] A review of Chinese research in the 1980s demonstrated that SJSR was by far the most frequently identified neurotic disorder in China,[21] whereas the diagnosis of depression was rarely used.[22] During certain periods, SJSR covered such a wide range of presentations, including schizophrenia, that clearly the diagnosis was being used in part to protect patients and their families from stigmatizing diagnoses.[18,19] Nonetheless, many patients did meet formal criteria for SJSR, which were increasingly well-defined through the 1980s.

In the now-classic example of, "the new cross-cultural psychiatry," Kleinman[11] studied 100 consecutive neurasthenia patients in a Chinese psychiatric outpatient clinic. Although he found that 87% of these patients were suffering from some sort of depressive disorder, he also found that the symptom presentations were very different from stereotypical "Western" cases—somatic symptoms were the most common chief complaints, and depressed mood was infrequently reported. He concluded that SJSR and MDD are both culturally shaped responses to social suffering, sharing commonalities but at the same time incomprehensible outside their specific cultural contexts.

This study led to numerous papers debating explanations for SJSR and somatization in China. Kleinman[23] himself proposed that the legacy of the Cultural Revolution might play a role, rendering certain psychological symptoms politically threatening. Of course, explanations contingent on historical events highlight the possibility of change over time. With the end of the Cultural Revolution and the opening of Chinese society, there is reason to anticipate that at least some of the cultural effects on depression and somatization might now be very different.[24]

Indeed, only a few years after the original study, Kleinman[25] reported on large changes underway during the 1980s, characterizing the period as one in which previously silenced emotions could now start to be expressed. Overlap with depressive disorders, coupled with the observation that the separate diagnoses did not provide clinically useful treatment information, led to a dramatic reduction in the use of SJSR[26] as a diagnosis or explanatory model. More recent epidemiologic studies suggest that rates of depressive disorders are increasing,[27–30] with adolescent figures comparable with those in North America.[31–33] The concerns of these patients may be shifting as well, to love and money rather than political conformity.[26]

These changes were well underway by the time the first cross-group comparisons were attempted. Yen and co-workers[34] found more somatic and fewer psychological symptoms among Chinese students seeking counseling compared with Chinese student controls. Yet, they also found fewer somatic symptoms in a Chinese student sample compared with Chinese-American and Euro-American student samples. They concluded that the Chinese emphasis on somatic symptoms is specific to people seeking help, with somatic symptoms being strategically chosen to more effectively access resources from the Chinese health care system.

The first direct comparison of clinical patients found that a somatic chief complaint was much more common in a depressed Malaysian Chinese sample compared with a depressed Euro-Australian sample.[20] Chinese respondents had higher endorsement rates for somatic symptoms on questionnaire compared with Euro-Australians;

Euro-Australian respondents had higher endorsement rates for psychological symptoms compared with Malaysian Chinese. Indeed, the latter effect was stronger, supporting the idea that "Western psychologization" is a cultural phenomenon deserving just as much investigation. A follow-up study in Australian primary care settings found these differences lessen as Chinese-Australians adapt to mainstream Australian society.[35]

Ryder and associates[36] used clinical interviews, structured interviews, and questionnaires in Chinese and Euro-Canadian psychiatric outpatients. There was again support for greater somatic symptom reporting in the Chinese sample, and even stronger support for greater psychological symptom reporting in the Euro-Canadian sample. Levels of "externally oriented thinking" (EOT), higher in the Chinese sample and predictive of somatic symptoms in both samples, partially explained the relation between cultural group and somatic symptom emphasis. Although numerous explanations of Chinese somatization have been proposed, they have rarely been tested empirically.[36,37]

Although cultural variation in symptom presentation continues despite rapid changes in Chinese society, these studies also demonstrate that it is rare for patients in either group to solely report one set of symptoms, either somatic or psychological, at the expense of the other. Chinese somatization, at least over the past decade, seems to be a matter of symptom emphasis rather than an utterly different way of presenting distress. At the same time, the explanatory value of EOT suggests that observed group differences might be more than strategic presentation of symptoms. It is to potential explanations for Chinese somatization that we now turn.

Pathologizing Explanations of Chinese Somatization

The first generation of explanations offered for Chinese somatization tended to assume that psychological symptom presentation was the norm for depression. Indeed, psychoanalysts introduced the term "somatization" to refer to a defense mechanism in which anxious affect is permitted to reach consciousness only through visceral expression.[38] This view implies that something else—a psychological experience closer to the true problem—is being somatized. Such a view in turn implies that a tendency to emphasize somatic symptoms represents an immature defense.[39] In other words, cultural contexts that foster such avoidance of threatening content are therefore less psychologically sophisticated.

A different hierarchy was proposed several decades ago based on linguistics rather than psychoanalysis. In this view, languages differ in terms of their capacity to describe emotions and other abstract psychological constructs in detail: The structure of a vocabulary directly reflects the emotional life of the population using that vocabulary.[40] English—predictably—ranks at the top, and Chinese is much lower down. Chinese patients might have depression, but lacking the language to describe it they rely instead on somatic metaphors.[41]

Both approaches have been criticized for proposing Eurocentric hierarchies that privilege classical mind–body dualism with its emphasis on the primacy of the mind.[42,43] This view corresponds with descriptions of individualistic values and the independent self-construal, emphasized in cultural contexts with origins in Western Europe. Because the most important features of personal identity are situated in the mind, a good self should be able to appraise these features and communicate them to others.[44] Much of the world's population, by contrast, does not hold such a model of the self.[45]

Strategic Explanations of Chinese Somatization

A number of additional explanations for Chinese somatization posit that the fundamental experience of depression is not so different across cultural contexts. Instead, a somatic symptom emphasis reflects the need for different strategies to navigate different contexts. The Chinese language does indeed have an adequate number of words to describe psychological states,[37,46] and somatic metaphors are often used as part of a culturally shaped communication style.[47] European languages also have such expressions; English includes expressions such as heartache, burning anger, blind panic, and butterflies in the stomach.[24,48] Somatic metaphors for emotions convey rich meaning, and do so across a wide range of cultural contexts.

Such metaphors are evocative in their own right, but can also help people talk indirectly about threatening ideas. Goffman[49] characterizes psychiatric stigma as a sense that people with mental illness have a spoiled identity, one that also carries over to those who interact with them. There is thus considerable pressure, especially from friends and family, not to be labeled in this way; moreover, such labeling can generate a looping effect in which the consequences of stigma worsens the illness.[50–53] Somatization allows psychologically distressed people to be sick without stigma.[54]

Psychiatric stigma in Chinese populations can be inferred from studies showing a help-seeking delay.[43,55–57] The elapsed time is spent pursuing traditional and self-care approaches of various types.[58] When psychosocial attributions are made, there is a tendency to prefer help from friends rather than physicians.[43] There is also a preference for nonpsychiatric medical practitioners rather than psychiatrists when professional help is deemed necessary.[58] Chinese families are particularly likely to shield the afflicted family member from the community when the need for professional help arises.[59]

Along with avoidance of psychiatric stigma, presentation of somatic symptoms can also be understood as "ticket behavior," emphasizing symptoms that provide access to care. Somatic symptoms are commonly reported in primary care across a range of countries, including Western Europe and North America.[60] Moreover, many patients who present initially with somatic symptoms in primary care settings go on to endorse psychological symptoms when asked about them directly.[23] Chinese people may simply have an even greater tendency to seek help from general medical practitioners when distressed, and emphasize those somatic symptoms perceived as relevant to a medical setting.[58] Is it possible, however, that perception of relevance actually magnifies the experience of the symptom itself?

An Attentional Explanation of Cultural Variation

Pathologizing explanations of Chinese somatization imply that culture shapes subjective experience of depressive symptoms. Strategic explanations instead emphasize various ways of navigating the social world, at times explicitly repudiating the ethnocentric assumptions of older approaches.[37,43] These strategies are not necessarily conscious, but they involve a reasonable approach to the social world. One communicates to specific others using available terms, idioms, metaphors, and so on, that best fit the purpose at hand—pursuing positive ends (eg, social support, symptom relief) while avoiding negative ones (eg, criticism, shame). In this view, "somatization is basically a communicative act."[61]

Implicit in this contrast of hierarchical and strategic explanations is the idea that only the former approach really involves variation in the subjective experience of symptoms. The latter approach is compatible with the idea that depression itself is the same around the world, but different people choose to emphasize different symptoms for culturally shaped reasons. Strategy does not necessarily preclude deep shaping of experience; however, Kleinman and Kleinman[23] argue that the Cultural Revolution profoundly shaped the emotional lives of people who lived through it.[23] If it is indeed possible for such strategies to change symptom experience itself, and not just how they are described or enacted, by what mechanisms might this take place?

Researchers have described characterological tendencies to attend to the body or away from thoughts and feelings, albeit with a tendency to pathologize them. For example, somatosensory amplification is defined as bodily hypervigilance, focus on weak and infrequent sensations, and tendency to assume that sensations signify problems.[62,63] The result is increased somatic symptom reporting without increased coherence between self-report and measureable physiologic change.[64,65] Others have proposed that somatization might be caused by difficulties in processing and expressing affect.[66] Alexithymia—literally, "no words for feelings"—is characterized by difficulty identifying feelings, difficulty describing feelings, and externally EOT. High scores on this trait are linked to various psychological and psychosomatic problems, including a tendency to identify negative emotional arousal as physical symptoms.

As an explanation for cultural differences in symptom presentation, alexithymia risks pathologizing particular groups.[67] Indeed, the original descriptions of alexithymia come from psychoanalysis, and both difficulty identifying feelings and difficulty describing feelings clearly describe pathology.[68] EOT, in contrast, represents a lack of interest in and attention to one's own emotional life, resembling a culturally shaped set of values about emotions rather than a particular impairment. If EOT differs from the other 2 components in helping to explain Chinese somatization and in relating to cultural values, we would have preliminary evidence that culture might be shaping the attentional processes involved in somatic symptom presentation.

Indeed, we observe this pattern in recent research. Greater alexithymia levels are found in Chinese versus Euro-Canadian samples,[69] a difference largely driven by EOT—which alone mediates cultural group differences in somatic symptom presentation.[36] Moreover, cultural variation in EOT comparing Euro-Canadian and Chinese-Canadian students is mediated by adherence to "Western" values.[70] EOT, but not other components of alexithymia, is also associated with these values in a Chinese psychiatric outpatient sample. (Dere J, Tang Q, Zhu X, et al. The cultural shaping of alexithymia: values and externally oriented thinking in a Chinese clinical sample. Submitted for publication.) Chinese cultural contexts encourage focus away from the internal world of emotions to the practical details of the external world, in turn shaping symptom presentation.

It is not necessary to assume that deep cultural variation in symptom presentation reflects stereotypes about the best way of presenting symptoms. Instead, we can consider how attentional processes encourage a focus on certain symptoms, processes that ultimately reflect different value priorities. In this view, depressed people living in Chinese cultural contexts who engage in EOT for culturally meaningful reasons are not dysfunctional, but nonetheless experience somatic symptoms as more salient and more important than psychological symptoms. Depressed people living in North American cultural contexts, meanwhile, find psychological experiences particularly salient and central to the sense that one has conveyed that experience to others.

Our consideration of the research literature on culture and depression has taken us to a point where deeper interpretation leading to a future research agenda is needed. We believe, however, that one cannot make much progress in that direction without a clear view of what "culture" actually is, what it means. Beyond the biopsychosocial model, in which 3 domains all contribute toward understanding mental health, we propose a single multilevel system—the culture–mind–brain—in which the 3 components are fundamentally inseparable. We briefly introduce this perspective and then use it to consider the implications of our attentional approach to Chinese somatization.

DEPRESSION AND THE CULTURE–MIND–BRAIN

In briefly presenting our emerging model of culture–mind–brain, we begin with an attempt to better describe what "culture" represents. Although we do not expect to provide a final definition—it may be impossible to do so—we believe a working definition is necessary at this point before continuing. Then, we turn to a summary of culture–mind–brain, considering implications for mental health. In closing, we reflect on the position of the body in such a system, important for any work on somatization. Note that we do not see this perspective as brand new, but rather as representing an emerging integration that extends back along several lines of thought on culture, psychology, and mental health. We also believe it points forward to new research and new ways of thinking about treatment, ideas to which we shall return.

What Is Culture?

Our starting point in understanding culture is the 'cultural psychology' approach of Shweder,[71] Markus and Kitayama,[44] Heine and Norenzayan,[72] and many others. We emphasize this approach because of its conception of how culture and psychology interrelate, and because this conception points to specific ways of conducting research. Mainstream psychiatric and psychological research tends to use "culture" as a synonym for ethnic group or nationality, and has done so for a long time. There are advantages, certainly—research designs are more straightforward and results are easier to discuss with clearly identified groups.

The danger here is a slippage from the pragmatic use of such groups for research purposes to the assumption that one is identifying fixed group characteristics. One runs the risk of stereotyping while evading important questions about why group differences are observed. "Culture" becomes a black-box explanation for observed differences, rather than a complex phenomenon that itself demands explication.[1] The last couple of decades brought a salutary shift away from this approach, defining culture in terms of beliefs and practices that pertain to a group, rather than as synonymous with the group itself.[73] Along with this general perspective come specific methods researchers can use to explore and unpack how culture shapes psychological processes, including those implicated in psychopathology.

Researchers also increasingly attend to heterogeneity among group members. Rather than treating each member as a perfect representative of that group, specific aspects of the cultural context shape different people in different ways. There is a sense in which sets of beliefs and practices are common to a group—even rejection of a norm is still shaped in certain ways by that norm, and others see this rejection in light of that norm.[4,74] There is another sense, equally important, in which beliefs and practices are distributed throughout a cultural group, rather than replicated in each member.

By emphasizing both beliefs and practices, we are arguing for a view of culture as, at the same time, "in the head" and "in the world."[1] Indeed, attempts to make a clear distinction here might represent a legacy of dualistic thinking. The idea of cultural scripts bridges these perspectives, reflecting meaning structures while guiding behavioral practices.[75] People perform "acts of meaning,"[76] behaviors that only make sense within a given cultural meaning system, shared at least in part by actor and observer.[74] Moreover, enacting these behaviors further shapes the meaning system.[77]

What do we mean here by "cultural script"? First, "scripts" refer to organized units of culturally salient knowledge, such as knowledge about the ways in which one communicates distress. This information is based on observation as well as formal learning; it may be implicit and thus not accessible via verbal recall. Second, scripts serve as mechanisms for rapid, automatic retrieval of information and recognition of patterns. Information stored in scripts is easily primed and activated, and is processed in tightly organized packages regardless of the script's apparent complexity. Finally, once scripts are enacted they are observable by others as behavior and become elements of the larger cultural context.[1]

Kleinman and Kleinman's[23] description of the Cultural Revolution's impact on symptom presentation in China can be understood this way. Cultural scripts emerged in which certain experiences were freighted with profoundly dangerous political significance. Some depression symptoms became closely bound with ideas of decadence, laziness, or antiproletarian attitudes.[21] For example, "hopelessness" signaled an indictment of communist society. The sufferer would know that others could perceive it this way, and might even do so themselves. They would then follow the script by not expressing such attitudes; others would play their roles too, reinforcing behaviors conforming to the script while making it difficult to express proscribed ideas. Somatic symptoms and SJSR would be easily understood as part of longstanding cultural scripts linking them to bodily and brain dysfunction.[78]

The Culture–Mind–Brain

The core claim of cultural psychology is not simply that "culture matters," but rather that culture and mind "make each other up."[79] This process is an integral part of socialization, in that the mind develops in cultural contexts that are themselves composed of minds. Children develop psychological systems designed to regulate thoughts, feelings, and actions in ways deeply shaped by the environment, and they also impact and help to shape that environment.[80,81] One must find ways of thinking and studying the psychological and the cultural so that neither is seen as the ultimate source of the other.[82]

Departing from traditional cultural psychology, we add brain to our conception of mutual constitution. It is now untenable to propose models of mental health that have no room for the brain and the ways in which it is shaped by the genome and, in turn, by evolutionary processes. Rather than replacing mind with brain, mind is retained as a separate level that is experiential, tool using, and social—deeply interconnected with the surrounding world and with other minds.[83,84] Incorporating the brain also keeps with the emerging subdiscipline of cultural neuroscience, which is documenting ways in which the environment shapes the highly plastic brain so that brain function reflects cultural variation.[85,86]

Indeed, the human brain seems to be adapted quite specifically for the acquisition of culture, and responds to cultural inputs with marked plasticity, especially early in development.[87] At the same time, the brain does not contain an infinite number of possibilities for human life. Biology places constraints on culture. There are a great number of possible ways in which culture can be configured, but the number is finite; the number of impossible configurations is practically infinite.[88–90] We should therefore expect a large but finite number of ways in which humans in different contexts respond to basic life predicaments, such as loss of status, resources, or relationships.

As with psychopathology in general, we see depression as an emergent property of culture–mind–brain. The implication is that while changes at 1 level affect all levels, ultimate cause cannot be assigned to any given level. This idea can be approached by considering different levels of complexity in the brain: "A disordered brain circuit does not require malfunctioning neurons, nor does a disordered neuron require malfunctioning molecules, although neither makes sense in the absence of neurons or molecules."[1] A brain-level change cascades through the system and affects the other levels—so too a mind-level change, or a culture-level change.

For example, the Cultural Revolution might have disrupted local social networks to cause profound chronic stress, with consequences for the brain,[91] pointing in turn to further consequences for mind and culture. Today, rapid modernization in China might be exerting its own effects on mind and brain. A mind-level intervention, such as cognitive-behavior therapy, is understood according to cultural scripts about appropriate ways of dealing with depression. If delivered in a culturally appropriate manner, the treatment not only changes thoughts, behaviors, and feelings, but also the brain.[92] None of these possibilities are surprising when culture–mind–brain is considered as a single system.

Situating the Body

Where does the body, so important for understanding somatic symptoms, fit into this model? We see "the body" as existing across all levels of culture–mind–brain. At the brain level, the body continually relays and receives signals to and from the brain, which monitors these sensory inputs, integrates them, and maintains a dynamic representation of the state of the body.[93,94] This interoceptive information is processed by the same brain areas that detect and evaluate hedonic changes and contribute to construction of the subjective experiences of emotion,[95–97] suggesting that neural representations of the body and emotions are intertwined.

At the mind level, emergent conscious representation of the body integrates sensory and hedonic inputs with conceptions of normative and non-normative bodily responses. These conceptions continually evolve based on personal and inferred experience, and are situation specific—for example, feeling exhausted is normal after a hard day's work or during a cold. Current feelings are compared with memories and expectations of typical bodily responses to a given situation. Once activated, these conceptions direct attention to particular bodily feelings. Conceptions that are highly salient in a given situation may even trump physiologic changes.[98,99] Notably, depression and somatization impair monitoring of one's bodily state by focusing attention on highly salient conceptions of the body.[100,101]

At the culture level, sufferers draw on the large but finite pool of possible responses to profound distress,[102] which includes numerous bodily reactions. Activated scripts draw attention to some responses and away from others.[1] More than shaping how these responses are described, attention magnifies or minimizes them, changing how they are experienced. Salient responses become particularly prominent and are drawn into the web of associations provided by the cultural script—what it means to have this response, whether it should be shared with others, and so on. In short, they become symptoms.

Thus, the assumption that somatic and psychological symptoms are in fact distinct reflects a particular cultural worldview rather than an underlying neural mapping of somatic and hedonic signals. Inherently integrated streams of somatic and psychological experiences are identified as related by people who conceptualize them as related. Others might conceptualize them as distinct, and so experience them as such. Somatization reflects culturally based tuning of these signals toward an amplification of somatic signals and reduced sensitivity to affective or cognitive signals. The result is neither closer nor further from the brain-level signals than the "Western" tendency to clearly separate the signals and prioritize the psychological. Both represent effects of activated cultural scripts.

ATTENTION TO SYMPTOMS IN THE CULTURE–MIND–BRAIN

We return now to Chinese somatization to reflect on how a culture–mind–brain approach pushes our thinking forward. While reviewing previous research, we used the standard diagnostic terminology shared by these studies. Here, in considering new directions, we prefer to use "profound distress" rather than using a specific diagnostic label, although we certainly believe that people meeting criteria for MDD—or SJSR—would fit under that general rubric. The aim is to take a step back from some of the cultural baggage that comes with specific diagnostic labels, especially when the key label includes the name of a symptom where the presentation and even meaning are under discussion.

The Social Life of Symptoms

Profound distress, however defined, does not emerge as a rational ordering of certain symptoms that need to be described to the right people, but rather as a chaotic mix of sensations, emotions, thoughts, and behaviors. Sufferers try to account for this chaos and cannot focus on everything at once; indeed, the more intense the experience, the greater the need to explain it and the more reliance upon scripts to do so.[103] People have access to cultural scripts relevant to profound distress and assume that others have access to them as well.[104]

One consequence of having a deeply social mind is awareness that one acts meaningfully in front of real and imagined audiences. Behaviors are watched and interpreted by others, thoughts are potentially shared or concealed from others, occupational impairment impacts on and may be judged by others, and so on. Indeed, there is evidence that depression can spread through populations, like an infectious disease but via mechanisms of social influence.[105] More than just encouraging help-securing or stigma-avoiding presentations, the real and imagined presence of others shapes our choice of scripts, the emotions that get expressed, and the symptoms that emerge.[1,106,107]

It is only through this process of socially and culturally shaped winnowing of chaotic experience to a specific set of symptoms that categories of "somatic" and "psychological" start to emerge. This distinction serves important functions. Sufferers may at times become consciously aware of the demands of a particular situation and choose to emphasize certain categories of experience. We believe it more likely, however, that, help-securing or stigma-avoiding presentations often seem strategic because they tend to work, in the aggregate, for many people facing similar situations in the same cultural context—and as such, these strategies get incorporated into cultural scripts.

Acute episodes pass, but leave a legacy in culture–mind–brain. The brain learns to process interoceptive information in new ways, with increased sensitivity to negative cues coupled with decreased coherence between experiences, communicative acts, behavioral expressions, and measurable physiologic changes.[100] Still-activated cultural scripts join with personal narratives about one's own failings, increasing likelihood for further distress and possibly future episodes.[108] Former sufferers have to adapt to the knowledge that they are capable of great disturbance and impairment while navigating the revised views of others as well. Actual experiences of profound distress in turn shape relevant cultural scripts: Sufferers typify these scripts, but also transcend them through their own specific narratives. If many sufferers add similar extra-script details, the script itself shifts.

From Conscious Strategy to Core Experience

We propose that attentional mechanisms are central to Chinese somatization—and "Western psychologization"—and that these mechanisms are deeply shaped by the social world. Rather than superseding previous efforts to explain why somatic symptoms might be emphasized in China, we retain their best aspects. We agree that social positioning strategies, such as those that facilitate help and avoid stigma, are important; however, we see these strategies as very often deeply experienced while acknowledging that they may at times be consciously chosen.

We also agree with Kleinman and Kleinman[24] that important historical and political contingencies can profoundly affect the cultural environment and thereby shape both the experience and expression of symptoms. Rapid modernization and urbanization may well be exerting similar effects in China presently.[78] The question remains, however—what are the means by which a social positioning strategy, such as how one talks to a friend about a problem, or a physician about a symptom, shapes the problem or symptom itself? We briefly review 3 possibilities.

Regulation can be implicit

People use effortful control to regulate emotions when needed under particular circumstances, but there is a tendency to assume that the default state, the normal and healthy state, is emotional expression. Research has demonstrated, in contrast, that suppression is not necessarily problematic and may in fact reflect culturally normative functioning. Depression in Euro-American cultural contexts is generally characterized by dampened emotional reactivity to negative or positive stimuli.[109] In Chinese-American cultural contexts, this effect is not observed—on some measures there is evidence of more reactivity in depressed people, even when the stimulus is positive.[110,111]

Emotional suppression is not necessarily a problem, but rather can make sense in particular contexts to fit cultural norms and expectations. That does not mean emotional suppression is consciously chosen as a strategy to that end. In fact, emotional experience can be—and often is—regulated implicitly. Implicit regulation happens when people learn to employ the same regulatory strategy repeatedly, making its use automatic, effortless, and less costly to psychosocial functioning.[112–115] This learning includes personal experience, but also social learning through direct observation of others or hearing relevant stories about others. Emotions and their constituents, including somatic sensations, thereby shift in ways that make sense for the situation without any effortful control.

Complicating matters, profound distress does more than generate emotional states in need of regulation. Regulatory processes are also adversely affected. The cultural norm hypothesis posits that MDD is associated with regulatory patterns that differ from local norms.[110,111] Profound distress in North American cultural contexts represents failure to adhere to scripts promoting open or exaggerated emotions[116]; profound distress in Chinese cultural contexts represents failure to adhere to scripts promoting moderated emotions.[117] Cultural scripts shape how distressed people attend to particular experiences while, at the same time, these people interpret some of these experiences as violations of scripts. In either case, we suspect that the attendant distress would make constant effortful and strategic regulation very difficult to maintain. The result is a combination of regulatory approaches, explicit and implicit, executed with varying degrees of success.

Expression shapes experience
In considering the gap between private experience of symptoms and their public expression, there is a tendency to assume that the former governs the latter. Where there is discrepancy, it is because the sufferer has chosen to conceal or distort their private experience. Emotion researchers going back to William James, in contrast, have long held that experience and expression shape one another; the experience of profound suffering is likely to be constructed at least in part on how the sufferer behaves and describes this experience to others. Sadness makes us frown, but frowning also makes us sad.[118,119] A cultural context that discourages certain public expressions will thereby shape private experience as well.

There is no single "true" report
Much of the debate on Chinese somatization involves consideration of which symptoms are true symptoms. Some approaches assume that psychological symptoms were both true and best; others assume that public symptom presentation reflects either private experience or strategic distortion. Such concerns are relevant to clinical practice as well, where "accuracy" of patient reports and their interpretation by the clinician is critical to effective diagnosis. We have argued, however, that contextual features profoundly shape both experience and expression of symptoms. Contextual features of the recall situation further complicate this picture. Just as we do not have perfectly accurate memories, symptom reports are never—strictly speaking—true.

Instead of thinking of these seeming distortions as noise or measurement error, we should consider them as valuable data. Similarly, lack of coherence between different aspects of an emotional problem does not reflect reporting errors. There is no reason to assume that somatic and psychological symptom clusters should closely align in any given sufferer. As emotion researchers have learned, we should not assume certain modes of assessment are "truer" than others. Self-disclosure or inner experience, behavior or cognition or physiologic response, each contribute to understanding and all are vulnerable to noise. Nor is the true response the average or aggregate across these signals; rather, it is the pattern across all signals, including inconsistencies.[120–122]

Summary
We believe that the application of a culture–mind–brain perspective to Chinese somatization opens up new possibilities for the study of longstanding questions in cultural psychiatry. There is the potential here to break down the false dichotomy between personal experience and public expression of symptoms. For anthropologists and cultural psychiatrists, who have long argued that the social world does indeed deeply shape personal experience, we suggest specific mechanisms by which this shaping might take place. That said, much of the supportive evidence is indirect. Although the processes and mechanisms we describe are plausible, and grounded in research, we await studies that apply our proposed approach to specific questions. A move toward the multimethod and interdisciplinary work required to systematically pursue culture and mental health research in this way is the necessary next step.

BROADER IMPLICATIONS FOR RESEARCH AND TREATMENT

For decades, psychiatrists and other mental health professions have spoken of the biopsychosocial approach, invoking it as a reminder that the biological, the psychological, and the social all contribute to our understanding of mental health. The approach we advocate here, building on developments in cultural psychiatry, anthropology, and cultural psychology, incorporates the same 3 broad domains. We believe the critical distinction is the idea of mutual constitution: We are making claims beyond the straightforward idea that each of 3 domains carries a proportion of the explanatory weight. To the extent that culture, mind, and brain can be said to "make each other up," effectively making for a single multilevel system, we have to adjust our views of mental illness and its treatment in fundamental ways.

Although the need for a new perspective following broadly these principles has been discussed within cultural psychiatry for decades,[123,124] we believe that with some exceptions this need has not had much influence on the psychiatric mainstream. One reason may be the current ascendancy, and in many ways remarkable successes, of genetics and neuroscience research. A second reason, intertwined with the first, may be that there is often a tendency to pit the biological and the cultural against one another. In viewing culture, mind, and brain as deeply interconnected, and ultimately unitary, we hope to challenge the assumption that we can take any part of this system seriously while dismissing the other parts.

A third, pragmatic, reason may be that taking seriously deeply argued cultural critiques of psychiatry requires us to rethink how we conduct research or deliver treatment, and may even imply that such pursuits are extremely difficult or no longer scientific. We believe, in contrast, that there is little lasting purpose to a culture–mind–brain approach unless it points the way to feasible research programs. As we have argued elsewhere,[1,4,80] there are in fact a plethora of methods available in various subdisciplines of psychology. Other disciplines have much to contribute here as well; the study of culture and mental health is inherently interdisciplinary.[24]

Many such methods are familiar to consumers of the psychiatric and behavioral sciences literatures—questionnaires and interviews, social experiments, physiologic readings, ethnographies. Others are newly emerging, with several particularly well-suited to the complex task of studying people in context—situation sampling, in vivo behavioral observation, examination of cultural products.[4] Moreover, although we anticipate most future work will continue focusing on 1 level while incorporating, we hope, awareness of the others, several recent studies showcase the potential for integration across levels; even, in a few cases, incorporating aspects of all 3 levels.[125,126] Application of a culture–mind–brain approach to Chinese somatization is but a small example of the potential.

A culture–mind–brain approach to mental health also impacts treatment. What are we to make of applied research that adapts well-established treatments for particular cultural contexts? There is insufficient space here to consider the many issues pertaining to cross-cultural adaptations of treatments. Although such adaptations can be deeply problematic, often little more than cultural dressing up of "Western" approaches, we see reason for optimism in efforts to carefully integrate culturally specific approaches. For example, there is ongoing work in China to incorporate Daoist perspectives into cognitive-behavior therapy for depression, and in Canada to develop culturally appropriate group cognitive-behavior therapy for Chinese migrants, with some supportive evidence.[127,128] Meta-analysis collapsing across groups provides at least some preliminary evidence that integrating cultural specificity into the design of treatment programs improves outcomes.[129]

Treatments developed in this way can potentially incorporate cultural research on mental health in ways that include these findings into how we work with individual patients. The move toward "unpacking culture," explicating processes underlying group differences while incorporating group heterogeneity, can also help us clinically. If we know that a particular script tends to shape symptom presentation in a particular way, we can better understand those patients for whom the script is not operating, and who thus might present symptoms in a different way. We cannot use culturally specific treatments in a "cookbook" manner, but rather must adapt them for actual people embedded in actual contexts.

There are implications for the "cultural competence" necessary to flexibly use suitable treatment programs. If people are deeply embedded in their local social worlds, it does not make much sense to proceed with a cookbook approach either to acquiring cultural competence or to delivering particular treatments. We have argued that "cultural groups" are best understood as pragmatic constructs for particular purposes.[1] Even understood this way, many North American clinicians could potentially encounter patients from dozens of groups. Ethnoracial blocs such as "Hispanic" or "Asian," most often used in the United States, are much too heterogeneous to support a cultural competence approach based on deep knowledge of the patient in context.[130]

What then is cultural competence? We believe that a culture–mind–brain approach to mental health requires that clinicians think about patients in their local worlds, learning from and with patients how they fit into these contexts. Doing so requires attention to available and activated scripts—what the patient believes, their intersubjective[74] beliefs about what others believe, how they act in the world as a result, and how others respond. Although no one can be expected to understand the countless ways in which a deeply interconnected system might work, a culture–mind–brain approach demands, at a minimum, openness to a wide range of potential information sources. Familial risks and psychopharmacologic mechanisms remain important, no more and no less than political conflict in the country of origin or religious beliefs about the meaning of suffering.

This general approach to cultural competence raises a further question—how is this different from clinical competence? Is not attention to these things part of being a good clinician? We agree. Yet, we believe there is value in keeping the 2 ideas separate, while maintaining that you cannot effectively have one without the other. The problem with maintaining a sole focus on clinical competence is that we can proceed sensitively, but without realizing the extent to which we are products of our own cultural contexts. Moreover, clinicians can fail to recognize how much they are shaped by their particular, and in some ways peculiar, local worlds—the ethos of medicine, psychiatry, and psychology.[131]

Returning to our opening examples, clinicians working with both Mrs Liu and Ms Chan would not get any closer to the "essence of Chinese-ness." Indeed, an important part of their learning experience should be realizing this. Attending to cultural context includes noticing how different these 2 patients are, not just how similar. At the same time, working with these patients might teach the clinician to attend more carefully to different ways in which somatic metaphors might convey profound distress. The clinician might become more adept at considering how different explanatory models shape acceptability of a treatment, and at proposing treatment options in ways that resonate with their patients. As part of that process, we hope they will notice that their own views of distress and its amelioration are shaped by their social position, in cultural context, at a particular historical moment.

Clinicians and researchers should come to perceive their own lives as culturally shaped ways of being in the world.[130] We need to understand our own contexts both to remain grounded in them while also defamiliarizing ourselves, seeing how we live as one way of living. Encountering cultural difference, through personal experience, clinical work, or research, then becomes part of understanding very different lives. Working cross-culturally can help us to do this, especially when accompanied by supervision or consultation, provided we do not assume that a guidebook and a few cases will teach us rules about how a particular cultural context operates. Cultural competence does not lead to easy answers, but vastly expands the possibilities we can imagine and then the questions we can ask.

SUMMARY

We have presented a view of culture and mental health that builds on work in cultural psychiatry, anthropology, and cultural psychology, and applied it to research on culture and depression. In particular, we have returned to the well-known topic of Chinese somatization. A culture–mind–brain approach to these questions helps us think about them in a way that points toward new research. We have applied this approach to thinking about a single set of questions, relevant to a single (DSM-based) diagnosis, in a single cultural group. The potential, however, is to rethink how we conceptualize mental health in ways consistent with cultural psychiatry's general perspective over the past several decades, while incorporating rather than rejecting the many recent advances in brain and behavior sciences. In so doing, we gain a more expanded and nuanced view of the global landscape of mental health, accompanied by a more expanded and nuanced view of individual patients.

REFERENCES

1. Ryder AG, Ban LM, Chentsova-Dutton YE. Towards a cultural— clinical psychology. Social and Personality Psychology Compass 2011;5:960–75.
2. Weissman MM, Bland RC, Canino GJ, et al. Cross-national epidemiology of major depression and bipolar disorder. JAMA 1996;276:293–9.
3. Andrade L, Caraveo-Anduaga JJ, Berglund P, et al. The epidemiology of major depressive episodes: results from the International Consortium of Psychiatric Epidemiology (ICPE) Surveys. Int J Methods Psychiatric Res 2003;12:3–21.
4. Ryder AG, Dere J, Sun J, et al. Personality disorders. In: Leong FT, Comas-Diaz L, Hall GCN, et al, editors. APA handbook of multicultural psychology. Washington, DC: American Psychological Association; in press.
5. Nesse RM. Is depression an adaptation? Arch Gen Psychiatry 2000;57:14–20.
6. Shweder RA. The cultural psychology of the emotions. In: Handbook of emotions New York: Guilford Press; 1993. p. 417–31.
7. Eid M, Diener E. Norms for experiencing emotions in different cultures: inter- and intranational differences. J Pers Soc Psychol 2001;81:869–85.
8. Mesquita B, Karasawa M. Different emotional lives. Cogn Emot 2002;16:127–41.
9. Scollon C, Diener E, Oishi S, et al. Emotions across cultures and methods. J Cross Cult Psychol 2004;304–26.
10. Kirmayer LJ. Cultural variations in the clinical presentation of depression and anxiety: implications for diagnosis and treatment. J Clin Psychiatry 2001;62:22–30.
11. Kleinman A. Neurasthenia and depression: a study of somatization and culture in China. Cult Med Psychiatry 1982;6:117–90.
12. Parker G, Gladstone G, Chee KT. Depression in the planet's largest ethnic group: the Chinese. Am J Psychiatry 2001;158:857–64.

13. Murray CJL, Lopez AD. The global burden of disease: a comprehensive assessment of mortality and disability from diseases, injuries, and risk factors in 1990 and projected to 2020. Cambridge: Harvard University Press; 1996.

14. Kessler RC, McGonagle KA, Zhao S, et al. Lifetime and 12-month prevalence of DSM-III-R psychiatric disorders in the United States. Results from the National Comorbidity Survey. Arch Gen Psychiatry 1994;51:8–19.

15. Hwu HG, Yeh EK, Chang LY. Prevalence of psychiatric disorders in Taiwan defined by the Chinese Diagnostic Interview Schedule. Acta Psychiatr Scand 1989;79:136–47.

16. Beard G. Neurasthenia, or nervous exhaustion. The Boston Medical and Surgical Journal 1869;80:217–21.

17. Liu S. Neurasthenia in China: modern and traditional criteria for its diagnosis. Cult Med Psychiatry 1989;13:163–86.

18. Lin TY. Neurasthenia revisited: its place in modern psychiatry. Cult Med Psychiatry 1989;13:105–29.

19. Yang H. The necessity of retaining the diagnostic concept of neurasthenia. Cult Med Psychiatry 1989;13:139–45.

20. Parker G, Cheah YC, Roy K. Do the Chinese somatize depression? A cross-cultural study. Soc Psychiatry Psychiatr Epidemiol 2001;36:287–93.

21. Cheung F. Health psychology in Chinese societies in Asia. In: Jansen M, Wenman J, editors. The international development of health psychology. Readings (UK): Harwood Academic Press; 1991. p. 63–74.

22. Lee S. Cultures in psychiatric nosology: the CCMD-2-R and international classification of mental disorders. Cult Med Psychiatry 1996;20:421–72.

23. Kleinman A, Kleinman J. Remembering the cultural revolution: alienating pains and the pain of alienation/transformation. In: Lin T-Y, Tseng WS, Yeh E, editors. Chinese societies and mental health. Hong Kong: Oxford University Press; 1995. p. 141–55.

24. Ryder AG, Ban LM, Dere J. Culture, self, and symptom: perspectives from cultural psychology. In: Hansen T, Berlinger P, Jensen de Lopez, K, editors. Self in culture in mind: conceptual and applied approaches. Aalborg (Denmark): Aalborg University Press; in press.

25. Kleinman A. Social origins of distress and disease: depression, neurasthenia, and pain in modern China. New Haven (CT): Yale University Press; 1986.

26. Lee S. Diagnosis postponed: shenjing shuairuo and the transformation of psychiatry in post-Mao China. Cult Med Psychiatry 1999;23:349–80.

27. Dennis C. Mental health: Asia's tigers get the blues. Nature 2004;429:696–8.

28. Lee S, Tsang A, Zhang M-Y, et al. Lifetime prevalence and inter-cohort variation in DSM-IV disorders in metropolitan China. Psychol Med 2007;37:61–71.

29. Phillips MR, Zhang J, Shi Q, et al. Prevalence, treatment, and associated disability of mental disorders in four provinces in China during 2001–05: an epidemiological survey. Lancet 2009;373:2041–53.

30. Zhou TX, Zhang SP, Jiang YQ, et al. Epidemiology of neuroses in a Shanghai community. Chinese Mental Health Journal 2000;14:332–4.

31. Liu X, Kurita H, Guo C, et al. Behavioral and emotional problems in Chinese children: teacher reports for ages 6 to 11. J Child Psychol Psychiatry 2000;41:253–60.

32. Liu X, Tein J-Y, Zhao Z, et al. Suicidality and correlates among rural adolescents of China. J Adolesc Health 2005;37:443–51.

33. Yang Y, Li H, Zhang Y, et al. Age and gender differences in behavioral problems in Chinese children: parent and teacher reports. Asian Journal of Psychiatry 2008;1: 42–6.

34. Yen S, Robins CJ, Lin N. A cross-cultural comparison of depressive symptom manifestation: China and the United States. J Consult Clin Psychol 2000;68:993–9.
35. Parker G, Chan B, Tully L, et al. Depression in the Chinese: the impact of acculturation. Psychol Med 2005;35:1475–84.
36. Ryder AG, Yang J, Zhu X, et al. The cultural shaping of depression: somatic symptoms in China, psychological symptoms in North America? J Abnorm Psychol 2008;117:300–13.
37. Cheung MCF. Facts and myths about somatization among the Chinese. In: Lin T-Y, Tseng WS, Yeh EK, editors. Chinese societies and mental health. Hong Kong: Oxford University Press; 1995. p. 156–80.
38. Craig T, Boardman A. Somatization in primary care settings. In: Bass C, editor. Somatization: physical symptoms and psychological illness. Oxford: Blackwell; 1990. p. 73–104.
39. Draguns JG, Bond MH. Abnormal behaviour in Chinese societies: clinical, epidemiological, and comparative studies. In: The handbook of Chinese psychology. New York: Oxford University Press; 1996. p. 412–28.
40. Leff J. The cross-cultural study of emotions. Cult Med Psychiatry 1980;1:317–50.
41. Leff JP. Psychiatry around the globe: a transcultural view. London: Gaskell; 1988.
42. Beeman WO. Dimensions of dysphoria: the view from linguistic anthropology. In: Kleinman A, Good B, editors. Culture and depression: studies in the anthropology and cross-cultural psychiatry of affect and disorder. Berkeley: University of California Press; 1985. p. 216–43.
43. Cheung FM, Lau BW, Wong SW. Paths to psychiatric care in Hong Kong. Cult Med Psychiatry 1984;8:207–28.
44. Markus HR, Kitayama S. Culture and the self: implications for cognition, emotion, and motivation. Psychol Rev 1991;98:224–53.
45. Henrich J, Heine SJ, Norenzayan A. The weirdest people in the world? Behav Brain Sci 2010;1–23.
46. Chang WC. A cross-cultural study of depressive symptomology. Cult Med Psychiatry 1985;9:295–317.
47. Lee S, Kleinman A. Are somatoform disorders changing with time? The case of neurasthenia in China. Psychosom Med 2007;69:846–9.
48. Lakoff G, Kövecses Z. The cognitive model of anger inherent in American English. In: Holland D, Quinn N, editors. Cultural models in language and thought. Cambridge: Cambridge University Press; 1987. p. 195–221.
49. Goffman E. Stigma: notes on the management of spoiled identity. Englewood Cliffs, NJ: Prentice-Hall; 1963.
50. Barney LJ, Griffiths KM, Jorm AF, et al. Stigma about depression and its impact on help-seeking intentions. Aust N Z J Psychiatry 2006;40:51–4.
51. Link BG, Struening EL, Rahav M, et al. On stigma and its consequences: evidence from a longitudinal study of men with dual diagnoses of mental illness and substance abuse. J Health Soc Behav 1997;177–90.
52. Markowitz FE. The effects of stigma on the psychological well-being and life satisfaction of persons with mental illness. J Health Soc Behav 1998;335–47.
53. Boyd Ritsher J, Otilingam PG, Grajales M. Internalized stigma of mental illness: psychometric properties of a new measure. Psychiatry Res 2003;121:31–49.
54. Goldberg DP, Bridges K. Somatic presentations of psychiatric illness in primary care setting. J Psychosom Res 1988;32:137–44.
55. Ryder AG, Bean G, Dion KL. Caregiver responses to symptoms of first-onset psychosis: a comparative study of Chinese-and Euro-Canadian families. Transcultural Psychiatry 2000;37:225–36.

56. Kleinman A. The cultural meanings and social uses of illness. A role for medical anthropology and clinically oriented social science in the development of primary care theory and research. J Fam Pract 1983;16:539–45.
57. Lin T-Y, Tardiff K, Donetz G, et al. Ethnicity and patterns of help-seeking. Cult Med Psychiatry 1978;2:3–13.
58. Cheung FM, Lau BW. Situational variations of help-seeking behavior among Chinese patients. Compr Psychiatry 1982;23:252–62.
59. Kirmayer LJ. Cultural variations in the response to psychiatric disorders and emotional distress. Soc Sci Med 1989;29:327–39.
60. Simon GE, VonKorff M, Piccinelli M, et al. An international study of the relation between somatic symptoms and depression. N Engl J Med 1999;341:1329–35.
61. Raguram R, Weiss MG, Channabasavanna SM, et al. Stigma, depression, and somatization in South India. Am J Psychiatry 1996;153:1043–9.
62. Barsky AJ, Cleary PD, Klerman GL. Determinants of perceived health status of medical outpatients. Soc Sci Med 1992;34:1147–54.
63. Barsky AJ, Wyshak G, Klerman GL. The somatosensory amplification scale and its relationship to hypochondriasis. J Psychiatr Res 1990;24:323–34.
64. Pennebaker JW, Watson D. Blood pressure estimation and beliefs among normotensives and hypertensives. Health Psychol 1988;7:309–28.
65. Pennebaker JW, Brittingham GL. Environmental and sensory cues affecting the perception of physical symptoms. Adv Environmen Psychol 1982;4:115–36.
66. Sayar K, Kirmayer LJ, Taillefer SS. Predictors of somatic symptoms in depressive disorder. Gen Hosp Psychiatry 2003;25:108–14.
67. Dion KL. Ethnolinguistic correlates of alexithymia: toward a cultural perspective. J Psychosom Res 1996;41:531–9.
68. Kirmayer LJ. Languages of suffering and healing: alexithymia as a social and cultural process. Transcultural Psychiatry 1987;24:119–36.
69. Zhu X, Yi J, Yao S, Ryder AG, et al. Cross-cultural validation of a Chinese translation of the 20-item Toronto Alexithymia Scale. Compr Psychiatry 2007;48:489–96.
70. Dere J, Ryder AG, Falk CF. Unpacking cultural differences in alexithymia: the role of cultural values among Euro-Canadian and Chinese-Canadian students. J Cross Cult Psychol, in press.
71. Shweder RA. Cultural psychology: what is it? In: Stigler JW, Shweder RA, Herdt G, editors. Cultural psychology: essays on comparative human development. Cambridge: Cambridge University Press; 1990. p. 1–4.
72. Heine SJ, Norenzayan A. Toward a psychological science for a cultural species. Perspect Psychol Sci 2006;1:251–65.
73. Betancourt H, López SR. The study of culture, ethnicity, and race in American psychology. Am Psychol 1993;48:629–37.
74. Chiu CY, Gelfand MJ, Yamagishi T, et al. Intersubjective culture: the role of intersubjective perceptions in cross-cultural research. Perspect Psychol Sci 2010;5:482–93.
75. DiMaggio P. Culture and cognition. Annu Rev Sociol 1997;23:263–87.
76. Bruner JS. Acts of meaning. Cambridge: Harvard University Press; 1990.
77. Kashima Y. Conceptions of culture and person for psychology. J Cross Cult Psychol 2000;31:14–32.
78. Lee S. Estranged bodies, simulated harmony, and misplaced cultures: neurasthenia in contemporary Chinese society. Psychosom Med 1998;60:448–57.
79. Shweder RA. Thinking through cultures: expeditions in cultural psychology. Cambridge: Harvard University Press; 1991.

80. Ryder AG, Sun J, Zhu X, et al. Depression in China across the lifespan: integrating developmental psychopathology and cultural-clinical psychology. J Clin Child Adolescent Psychol, in press.

81. Kitayama S, Mesquita B, Karasawa M. Cultural affordances and emotional experience: socially engaging and disengaging emotions in Japan and the United States. J Pers Soc Psychol 2006;91:890–903.

82. Shweder RA. The confessions of a methodological individualist. Culture & Psychology 1995;1:115–22.

83. Vygotsky L. Mind in society: the development of higher psychological processes. Cambridge: Harvard University Press; 1978.

84. Kirmayer LJ. The future of critical neuroscience. In: Choudhury S, Slaby J. Critical neuroscience: a handbook of the social and cultural contexts of neuroscience. Oxford: Wiley-Blackwell; 2012. p. 367–83.

85. Chiao JY. Cultural neuroscience: a once and future discipline. Prog Brain Res 2009;178:287–304.

86. Kitayama S, Uskul AK. Culture, mind, and the brain: current evidence and future directions. Annu Rev Psychol 2011;62:419–49.

87. Wexler BE. Brain and culture: neurobiology, ideology, and social change. Cambridge: The MIT Press; 2008.

88. Gilbert P. Evolutionary approaches to psychopathology and cognitive therapy. J Cogn Psychother 2002;16:263–94.

89. Mealey L. Evolutionary psychopathology and abnormal development. In: Burgess RL, MacDonald K, editors. Evolutionary perspectives on human development. Thousand Oaks, CA: Sage; 2005. p. 381–405.

90. Öhman A, Mineka S. Fears, phobias, and preparedness: toward an evolved module of fear and fear learning. Psychol Rev 2001;108:483–522.

91. Kendler KS, Thornton LM, Gardner CO. Stressful life events and previous episodes in the etiology of major depression in women: an evaluation of the" kindling" hypothesis. Am J Psychiatry 2000;157:1243–51.

92. DeRubeis RJ, Siegle GJ, Hollon SD. Cognitive therapy versus medication for depression: treatment outcomes and neural mechanisms. Nat Rev Neurosci 2008; 9:788–96.

93. Craig AD. How do you feel? Interoception: the sense of the physiological condition of the body. Nat Rev Neurosci 2002;3:655–66.

94. Damasio A. Feelings of emotion and the self. Ann N Y Acad Sci 2003;1001:253–61.

95. Craig AD. Interoception and emotion: a neuroanatomical perspective. In: Lewis M, Haviland-Jones JM, Feldman-Barrett L, editors. Handbook of emotion. New York: Guilford Press; 2008. p. 272–88.

96. Blood AJ, Zatorre RJ. Intensely pleasurable responses to music correlate with activity in brain regions implicated in reward and emotion. Proc Natl Acad Sci U S A 2001;98:11818–23.

97. Damasio AR, Grabowski TJ, Bechara A, et al. Subcortical and cortical brain activity during the feeling of self-generated emotions. Nat Neurosci 2000;3:1049–56.

98. Mauss IB, Wilhelm FH, Gross JJ. Is there less to social anxiety than meets the eye? Emotion experience, expression, and bodily responding. Cogn Emot 2004; 18:631–42.

99. Bogaerts K, Millen A, Li W, et al. High symptom reporters are less interoceptively accurate in a symptom-related context. J Psychosom Res 2008;65:417–24.

100. Paulus MP, Stein MB. Interoception in anxiety and depression. Brain Struct Funct 2010;5–6:451–63.

101. Gardner RM, Morrell JA, Ostrowski TA. Somatization tendencies and ability to detect internal body cues. Percept Mot Skills 1990;71:364–6.
102. Shorter E. From paralysis to fatigue: a history of psychosomatic illness in the modern era. New York: Maxwell Macmillan; 1992.
103. Philippot P, Rimé B. The perception of bodily sensations during emotion: a cross-cultural perspective. Polish Psychological Bulletin 1997;28:175–88.
104. Ban LM, Kashima Y, Haslam N. Does understanding behavior make it seem normal? Perceptions of abnormality among Euro-Australians and Chinese-Singaporeans. J Cross Cult Psychol 2010. DOI: 10.1177/0022022110385233.
105. Rosenquist JN, Fowler JH, Christakis NA. Social network determinants of depression. Mol Psychiatry 2011;16:273–81.
106. Chentsova-Dutton YE, Tsai JL. Self-focused attention and emotional reactivity: the role of culture. J Pers Soc Psychol 2010;98:507–19.
107. Lam KN, Marra C, Salzinger K. Social reinforcement of somatic versus psychological description of depressive events. Behav Res Ther 2005;43:1203–18.
108. Wichers M, Geschwind N, van Os J, et al. Scars in depression: is a conceptual shift necessary to solve the puzzle? Psychol Med 2010;40:359–65.
109. Bylsma LM, Morris BH, Rottenberg J. A meta-analysis of emotional reactivity in major depressive disorder. Clin Psychol Rev 2008;28:676–91.
110. Chentsova-Dutton YE, Chu JP, Tsai JL, et al. Depression and emotional reactivity: variation among Asian Americans of East Asian descent and European Americans. J Abnorm Psychol 2007;116:776–85.
111. Chentsova-Dutton YE, Tsai JL, Gotlib IH. Further evidence for the cultural norm hypothesis: positive emotion in depressed and control European American and Asian American women. Cult Divers Ment Health 2010;16:284–95.
112. Cheung RYM, Park IJK. Anger suppression, interdependent self-construal, and depression among Asian American and European American college students. Cultur Divers Ethnic Minor Psychol 2010;16:517–25.
113. Mauss IB, Evers C, Wilhelm FH, et al. How to bite your tongue without blowing your top: implicit evaluation of emotion regulation predicts affective responding to anger provocation. Pers Soc Psychol Bull 2006;32:589–602.
114. Mauss IB, Bunge SA, Gross JJ. Culture and automatic emotion regulation. In: Vandekerckhove M, von Scheve C, Ismer S, et al, editors. Regulating emotions: culture, social necessity, and biological inheritance. Malden (MA): Wiley-Blackwell; 2008. p. 39–60.
115. Soto JA, Perez CR, Kim Y-H, et al. Is expressive suppression always associated with poorer psychological functioning? A cross-cultural comparison between European Americans and Hong Kong Chinese. Emotion 2011. [Epub ahead of print].
116. Bellah RN, Sullivan WM, Tipton SM, et al. Habits of the Heart. Berkeley: University of California Press; 1985.
117. Russell JA, Yik MSM. Emotion among the Chinese. In: Bond MH, editor. The handbook of Chinese psychology. Hong Kong: Oxford University Press; 1996. p. 166–88.
118. Larsen RJ, Kasimatis M, Frey K. Facilitating the furrowed brow: an unobtrusive test of the facial feedback hypothesis applied to unpleasant affect. Cogn Emot 1992;6:321–38.
119. McIntosh DN. Facial feedback hypotheses: evidence, implications, and directions. Motiv Emot 1996;20:121–47.
120. Mauss IB, Levenson RW, McCarter L, et al. The tie that binds? Coherence among emotion experience, behavior, and physiology. Emotion 2005;5:175–90.

121. Fernandez-Dols JM, Sanchez F, Carrera P, et al. Are spontaneous expressions and emotions linked? An experimental test of coherence. J Nonverbal Behav 1997;21: 163–77.

122. Ruch W. Will the real relationship between facial expression and affective experience please stand up: the case of exhilaration. Cogn Emot 1995;9:33–58.

123. Kleinman AM. Depression, somatization and the "new cross-cultural psychiatry." Soc Sci Med 1977;11:3–10.

124. Kirmayer LJ. Beyond the "new cross-cultural psychiatry": cultural biology, discursive psychology and the ironies of globalization. Transcult Psychiatry 2006;43:126–44.

125. Kim HS, Sherman DK, Mojaverian T, et al. Gene-culture interaction: oxytocin receptor polymorphism (OXTR) and emotion regulation. Soc Psychol Personal Sci 2011;2:665–72.

126. Kim HS, Sherman DK, Sasaki JY, et al. Culture, distress, and oxytocin receptor polymorphism (OXTR) interact to influence emotional support seeking. Proc Natl Acad Sci U S A 2010;107:15717–21.

127. Chang DF, Tong H, Shi Q, et al. Letting a hundred flowers bloom: counseling and psychotherapy in the People's Republic of China. J Mental Health Counsel 2005; 27:104–16.

128. Shen EK, Alden LE, Söchting I, et al. Clinical observations of a Cantonese cognitive-behavioral treatment program for Chinese immigrants. Psychotherapy: Theory, Research, Practice, Training 2006;43:518–30.

129. Griner D, Smith TB. Culturally adapted mental health intervention: a meta-analytic review. Psychotherapy: Theory, Research, Practice, Training 2006;43:531–48.

130. Ryder AG, Dere, J. Canadian diversity and clinical psychology: defining and transcending "cultural competence." CAP Monitor 2010;35:1, 6–12.

131. Kleinman A, Benson P. Anthropology in the clinic: the problem of cultural competency and how to fix it. PLoS Med 2006;3:e294.

Recovery from Depression

Nada L. Stotland, MD, MPH*

KEYWORDS
- Depression • Recovery • Remission • Treatment

Although depression has been recognized by physicians, philosophers, and poets since ancient times, full recovery from depression was ill-defined and largely ignored in clinical practice until quite recently. Treatment was considered adequate or successful if a patient's mood and function seemed to be significantly better after treatment than before. The only measures of improvement were the patient's reports of function and symptom reduction. Persistent or chronic symptoms were largely regarded as characterological and were labeled depressive personality.

Although effective antidepressant medications became available in the 1960s, there was strong resistance to the use of medication from the psychoanalytic community, which largely dominated academic psychiatry. Medication was considered to be a "band-aid" that merely covered over symptoms, depriving depressed patients of the opportunity and motivation to pursue and work through the unconscious conflicts that were believed to have caused their illness. Presumably the psychoanalytic process would not only alleviate symptoms, it would also eliminate or limit vulnerability to future episodes, which would be a close approximation to recovery. Failure to improve was believed to result from patients' own unconscious resistance rather than the failure of treatment to help them. However, the success or failure of psychoanalytic treatment in producing recovery from depression was never subjected to scientific scrutiny. In the light of current knowledge, it is likely that many patients did not recover from psychoanalysis alone.

Although persistent symptoms are still referred to as treatment-resistant, we no longer blame patients for their own misery. Today the goal of recovery, or remission, is mainstream psychiatry, in fact mainstream medicine. The July 27, 2011 *Journal of the American Medical Association* features, in its Medical News and Perspectives section, an article, "New Tool to Gauge Depression Remission."[1]

The current focus on recovery derives at least partly from the discovery that far fewer patients were achieving full return to premorbid mood and function than was realized. That recognition led the field to identify recovery, rather than improvement,

There was no external support for the work reflected in this article.
The author has no financial relationship with any company or organization related to the content of this article.
Department of Psychiatry, Rush Medical College, 2150 Harrison Street, Chicago, IL 60612, USA
* 5511 South Kenwood Avenue, Chicago, IL 60637-1713.
E-mail address: nadast@aol.com

Psychiatr Clin N Am 35 (2012) 37–49
doi:10.1016/j.psc.2011.11.007
0193-953X/12/$ – see front matter © 2012 Elsevier Inc. All rights reserved.

psych.theclinics.com

as a treatment goal and to actively pursue new treatment options more likely to result in full recovery.

A number of hopeful approaches have been identified:

- More standardized and aggressive treatment with antidepressants
- Treating residual or chronic symptoms as well as the full depressive syndrome
- Matching patients to specific medications at the outset of treatment by using pharmacogenetics, electroencephalography (EEG), or other tools
- Cognitive interventions to enhance positive thinking
- The treatment of cooccurring psychiatric and general medical disorders, including substance abuse
- The improvement of doctor-patient relationships and active involvement of patients in selecting and carrying out treatment modalities
- The power of combining psychopharmacologic and psychotherapeutic treatments.

Some of these approaches improve outcomes, but because the incidence of recovery was not reported in the past and because there is little or no knowledge about the odds of spontaneous recovery in undiagnosed and untreated patients, there is no way of knowing whether the percentage of overall outcomes has improved.

DEFINITIONS AND IMPLICATIONS

There are three concepts of recovery as pertains to serious mental illness:

- One concept roughly equates recovery with relief of symptoms and reflects an optimism that, with thoroughgoing and well-conceived treatment, patients can be restored to a premorbid level of functioning.
- The second concept would set the bar higher than premorbid functioning; recovery would mean the achievement not just of premorbid levels but of normative, or ideal, levels of mood and function.
- A contrasting concept of recovery sees recovery as a process rather than an end and aims to support the development of skills for living a healthy life with a chronic illness or perhaps even growing beyond illness. The latter concept arose from the so-called consumer movement, which focuses on psychotic illness, schizophrenia in particular.

The Evolution of the Recovery Concept

Up to 50 or 60 years ago, many people diagnosed with schizophrenia in the United States were relegated to a lifetime of being warehoused in large public hospitals. They were not offered psychosocial interventions and were considered unsuitable for the psychoanalytic or psychodynamic treatments that predominated. Few in the medical and mental health professions or the public were aware that many people with schizophrenia actually left those hospitals and functioned for the rest of their lives with or without recurrences. Manic-depressive illness was regarded in much the same way, except that it was understood that episodes of comparative rationality alternated with mania or depression.

Although return to a premorbid level of function was theoretically the goal of mental health treatment, there was no system for identifying the specifics of that level of function. There was no regularized system or scale for recording a patient's progress. The concept of "recovery" originated with the consumer movement. It was a response to the widespread belief among both mental health professionals and the general public that serious mental illnesses not only could not be cured, but invariably they robbed those who had them of anything resembling normal lives: education, friends, family, jobs.

Over the course of the last decade or two, activists among people diagnosed with severe and persistent mental illnesses began to call themselves consumers. They refused to be resigned to a lifetime of disability and exclusion. They have been encouraged by accounts of similarly diagnosed individuals who have achieved considerable success in their careers and their relationships, and they are joined by many advocates in the mental health professions.

Most unipolar depression was not really included in this phase of the recovery movement. The focus on recovery from depression seems to come instead from studies of antidepressant efficacy. It became apparent that standard treatments were not sufficient for recovery in many patients and that many others improved without achieving full recovery.[2]

Three new and related developments in the concept of recovery are interesting and important:

- The focus on positive changes in a patient's condition rather than the relief of negative signs and symptoms.
- Measuring days at work, productivity, or the percentage of days without depression may be more useful from a research and public health standpoint than the measurement of mood or other symptoms alone.
- The teasing apart of different signs and symptoms in the course of remission or recovery, because all may or may not change or improve at the same rate.

The definition of depression includes signs and symptoms of mood, energy, concentration, appetite, sleep, libido, guilt, hopelessness and helplessness, and others. Decades ago it was believed that specific depressive symptoms generally improved before the patient subjectively felt better. This belief enabled the clinician to ask discouraged patients about particular signs and symptoms and, if the symptoms had improved, to reassure them that recovery (as then understood) was underway. The patient's overall level of function, however, was not usually addressed except as it pertained to the ability, in the case of patients so disabled by depression that they could not function, to return to work and/or family responsibilities.

In the *Diagnostic and Statistical Manual of Mental Disorders, Fourth Edition,* level of function is relegated to a separate category called Axis V.[3] However, function is of paramount importance to patients and their families and employers. Information about differing rates of improvement for different signs and symptoms can still help patients and clinicians identify the first signs of recovery and anticipate its ongoing course. Aikens and colleagues[4] followed 573 depressed patients treated with selective serotonin reuptake inhibitors. They discovered that mood improvement did not change at the same rate as either somatic complaints or hopefulness. Pain decreased earlier in treatment, whereas hopefulness improved more gradually. Affect and job and social functioning improved along with mood. Clearly, the concept of recovery as a unitary phenomenon is too narrow for optimal utility in either research or clinical care.

The Challenge of Defining Recovery

With regard to recovery from depression, there is neither a way to determine a baseline (in most patients) nor a definition of a normal mood state. For a single, acute, discrete episode of depression in a previously highly functioning and euthymic individual, recovery would presumably mean a return to the state before the episode. However, clinical practice seldom confronts us with such clear cases. What does euthymic mean—other than the absence of depression and mania? How content, stable, or happy is a normal person supposed to be? Probably most patients were not perfectly happy or content before developing symptoms severe enough to bring them to our offices, clinics, and hospitals.

For many people, life circumstances are tough; their children or parents do not behave as they or we would like, their jobs are not fulfilling, their bosses are demanding and unfair, they do not have as much money as they need or think they need. Many have suffered losses and other traumas. How resilient is a normal person supposed to be under these circumstances? Does euthymia mean maintaining a good mood whatever the circumstances? If the whole idea is to reach beyond the relief of symptoms, who can we point to as the exemplar of euthymia? For the clinician, what is the end point of treatment? Given that life circumstances are seldom optimal and that some degree of dissatisfaction or negative mood may be nearly universal, it may be that the most useful therapeutic goal would be resilience—the ability to withstand change and difficulty—rather than euthymia. Fortunately, resilience is another topic of great current interest and study. Unfortunately, it is just as difficult to define as recovery.

WHY DOES RECOVERY MATTER?
Depression in Children

When depression begins in childhood or adolescence, it comes to seem like a trait rather than a state and is not recognized as a disease. The consequences can be disastrous. The child is withdrawn or irritable and unable to make friends or even work effectively with other children. In the classroom, the depressed child, in contrast with children whose psychiatric problems cause disruptive behavior, does not make trouble and therefore does not engage the teacher, who would otherwise alert parents to the need for diagnosis and treatment. The child does not have the energy or confidence to master basic educational skills. The child eats and sleeps poorly and is at increased risk of infection and other conditions. The depressed child may be hyperactive or hypoactive but does not engage in constructive muscular exercise and acquire basic athletic skills.

The hopelessness and helplessness intrinsic to depression also keep the child from developing the self-efficacy and self-confidence necessary for trying new activities and mastering new skills. The child may not form the life aspirations that motivate learning. The child's depression may engender depression, whether clinical or subclinical, in parents, lessening the likelihood that they will recognize their child's illness and respond appropriately. In fact, the child's depression may result from a vulnerability shared with depressed parents. Children of depressed parents are highly likely to have mood and anxiety disorders and behavior problems that develop early, persist into adulthood, and cause life impairment. When mothers remit, children improve. When they do not remit, children get worse.[5]

Thus, depression warps development and keeps the developing individual from developing the tools, skills, and support networks that are necessary for recovery. The combination of misery and lack of attention from adults caused by depression can even result in childhood or adolescent suicide.

For all these reasons, recovering in adulthood from childhood depression, whether chronic, recurrent, or even a single episode, can be an uphill battle. The aftermath of early depression can include a lackluster education, a lack of career direction, a dearth of social skills and contacts, and memories of isolation and unhappiness. The ongoing human cost of residual depressive symptoms has now been recognized.[6] It would seem that intense remediation is necessary to help the adult with a childhood history of depression reawaken innate interests and talents that have been obscured by developmental deprivation. There is no adult premorbid level of function. This issue has received little or no attention.

Comorbidity

A PubMed search for "recovery from depression" yields more articles about depression as a factor in recovery from a wide range of general medical conditions, especially stroke, than about recovery from depression as a mental disorder. In Cramer's study of stroke patients, fluoxetine not only treated patients' depression, but also enhanced motor recovery.[7]

Depression is not only a factor in recovery from various general medical conditions, it is also a factor in their genesis. (Please see also the article by Rackley and Bostwick elsewhere in this issue.) In a study reported in the journal *Stroke*, depression was identified in the histories of 80,574 women aged 54 to 79, using either physician charting, patient mental health questionnaire, or antidepressant medication. The investigators' conclusion was that "depression is associated with a moderately increased risk of subsequent stroke."[8]

The most common somatic symptom of depression is pain in the abdomen, head, or back. Although pain is a common symptom, it is seldom included in abbreviated checklists for the diagnosis of depression or in depression symptom lists aimed at the public. Somatic pain is associated with a poorer prognosis.[8] The resolution of pain seems to be important for recovery, and that pain is often the first symptom to improve with treatment.[9]

Whereas there are data about the impact of depression on the course of several general medical conditions (cancers, stroke, diabetes), there is little information on the impact of general medical conditions on recovery from depression. Similarly, it is not known how the resolution of environmental precipitants and causes affects the course of depression. A study in Mexico concluded that helping depressed women out of poverty significantly decreased the incidence of depression.[10]

Depression is also very commonly comorbid with other psychiatric disorders. Anxiety, for example, is so commonly associated with depression that it is difficult to decide which, if either, is the primary diagnosis. Within step one of STAR*D (Sequenced Treatment Alternatives to Relieve Depression) treatment, 53.2% of patients had anxious depression, predicting poorer outcome than those not anxious.[11] Of patients in the STAR*D study, 29.4% had concurrent substance abuse disorders. This subset had more severe depressive symptoms, a higher risk of suicide, and more frequent anxiety disorders.[12,13] Eating disorders and depression are both more common in women and frequently coexist. Mischoulon and colleagues[14] found that the course of depression in the context of an eating disorder was protracted and that antidepressant medication did not affect the likelihood of recovery or protect against relapse.

Insomnia is a symptom, not a disease, but it is a major factor in depression and recovery from depression. At least 25% of patients with depression have insomnia. Most are untreated or undertreated, and persistent insomnia is associated with more severe and long-lasting depression.[15–17]

CHALLENGES TO THE ACHIEVEMENT OF RECOVERY
Social and Personal Attitudes Toward Depression

Depression is both slippery and sticky. It is slippery because the word *depression* is used both to denote a disease and in common parlance to mean a feeling of sadness or discouragement that is occasioned by a negative life event or situation and that resolves with the resolution of that event or situation or by dint of conscious efforts at stoicism, distraction, or active intervention. This kind of "depression" happens at some time or other to everyone. It is normative. It does not require professional intervention. Depression is sticky because it is often recurrent and sometimes chronic.

The confusion between depression as a normative experience and depression as a disease is further complicated by the belief that it is natural or unavoidable to experience depressed feelings under certain circumstances. Of course this concept is true. However, depressed mood accompanied by other symptoms lasting more than 2 weeks, causing significant distress, and impairing the individual's ability to function is not normative. This confusion can undermine the natural inclination to seek help when one is disabled or in pain or to encourage others to seek help when they are in pain. One might say it leads to cultural therapeutic nihilism.

Contrast this attitude toward depression with cultural attitudes toward other "natural" medical sequelae of negative events. For example, a pedestrian's collision with a moving vehicle causes injury. We do not simply say, "Of course you are injured"; we feel compelled to obtain treatment for the injury. On the other hand, when a loss or disappointment precipitates depression, people are more inclined to observe, "Of course you are depressed," and leave it at that.

Although large public education campaigns including accounts by public figures of their own experiences with depression have significantly increased public acceptance of depression as a real and treatable disease, many people are still confused about the distinction between the ubiquitous experience of temporarily depressed mood and the disease of depression. They continue to blame the depressed individual for not soldiering on or behaving in ways that help to resolve the discouraged or sad moods everyone experiences. Deeply pious members of some religious groups regard depression as a punishment for sinful acts or thoughts, with resolution to be achieved by prayer and failure to recover as indicative of the need for more prayer. In either case, depressed individuals are blamed for their own depression, and attempts to find diagnosis and treatment are regarded as ways to avoid personal responsibility.

In any event, if depression is not a real disease there can be no genuine treatment for it, psychotherapy is regarded as self-indulgent discussions with a sympathetic listener, and the prescription of medication as a knee-jerk response or even a way for doctors and pharmaceutical companies to make money. At worst, antidepressant medication is thought to cause dangerous changes in brain function, to be addictive, and to turn people into zombies. To be surrounded by others, especially significant others, who hold and express these beliefs and discourage patients from seeking or maintaining treatment is a major obstacle to recovery. Thus, many or most patients fail to fill antidepressant prescriptions and, of those who do, many discontinue them before the prescribed end date. Patients in a British study reported that they only agreed to take antidepressants when every other approach had failed and they had "hit bottom."[18] Although most people eventually recover from a discrete episode of depression—not without personal and social cost—treatment increases the likelihood and speed of recovery.

Negative attitudes about antidepressants are by no means limited to the uninformed. Negative attitudes have been expressed by professionals and repeated in the media. In fact, the title of one article includes the words "crisis of confidence."[19] The interpretation—or misinterpretation—of research findings has led many to question or discount any therapeutic action of antidepressants and to conclude that antidepressants increase the risk of suicide.

The Impact of Trauma

Depression may occur with or without an identifiable precipitant. When the precipitant is a trauma of some kind, further exposure to that trauma seriously complicates recovery from depression. Sexual assault is one such case. These negative outcomes seem to result not only from the direct effects of trauma but also from patients' attempts to cope with them—by isolating themselves and decreasing their activities outside their homes, for example. Sexual assault victims can also easily be retraumatized by their contact with emergency room staff, police, lawyers, and the need to testify and be cross-examined in court.[20]

Age

Age is another factor. A study of all adult residents of one county in Norway revealed that the prevalence of depression increased from age 76 onward and that advancing age was associated with a decrease in recovery.[21]

Health Care Systems

In the United States, recovery from depression is complicated by our uncoordinated system, or nonsystem, of health care provision and the limitations of virtually all forms of health care insurance when it comes to psychiatric diagnosis and treatment. Third-party payers are reluctant to support further treatment after an individual's symptoms have improved. Often there is an arbitrary limitation on the number of treatment sessions. Recent health care legislation may mitigate this problem.

The need for psychosocial approaches to recovery from mania, or bipolar disorder, is more widely recognized than is the case for depression. Mania is such a disruptive condition that it is clear to everyone that the affected individual has caused embarrassment at the least as well as financial and other forms of ruin to themselves and their families and that their recovery depends not only on the suppression of future episodes but also on reparations to reputations, careers, and relationships. There has been little if any such focus for those trying to recover from depression. There are studies of the negative impact of parental depression on children, both before and after birth, but rarely is family intervention offered to the recovering parent. Health insurance companies are unlikely to be willing to fund more than the most basic maintenance treatment, not to mention reparative psychosocial interventions, after the resolution of acute or chronic symptoms. Psychosocial rehabilitation is very limited and is restricted to individuals recovering from psychotic illness or developmental disability. There are probably few clinicians aware of the need for reparative therapy for depression and prepared to offer it. Large employers, increasingly aware of the impact of depression on their businesses, may be willing partners in helping valued employees reintegrate into their jobs.

Many colleagues report that some health insurance companies do not cover psychotherapeutic treatment for depression, or they require a failed trial of pharmacotherapy before agreeing to reimburse for psychotherapy. Many others provide only split treatment or enact reimbursement scales that discourage combined treatments. Although a combination of psychotherapy and pharmacotherapy produces the best treatment outcomes for depression, many third-party payers refuse to cover combined psychotherapeutic and psychopharmacologic treatment provided by one professional, generally a psychiatrist. If payers cover both modalities, they require for reasons of economy that a nonphysician, generally a social worker or counselor of some kind, provide psychotherapy, while a physician, not necessarily a psychiatrist, writes prescriptions for antidepressants. This arrangement does not take into account the fact that changes in a patient's condition may stem from developments in the psychotherapeutic process or in the use or effects of medication. Most often the psychotherapist and prescribing physician are in different locations and on different schedules. Communication between them is difficult; the use of e-mail, which might be the easiest to accomplish, is limited by concerns about confidentiality.

Psychotherapy alone is adequate treatment for mild cases of depression and is efficacious in maintenance of remission. Some patients reluctant to take antidepressant medication would in principle welcome or at least accept psychotherapy. However, most efficacy research has been performed on the use of manual-based psychotherapies such as cognitive-behavioral therapy and interpersonal therapy. Experts in the provision of these kinds of psychotherapy seem to be few. These services may not be included in a patient's insurance plan, and a patient has no way of knowing from a list of included psychotherapists which are capable of performing these kinds of evidence-based treatments. Psychotherapy also takes more time than the receipt of a prescription, and therapists may not be available at times that do not interfere with a patient's job or other time-specific obligations.

CHANGING TREATMENT EXPECTATIONS, APPROACHES, AND OUTCOMES
Clinical Treatment Research

The massive STAR*D trials enrolled 2876 depressed patients from both mental health and primary care settings, assigned them to medication or psychotherapy treatment, and implemented a structured, sequential approach for those for whom the first treatment effort failed to provide remission. No one treatment proved more effective than another within this heterogeneous group of subjects. Patients with psychiatric or general medical comorbidity and those functioning more poorly at baseline were less likely to recover.[22] The study addressed not only the signs and symptoms of depression but also subjects' health-related quality of life (HRQOL). Not surprising, the severity of depressive symptoms was associated with lower HRQOL, but lower HRQOL was also associated with being African American or Hispanic, being separated or divorced, being unemployed, having less education, having public medical insurance, and having more general medical disorders.[23]

The interpretation of STAR*D findings is hotly debated. Most investigators appreciate the fact that the study was conducted with a large cohort of actual patients. Shern and Moran[24] applauded the 70% remission rate but raise concern over the attrition rate and the 30% of subjects who did not achieve remission. Gaynes and colleagues[25] noted that remission rates were generally not as high as had been expected and that, for patients who required but did not fully respond to two full-scale treatment trials, the likelihood of remission was low. Rush and colleagues[26] viewed the findings differently: they noted that 67% of patients who stayed with the study through four treatment steps achieved remission. They also noted, as did others, that full remission, as contrasted with partial response, meant a significantly lower relapse rate.[26] Both studies are correct; the remission rates for those who remained in the study over four treatment steps were 37.8%, 30.6%, 13.7%, and 13.0%, resulting in an overall rate of 67%.[27] The lack of information about the subjects who did not complete the study makes interpretation still more difficult.

Laboratory Findings

Several genetic and other physiological factors seem to be associated with treatment response. Study of these factors enhances our understanding of the biological mechanisms involved in depression and may enable us to individualize treatment prospectively. A study by Binder and colleagues[28] revealed that polymorphism in genes regulating the corticotrophin-releasing factor system is associated with anti-depressant treatment response.

Laje and colleagues[29] found associations between DNA findings and responses to specific antidepressants. A study by DeBattista and colleagues[30] demonstrated a relationship between referenced EEG findings and responses to antidepressant regimens. A new study by Kerestes and colleagues[31] demonstrates persistently abnormal prefrontal brain activity even after depression remission. A French study subjected mice to unpredictable chronic mild stress; this exposure resulted in reduced hippocampal neurogenesis and reduced the relationship between the hippocampus and the hypothalamic-pituitary-adrenal axis. The administration of fluoxetine restored this relationship by recruiting new neurons.[32]

Applications

The most obvious treatment implication for recovery from depression is to set full recovery as a treatment goal, to systematically measure progress toward that goal, and to change the treatment plan in accordance with treatment response. This expectation and this process, like other treatment decisions, needs to be shared with the patient at the outset. In fact, using the recovery model, the clinician does not simply "share" this expectation with the patient but arrives at it together with the patient. This assurance will foster another crucial factor in recovery: hope.

It is also important to ask patients how they feel about being or having been depressed and how it has affected their life and then to consider with them how they may integrate the experience and optimize their relationships, work contributions, other interests, and general life satisfaction. Individuals who recover from chronic, perhaps lifelong, depression find themselves in a welcome but strange new psychological world. They may need to grieve years of unhappiness and lost opportunities. They need to find ways to acquire the skills and experiences they would have had if they had not been depressed and to use those skills and experiences to build more satisfying, productive, and joyful lives.

Depression creates a vicious cycle; discouragement diminishes success, which increases discouragement. However, this cycle can turn in the opposite direction. Psychosocial interventions that lead to any improvement enhance the chances of full recovery. Just as negative life events and cognition laden with negative thoughts increase the risk of depression, enhancing the positive aspects of cognitive style and having positive life experiences improves resilience to depressive symptoms.[33] Psychodynamically oriented clinicians may be reluctant to give patients advice about their lives, but suggestions and encouragement, as well as formal cognitive therapy, can be important in reversing the vicious cycle.

Reassurance

Treatment cannot help people recover if they do not use it. The patient must co-own the treatment with the clinician.[34] Patients' perception that treatment was imposed upon, rather than chosen by, them was a powerful force for the creation of the recovery movement. The clinician must give the patient time to educate himself or herself and the family. Some people look down on or fear psychotherapy. Many people are reluctant to take medication, especially psychotropic medication, especially after symptoms improve or resolve. They need renewed assurance that antidepressants are safe and not addictive. This assurance has been weakened by more recent revelations that some people have serious symptoms in the course of discontinuing antidepressants, notably paroxetine. In the absence of comprehensive follow-up studies, it is difficult to know how common a problem this is. On the other hand, most people who have had an episode of depression dread the possibility of another such episode. Those whose most recent episode is not their first should, of course, be advised of the likelihood of recurrences and are more likely to wish for maintenance treatment.

Several issues raised in this article hover on the border between research and clinical application. One issue just mentioned is the role of families. Given an environment where many people doubt the validity of the diagnosis and the effectiveness of treatment—even believing that treatment is dangerous—family members can have a powerful and reassuring impact on patients' own attitudes towards diagnosis and treatment. The evaluation of a patient with depression can include questions about family relationships and specifically about the attitudes of the family members most important to the patient. The responses to these questions can point the clinician in the direction of individual psychodynamic work on family issues and/or treatment sessions with the family. In some cases it may become apparent that the patient's depression is fostered by members of the family or is a significant component of basic family dynamics. In these cases, full-scale family treatment may be indicated.

The work of the recovery movement in schizophrenia, as referenced previously, indicates that the concept and process of recovery is in itself therapeutic. This approach includes several steps, which may occur in any sequence. First, the clinician and patient must discuss and agree on the treatment goals and techniques. Most clinicians are trained to assume that the generic relief of symptoms is the goal of treatment, but patients' goals may be different. Some patients may simply want to regain the mood and function with which they were satisfied before a bout of depression, but others want to do better at work, to find a mate, to be better parents, or to enjoy other life satisfactions. Second, the clinician and patient consistently review progress toward the goals or any changes in goals. Third, individuals recovered or recovering from depression may be a crucial source of encouragement, advice, support, and hope to the patient. Because the current recovery movement is largely centered on psychotic illness, depressed patients may be more likely to find peer support in peer groups and advocacy organizations focused on depression rather than on recovery.

Positive psychology is the concept of addressing psychological well-being not as the absence of pathology but as a model of optimal mood, function, satisfaction, productivity, and self-fulfillment. Although positive psychology is by definition not focused on pathology, it may well have useful implications for the treatment of, particularly recovery from, depression. In fact, positive psychology could be viewed as a fourth essential of recovery, encompassing the ascertainment and support of the patient's strengths, values, self-image, and general health. Self-care—eating well, getting enough sleep, exercising, spending time in fulfilling activities and with friends and loved ones—is an important component of recovery from depression. Happiness is a more controversial goal. Some religions share with Sigmund Freud the notion that life is inherently difficult and at times painful. Perhaps happiness is best defined as a reasonable level of comfort with oneself and one's own situation.

DIRECTIONS FOR FUTURE RESEARCH

The ideas outlined just previous have not been subject to empirical investigation. It is likely that such investigation will provide powerful tools for individuals attempting to recover from depression and for the clinicians dedicated to helping them.

The assertion that depression leaves long-lasting negative sequelae deserves further study. What happens to people after they recover from acute or chronic depression? What factors improve outcomes? How do people integrate the experience of depression into their self-perceptions and plans for their future? And how do we conceptualize and measure recovery? At least one new tool for assessing depression remission has been developed.[35]

Most research has been performed on subjects with acute episodes of depression. It is not known how many cases are chronic or how to predict with accuracy whether depressive symptoms will become chronic. Studies of resilience are focused on those who function well despite adversity but may also yield information about those who do not. Some among the latter will prove to be depressed.

The STAR*D study, as outlined previously, has both positive and negative implications for recovery from depression. Because treatment was limited to specific medications, it is not known whether outcomes would have been better if clinicians had been free to choose medications for each patient. Because recovery from depression in the current sense is a fairly new concept, there is no way of knowing whether more patients are achieving recovery now than in the past. STAR*D and other studies do offer the prospect that more patients can achieve recovery in the future.

The United States Food and Drug Administration requires only short-term studies before allowing antidepressant medications to be prescribed. Long-term follow-up of studies is badly needed to determine which therapy or combinations of therapies provide the best chances for long-term recovery. In fact, there is very little information to offer patients about the effects of antidepressant medication over many months and years.

The ongoing search for genetic and other factors that will help us match each patient to the treatment most likely to be effective should include long-term follow-up including not only symptom change but also life function and satisfaction.

Now that significant relationships between depression and major general medical disorders such as cardiovascular disease (including stroke) have been identified, we need to know whether recovery from depression changes the course of other diseases, both general medical and psychiatric.

SUMMARY

Full recovery from depression, as contrasted with symptom improvement, is a relatively new concept and therapeutic goal. It is an important goal, because the failure to achieve this goal leaves many patients with less productive and fulfilling lives, it leaves some children with lasting deficits, and it deprives families and societies of loved ones' and employees' care and investment. As a new therapeutic concept, recovery from depression is not as easy to define as it might seem; many or most patients were not euthymic before an episode of depression or have had some level of depression throughout their lives. There is no measurable definition of euthymia.

In addition to definitional difficulties, we need to study and address other barriers to the achievement of recovery from depression. All the barriers to the diagnosis and treatment of depression are barriers against recovery: negative social and professional attitudes, comorbidity, lack of access to demonstrably efficacious professional and social services, and inability to match patients with the antidepressants most likely to help them. Efforts to address many of these knowledge and attitude gaps are already underway. Long-term studies are needed, both observational and experimental. Most published studies encompass only weeks or at best months of follow-up, but recovery must be sustained to be meaningful.

As noted previously, there has been little or no attention to the developmental impact of depression. The restoration of premorbid function is not sufficient when depression has hindered a patient's ability to form satisfying relationships and choose and perform satisfying work. We need to learn how to remediate patients whose history of depression has stifled their talents and aspirations.

Studying these issues will not be easy, but millions of individuals with depression, and their physicians, will profit by it; it will be well worth the effort.

REFERENCES

1. Voelker, R. New tool to gauge depression remission focuses on good feelings, not bad ones. JAMA 2011;306(4):363–4.
2. Pigott HE, Leventhal AM, Alter GS, et al. Efficacy and effectiveness of antidepressants: current status of research. Psychother Psychosom 2010;79(5):267–79.
3. American Psychiatric Association. Diagnostic and Statistical Manual of Mental Disorders. 4th edition. Washington (DC): American Psychiatric Association; 1994.
4. Aikens JE, Kroenke K, Nease DE Jr, et al. Gen Hosp Psychiatry 2008;30(1):26–31.
5. Weissman MM, Pilowsky DJ, Wickramaratne PJ, et al. Remissions in maternal depression and child psychopathology: a STAR*D-child report. JAMA 2006;295(12): 1389–98.
6. McIntyre RS, O'Donovan C. The human cost of not achieving full remission in depression. Can J Psychiatry 2004;49(3 Suppl 1);10S–6S.
7. Cramer SC. Listening to fluoxetine: a hot message from the FLAME trial of poststroke recovery. Int J Stroke 2011;6(4):315–6.
8. Pan A, Okereke O, Sun Q, et al. Depression and incident stroke in women. Stroke 2011;42(10):2770–5.
9. Leuchter AF, Husain MM, Cook IA, et al. Painful physical symptoms and treatment outcome in major depressive disorder: a STAR*D (Sequenced Treatment Alternatives to Relieve Depression) report. Psychol Med 2010;40(2):239–51.
10. Ozer EJ, Fernald LC, Weber A, et al. Does alleviating poverty affect mothers' depressive symptoms? A quasi-experimental investigation of Mexico's Oportunidades programme. Int J Epidemiol 2011. [Epub ahead of print].
11. Fava M, Rush AJ, Alpert JE, et al. Difference in treatment outcome in outpatients with anxious versus nonanxious depression: a STAR*D report. Am J Psychiatry 2008; 165(3):342–51.
12. Davis LL, Frazier E, Husain MM, et al. Substance use disorder comorbidity in major depressive disorder: a confirmatory analysis of the STAR*D cohort. Am J Addict 2006;15(4):278–85.
13. Howland RH, Rush AJ, Wisniewski SR, et al. Concurrent anxiety and substance use disorders among patients with major depression: clinical features and effect on treatment outcome. Drug Alcohol Depend 2009;1(1–3):248–60.
14. Mischoulon D, Eddy KT, Keshaviah A, et al. Depression and eating disorders: treatment and course. J Affect Disord. 2011;130(3):470–7.
15. Sunderajan P, Gaynes BN, Wisniewski SR, et al. Insomnia in patients with depression: a STAR*D report. CNS Spectr 2010;15(6):394–404.
16. Gulec M, Selvi Y, Boysan M, et al. Ongoing or re-emerging subjective insomnia symptoms after full/partial remission or recovery of major depressive disorder mainly with the selective serotonin reuptake inhibitors and risk of relapse or recurrence: a 52-week follow-up study. J Affect Disord 2011;134(1-3):257–65.
17. Brand S, Kirov R. Sleep and its importance in adolescence and in common adolescent somatic and psychiatric conditions. Int J Gen Med 2011;4:425–42.
18. Schofield P, Crosland A, Waheed W. Patients' views of antidepressants: from first experiences to becoming expert. Br J Gen Pract 2011;61(585):142–8.
19. Nierenberg AA, Leon AC, Price LH, et al. Crisis of confidence: antidepressant risk versus benefit. J Clin Psychiatry 2011;72(3):e11.

20. Najdowski CJ, Ullman SE. The effects of revictimization on coping and depression in female sexual assault victims. J Trauma Stress 2011;24(2):218–21.

21. Solhaug HI, Romuld EB, Romild U, et al. Increased prevalence of depression in cohorts of the elderly: an 11-year follow-up in the general population-the HUNT study. Int Psychogeriatr 2012;24(1):151–8.

22. Sinyor M, Schaffer A, Levitt A. The sequenced treatment alternatives to relieve depression (STAR*D) trial: a review. Can J Psychiatry 2010;55(3):126–35.

23. Daly EJ, Trivedi MH, Wisniewski SR, et al. Health-related quality of life in depression: a STAR*D report. Ann Clin Psychiatry 2010;22(1):43–55.

24. Shern DL, Moran H. STAR*D: helping to close the gap between science and practice. Psychiatr Serv 2009;60(11):1458–9.

25. Gaynes BN, Warden D, Trivedi MH, et al. What did STAR*D teach us? Results from a large-scale, practical clinical trial for patients with depression. Psychiatr Serv 2009; 60(11):1439–45.

26. Rush AJ, Warden D, Wisniewski SR, et al. STAR*D: revising conventional wisdom. CNS Drugs 2009;23(8):627–47.

27. Rush AJ, Trivedi MH, Wisniewski SR, et al. Acute and longer-term outcomes in depressed outpatients requiring one or several treatment steps: a STAR*D report. Am J Psychiatry 2006;163(11):1905–17.

28. Binder EB, Owens MJ, Liu W, et al. Association of polymorphisms in genes regulating the corticotrophin-releasing factor system with antidepressant treatment response. Arch Gen Psychiatry 2010;67(4):369–79.

29. Laje G, Perlis RH, Rush AJ, et al. Pharmacogenetics studies in STAR*D: strengths, limitations, and results. Psychiatr Serv 2009;60(11):1446–57.

30. DeBattista C, Kinrys G, Hoffman D, et al. The use of referenced-EEG (rEEG) in assisting medication selection for the treatment of depression. J Psychiatr Serv 2011;45(1):64–75.

31. Kerestes R, Ladouceur CD, Meda S, et al. Abnormal prefrontal activity subserving attentional control of emotion in remitted depressed patients during a working memory task with emotional distracters. Psychol Med 2012;42(1):29–40.

32. Surget A, Tanti A, Leonardo ED, et al. Antidepressants recruit new neurons to improve stress response regulation. Mol Psychiatry 2011;16(12):1177–88.

33. Haeffel GJ. Resilience to depressive symptoms: the buffering effects of enhancing cognitive style and positive life events. J Behav Ther Exp Psychiatry 2011;42(1):13–8.

34. Tibaldi G, Salvador-Carulla L, Garcia-Gutierrez JC. From treatment adherence to advanced shared decision making: new professional strategies and attitudes in mental health care. Curr Clin Pharmacol 2011;6(2):91–9.

35. Nease DE Jr, Aikens JE, Klinkman MS, et al. Toward a more comprehensive assessment of depression remission: the Remission Evaluation and Mood Inventory Tool (REMIT). Gen Hosp Psychiatry 2011;33(3):279–86.

Etiology of Depression: Genetic and Environmental Factors

Radu V. Saveanu, MD[a],*, Charles B. Nemeroff, MD, PhD[b]

KEYWORDS

• Trauma • Genes • Environment • Depression

Major depression is a common disorder, accounting for more disability than any other disorder worldwide. The rates of major depression in the United States rose markedly in the decade from 1991 to 2001, from 3.33% to 7.06%.[1] This increase is of considerable consequence, because depression is associated with significant morbidity, disability, increased medical comorbidities, and mortality.[2] It is the most significant risk factor for suicide, a leading cause of death worldwide, especially in adolescents, young adults, and the elderly.

Despite the prevalence and costly consequences of depression, there are still no validated, diagnostically useful biological tests to aid in the diagnosis of this disorder and very few that predict a response to established and effective treatments. Similarly, although some promising candidates are emerging, there are no biomarkers, such as alteration in gene expression or tumor marker, that are associated with improvement with antidepressant or psychotherapeutic treatments.

Of considerable concern is the recent realization, stemming from several large-scale treatment studies, that the efficacy and effectiveness of currently available antidepressants and psychotherapy are unacceptably low (eg, STAR*D).[3]

Dr Saveanu has indicated financial relationships with Novartis, Brain Resources, Inc (grants/research support).

Dr Nemeroff has indicated financial relationships with American Foundation for Suicide Prevention (AFSP), NovaDel Pharma (board of directors); Xhale, Tadeka (consultant); NIH, Agency for Healthcare Research and Quality (grants/research support); CeNeRx Bio Pharma, PharmaNeuroBoost (other financial interests); AFSP, CeNeRx Bio Pharma, National Alliance for Research on Schizophrenia and Depression, NovaDel Pharma, PharmaNeuroBoost, Anxiety Disorders Associate of America (scientific advisory boards); CeNeRx Bio Pharma, Concept Therapeutics, NovaDel Pharma, PharmaNeuroBoost, Revaax Pharma, Xhale (stockholder).

[a] Department of Psychiatry and Behavioral Sciences, Leonard M. Miller School of Medicine, University of Miami, 1695 Northwest 9th Avenue, #3100, Miami, FL 33136, USA
[b] Department of Psychiatry and Behavioral Sciences, Leonard M. Miller School of Medicine, University of Miami, 1120 Northwest 14th Street, Suite 1455, Miami, FL 33136, USA
* Corresponding author.
E-mail address: rsaveanu@med.miami.edu

Psychiatr Clin N Am 35 (2012) 51–71
doi:10.1016/j.psc.2011.12.001
0193-953X/12/$ – see front matter © 2012 Elsevier Inc. All rights reserved.

These studies highlight the paramount importance of understanding the pathogenesis and pathophysiology of depression.[3] The development of scientifically based, rational new treatments is dependent on a comprehensive understanding of the genetic and environmental contributions to depression and its associated neurobiology. Approximately one-third of the risk for the development of depression is inherited, and two-thirds is environmental.[4]

Many new findings and research directions have emerged that may have significant implications for clinical practice. In this article the authors review several major new discoveries relevant to the current understanding of brain alterations in depression, including gene-environment (G×E) interactions. The authors also demonstrate how molecular neurobiology and structural and functional brain imaging techniques have helped to inform understanding of these brain activities. The focus is on the association between adverse life events including childhood maltreatment, genetic variations, and the risk for developing major depression. Finally, the authors discuss how these G×E interactions and subsequent epigenetic modifications may inform treatment choices and modalities. The article begins with a brief review of the pathophysiology of depression.

PATHOPHYSIOLOGY OF DEPRESSION

The current view of the etiology of depression is best summarized as a prototypical G×E interaction model similar to that for other complex diseases such as cancer, hypertension, and diabetes. The focus within the model has been on three major monoamine systems—serotonin (5-hydroxytryptamine, 5HT), norepinephrine (NE) and dopamine (DA). The emerging new tools of molecular neurobiology and functional brain imaging have provided additional support for the involvement of these three systems.

Serotonin Alterations in Depression

Evidence from an impressive array of studies supports a preeminent role of the involvement of central nervous system (CNS) 5HT systems in depression. Postmortem, cerebrospinal fluid (CSF) and neuroendocrine studies demonstrate reduced activity of serotonergic neurons in depressed patients. New data from postmortem and positron emission tomography (PET) imaging studies demonstrate a reduction in the number of serotonin transporter (SERT) binding sites (the site of action of selective serotonin reuptake inhibitors, SSRIs) in the midbrain and amygdala of drug-free depressed patients, as well as a reduction in both presynaptic (in the midbrain) and postsynaptic (in the mesiotemporal cortex) 5HT receptor subtypes of depressed patients.[5-6] Previous studies demonstrated an increase in $5HT_2$ receptor density, perhaps due to a relative decrease in 5HT availability.

Involvement of 5HT circuits in depression is further supported by observations that depressed patients in remission after treatment with SSRIs, when challenged by an experimental maneuver that reduces CNS 5HT availability (ie, tryptophan depletion) exhibit a rapid return of depressive symptoms, in a few hours in many cases.[7]

Further support comes from the game-changing observation that individuals with the s allele of the promoter region of the SERT gene (SLC 6A4) are unusually vulnerable to the depressogenic effects of early life stress such as child abuse or neglect.[8] The SERT is a critical protein in regulating the availability of serotonin in the CNS. The s allele of the SERT gene is associated with reduced functional capacity of the SERT.

This finding suggests that, in vulnerable individuals, reduced 5HT availability is associated with the rapid emergence of depression, especially in those exposed to early life stress. **Box 1** summarizes the alterations in 5HT systems in depression.

Norepinephrine Alterations in Depression

NE-containing circuits are also considered to be involved in mood disorders.[9] Similar to drugs that increase 5HT availability, NE reuptake inhibitors such as nortriptyline and reboxetine are effective antidepressants. Moreover, neurochemical and neuroendocrine studies in depressed patients and postmortem findings support a role for NE dysfunction in depression; these data are summarized in **Box 2**. Alterations in noradrenergic circuits may also play a preeminent role in patients with treatment-resistant depression. Whether antidepressants that are believed to act on both 5HT and NE neurons are more effective than those that act solely on 5HT or NE neurons remains controversial, but recent metaanalyses suggest that if any advantage exists, it is relatively small.[10]

> **Box 3**
> **Alterations of dopaminergic systems in depression**
>
> - DA is the major neurotransmitter that mediates the ability to experience pleasure. Anhedonia is the inability to experience pleasure, a cardinal feature of depression.
> - A high rate of depression is seen in patients with Parkinson's disease, a disorder characterized by DA neuron degeneration.
> - Brain imaging and postmortem studies have revealed decreased dopamine transporter binding and increased postsynaptic D2/D3 receptor binding, all indicative of reduced DA neurotransmission.
> - Reductions in the major metabolites of DA have been reported in the CSF of depressed patients.
> - Increased MAO-A activity is found in the CNS system of depressed patients.
> - Drugs that increase DA neurotransmission such as MAOIs, DA reuptake blockers, and DA receptor agonists possess antidepressant properties.
>
> *Abbreviation:* MAOI, monoamine oxidase inhibitor.
>
> *Reprinted with permission from* FOCUS, (Copyright ©2008). American Psychiatric Association.

Dopamine Alterations in Depression

Although DA-containing neuronal pathways have been largely implicated in the pathophysiology of schizophrenia, much evidence now supports an important role for CNS DA circuits in depression. In fact, many investigators[11] suggest that suboptimal therapeutic responses to SSRIs and selective serotonin-norepinephrine reuptake inhibitors (SNRIs) may be due in part to their relative lack of effect on brain DA circuits.

Partly because of the low remission rates in clinical trials with SSRIs and SNRIs, a potential role for CNS DA circuits in depression has been postulated. This emergence of a DA hypothesis of depression is not surprising in view of the fact that the inability to experience pleasure, anhedonia, is considered by many to be the most important pathognomonic symptom of depression, and pleasure, whether associated with eating, social, or sexual behavior, is primarily mediated by activation of DA neurons. **Box 3** summarizes the evidence for the role of altered dopaminergic circuits in depression. Both postmortem tissue and PET imaging studies have revealed reduced DA transporter binding sites[12] and increased postsynaptic DA D2/D3 receptor density, indicative of a reduction in the synaptic availability of DA in depression. These findings suggest that treatments that enhance DA neurotransmission such as monoamine oxidase inhibitors, DA receptor agonists, or triple (5HT, NE, and DA) reuptake inhibitors (currently under investigation) may represent a novel approach to SSRI nonresponders.

There is some evidence for the involvement of other neurotransmitter systems in the pathogenesis of depression as well. These include the glutamate γ-aminobutyric acid, substance P, brain-derived neurotrophic factor (BDNF), thyrotropin-releasing hormone, corticotropin-releasing factor (CRF), somatostatin, leptin, and acetylcholine-containing neurons.[13] However, a comprehensive discussion of these systems is beyond the scope of this article.

THE NEUROANATOMY OF DEPRESSION

Although there is little doubt that various neurotransmitter systems are pathologically involved in depression, no single neurotransmitter system seems to be solely responsible. This is not surprising when one considers the panoply of symptoms that comprise the depressive syndrome, including depressed mood, loss of interest in usual activities, inability to experience pleasure, impaired concentration, disturbed sleep, decreased appetite, and suicidality. A more recent conceptual approach to the biology of depression is to consider it a disorder involving several critical brain regions and associated pathways.

Advances in brain imaging have allowed the identification of these brain regions and associated circuits. Structural brain imaging using magnetic resonance imaging has revealed altered volumes of several brain regions in patients with depression, most notably a reduction in hippocampal and caudate nucleus size and an increase in pituitary volume. It is now evident that some of the previously described changes in certain brain structures may be more likely caused by early life stress during a critical period in brain development than to depression per se.[14] PET studies led by Mayberg and colleagues[15] and Drevets[16] support the hypothesis that depression is characterized by abnormalities in limbic system–cerebrocortical circuits, more specifically, reduced activity in frontal cortical areas and hyperactivity in the amygdala and other limbic sites. The subgenual cingulate cortex (Cg25) seems of paramount importance; this brain area shows a striking decrease in activity in response to clinical improvement of depression after treatment with SSRIs, electro-convulsive therapy and other novel treatments and is a target for deep brain stimulation treatment of refractory depression.

STRESS, INFLAMMATION, AND THE NEUROENDOCRINE SYSTEM

Many patients with depression are known to hypersecrete cortisol (the major adrenocortical stress hormone).[17] The observations that patients with Cushing disease or syndrome often experience depression and anxiety and that healthy individuals exposed to stress increase production and secretion of glucocorticoids contributed to the modern stress-diathesis hypothesis of depression. According to this hypothesis, excess secretion of cortisol and other hormones of the hypothalamic-pituitary-adrenal (HPA) axis plays a significant role in the pathogenesis of depression. A variety of tests are available to measure the activity of the HPA axis.

Most frequently used in psychiatric patients is the dexamethasone suppression test (DST), in which small (1-mg) doses of the synthetic glucocorticoid dexamethasone are administered orally at 11 PM and plasma cortisol concentrations are measured at two or three time points the following day.[18] Dexamethasone acts primarily on the anterior pituitary corticotrophs to reduce the secretion of adrenocorticotropic hormone (ACTH), resulting in a decrease in the synthesis and release of cortisol from the adrenal cortex. Failure to suppress plasma cortisol concentrations after dexamethasone administration suggests impaired feedback regulation and hyperactivity of the HPA axis.

Many drug-free patients with depression fail to suppress cortisol secretion after administration of dexamethasone. Dexamethasone nonsuppression failed as a biological diagnostic test for depression because patients with other diagnoses exhibit DST nonsuppression, including those with eating disorders, Alzheimer disease, and bipolar disorder. In depressed patients, however, DST nonsuppression has generally been found to be associated with depression severity and, when persistent, with a significant risk for relapse. The major contribution of the DST was to serve as an impetus for subsequent studies exploring the pathophysiology of the HPA axis in depression.

In 1981, the long sought-after hypothalamic releasing hormone CRF, a 41 amino acid–containing peptide, was chemically characterized, greatly accelerating research on the HPA axis, stress, and depression. Neurons of the paraventricular nuclei of the

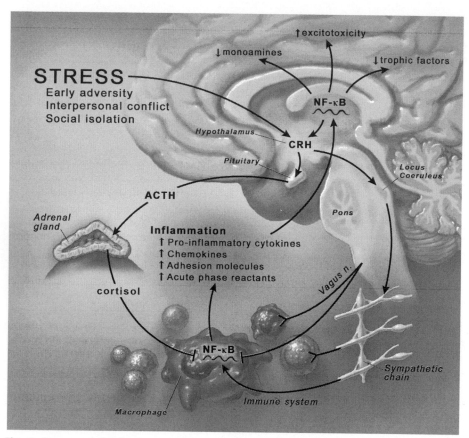

Fig. 1. Stress and the immune and neuroendocrine systems. CRH, corticotropin-releasing hormone. (*From* Miller HM, Maletic V, Raison CL. Inflammation and its discontents: the role of cytokines in the pathophysiology of major depression. Biol Psychiatry 2009;65:732–41; with permission.)

hypothalamus project to the median eminence where their nerve terminals secrete CRF into the hypothalamo-hypophyseal portal system. CRF is then transported in this specialized vascular system to the anterior pituitary where it acts on corticotrophs to increase ACTH secretion, thereby controlling HPA axis activity. Of paramount importance was the discovery that CRF is also widely distributed in extrahypothalamic brain areas where it functions, in concert with the hypothalamic CRF system, as a neurotransmitter coordinating the behavioral, autonomic, endocrine, and immune responses to stress (**Fig. 1**).

Synthetic CRF allowed the development of a CRF stimulation test, in which CRF is administered intravenously and plasma ACTH and cortisol concentrations are measured at 30-minute intervals over a 2- to 3-hour period. Normal, healthy volunteer subjects respond to CRF infusion with increased secretion of ACTH and cortisol, whereas depressed patients exhibit a blunted ACTH but normal cortisol response. Not surprising, the blunted ACTH response to CRF occurs in depressed DST nonsuppressors but not in depressed patients with normal DST suppression. The

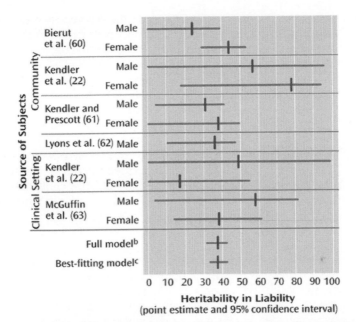

Fig. 2. Genetics of major depressive disorder. Note: aggregate valued across studies of heritability in liability to major depression. Reference citations are from the previously published source and are not included in the current article. (*Reproduced from* Sullivan PF, Neal MC, Kendler KS. Genetic epidemiology of major depression: review and meta-analysis. Am J Psychiatry 2000;157:1552–62. *Reprinted from* the American Journal of Psychiatry, copyright © 2000, American Psychiatric Association; with permission.)

dex-CRF test, which combines the DST and the CRF stimulation test, is arguably the most sensitive test of HPA axis activity.[19]

Many of the HPA axis alterations in depressed patients may result from chronic CRF hypersecretion. Depressed patients frequently exhibit elevated CSF CRF concentrations.[20] Further, postmortem studies of individuals depressed at the time of death or those who committed suicide have revealed a decreased density of CRF receptors in the frontal cortex, decreased expression of CRF_1 receptor mRNA, and increased CRF concentrations in a variety of cerebrocortical brain areas and the locus coeruleus compared with control subjects.[21] Successful treatment of depression reduces elevated CSF CRF concentrations.[22] Moreover, similar to continued DST nonsuppression, persistently elevated CSF CRF in symptomatically improved depressed patients is associated with early relapse of depression. These data are supported by animal studies showing that CRF administered directly into the CNS produces many signs and symptoms of depression including decreased appetite, weight loss, decreased sexual behavior, disrupted sleep, and altered locomotor activity.[23]

As noted earlier and illustrated in **Fig. 2**, approximately 30% to 40% of the risk of development of depression is believed to be heritable, with the remaining variability imparted by the environment. Exposure to stress, a process primarily regulated by CRF-containing neural circuits and the HPA axis, is known to precipitate depression in vulnerable individuals. Moreover, early life stress such as child abuse or neglect occurring during neurobiologically vulnerable periods of development is one of the major means whereby the environment influences the development of depression. Heim and colleagues[24] identified a number of abnormalities in individuals with early life stress histories including (a) increased CSF CRF concentration, (b) sensitization of the neuroendocrine stress response, (c) glucocorticoid resistance, (d) activation of the immune system, and (e) reduced hippocampal volume. These structural, neuroendocrine, and immunologic changes are similar to those seen in depression, but the authors believe that they precede the onset of depression.[24]

The authors' group has also demonstrated that depressed women with a history of prepubertal sexual abuse exhibit persistently increased HPA axis activity as evidenced by a blunted ACTH response to CRF infusion and both hypercortisolemia and increased ACTH secretion in response to a standardized laboratory stressor, the Trier Social Stress Test.[25] Using the dex-CRF test, the authors recently demonstrated increased HPA axis activity in adult men with major depression and a history of child abuse.[26]

Substantial evidence suggests that sustained activation of the immune system or chronic inflammation may be one of the underlying pathologic processes in depression.[27] Elevated levels of proinflammatory cytokines such as interleukin 6 (IL-6), interleukin 1 (IL-1), tumor necrosis factor–alpha (TNF-alpha), interferon-gamma, as well as C-reactive protein (CRP, an acute phase protein) are consistently reported in depressed patients.[28–30] There is a direct correlation between the severity of depressive symptomatology and the magnitude of cytokine elevation.[31–32] Proinflammatory cytokines (released during immune activation or inflammation) modulate many of the biological functions implicated in depression such as neuroendocrine function (CRF and HPA axis activation), neuroplasticity, and alterations in neurotransmitter metabolism (serotonin, NE, DA, glutamate, and so forth).[33–37] Patients with a variety of inflammatory medical disorders have an elevated incidence of depression, and depressed individuals are at significantly high risk of developing diabetes or cardiac disease (disorders associated with inflammation).[38]

Antiinflammatory agents may reduce depressive symptoms. Celecoxib (a COX-2 inhibitor that reduces the inflammatory response) had significant therapeutic effects in patients with depression when used as an augmentation strategy added to reboxetine treatment.[39] Etanercept, an agent used to treat psoriasis and a TNF-alpha (inflammatory cytokine) antagonist, showed significant antidepressant properties that were independent of improvement in psoriatic symptoms.[40]

With this background, the authors briefly review stress and inflammation. Chronic or overwhelming stress (ie, early life stress, abuse, neglect) leads to chronic activation of the immune system and prolonged production of multiple antiinflammatory markers. Whereas acute and brief activation of the immune system is necessary to restore health, chronic activation leads to significant dysregulation of the neuroendocrine system, causing changes the authors typically see in depression.

Kiecolt-Glaser and colleagues[41] found that chronic stress in caretakers of patients with dementia is associated with high concentrations of IL-6, CRP, and other inflammatory markers. Similar findings were observed in couples dealing with the chronic stress of marital discord. The authors' group has studied depressed men who had a history of early life stress and found that they exhibited both a baseline hyperinflammatory state and a hyperactive inflammatory response to stress.[42] Another study found that childhood maltreatment was associated with significant elevations in CRP concentrations 20 years later.[43]

There are a number of pathways by which chronic stress induces chronic activation of the immune system and the subsequent development of depression. These findings were recently reviewed by Currier and Nemeroff [27] and are summarized as follows.

Proinflammatory cytokines IL-1, IL-6, and TNF-alpha increase CRF production, which, as previously indicated, leads to hyperactivity of the HPA axis, a frequent finding in depression. IFN-alpha, IFN-gamma, and TNF-alpha up-regulate the human SERT and this up-regulation, at least theoretically, results in decreased synaptic serotonin availability and reduced serotonergic transmission. Several animal studies have demonstrated that IFN-alpha administration decreases CSF DA concentrations. In humans, decreased levels of CSF homovanillic acid (a measure of DA turnover) have been reported in depressed patients. Proinflammatory cytokines have been reported to produce prolonged glutamatergic activation that may contribute to depression. Increased hippocampal concentrations of TNF-alpha and IL-1 have been associated with reduced hippocampal neurogenesis, a finding reported in chronic depression. See **Fig. 1** for an illustration of the cascade of stress-related changes in neuroendocrine and immune systems.

GENES AND ENVIRONMENTAL INFLUENCES IN THE DEVELOPMENT OF DEPRESSION

In this section the authors provide further evidence for a preeminent role of environmental factors, namely early life adversity and genotype, in determining risk for depression.

Early Life Trauma and Depression

Traumatic experiences of childhood are, unfortunately, prevalent in our society and worldwide. The Children's Bureau, Administration of Children, Youth, and Families (2006) estimate there are about 3 million child maltreatment reports each year, of which nearly 1 million are substantiated. Among substantiated reports, 60% are classified as neglect, 20% as physical abuse, and 10% as sexual abuse. Studies have reported that about 20% to 25% of women and 8% to 9% of men experience sexual abuse in childhood.[44,45] Frequently, sexual abuse is accompanied by physical abuse, further complicating this unfortunate state of affairs. Approximately 28% of girls who are sexually abused between the ages of 6 and 16 years are also physically abused.[46] The prevalence of emotional abuse and neglect is likely much higher than that of sexual and physical abuse but more difficult to measure and quantify. In addition, a large percentage of children lose one or both parents or live with a parent who is not able to provide continuous care.

A number of studies have shown that onset of mood disorders such as depression is undoubtedly impacted by stressful life events that occur in childhood.[47–50] In one community-based study of approximately 2000 women of various socioeconomic levels, those with a history of childhood physical or sexual abuse had an increased risk of depression and anxiety and were more likely to have abused drugs or attempted suicide than women without such a history.[47] Women with a history of childhood abuse have a four-fold increased risk of developing depression as opposed to women with no history of abuse.[48] Individuals with a history of childhood abuse are not only at higher risk for developing posttraumatic stress disorder (PTSD),[51] but also panic disorder, generalized anxiety disorder, bipolar disorder, and schizophrenia.[51–53]

Early life trauma has also been shown to impact the clinical course of depression. Patients with depression who have a history of childhood trauma have (a) lower rates of remission and recovery, (b) longer episodes of depression, (c) a more chronic disease course, and (d) earlier onset of depressive symptoms.[54–56]

However, research has shown that many victims of early life adversity do not develop depression or any other psychiatric illness. McGloin and Windom[57] found that 48% of children with documented histories of abuse or neglect did not fulfill criteria for an adult psychiatric disorder. What makes these individuals different?

Collishaw and colleagues[58] studied individuals who were resilient to the negative effects of childhood maltreatment. They found that a significant number of individuals who had early life abuse showed no evidence of psychiatric sequelae in adult life. Their resilience seems to be associated with perceived positive parental care, personality style, and the quality of peer and love relationships. The resilience of these individuals may be related to the timing of the early life adversity. There is now evidence that there are sensitive or critical periods in childhood when traumatic events may have particularly deleterious effects on development. This evidence points to an area that clearly needs further study and potentially has huge treatment implications.

Gene-Environment Interactions

There is a strong relationship between genetic predisposition to depression and the impact of early traumatic experiences during critical phases of development. Even though early life stress increases risk of depression, there are important differences in the way individuals respond to the same stressful event, and these differences may be explained in part by genetic factors. A variety of genetic polymorphisms seem to exert control over the degree of sensitivity to adverse events in early life. To demonstrate this phenomenon, several such G×E interactions are described.

Among the first to identify a G×E interaction were Caspi and colleagues.[8] They found a significant association between the promoter region of the SERT gene (5-HTTLPR), stress, and depression. Individuals with the s allele are unusually vulnerable to the depressogenic effects of early life stress (child abuse or neglect). Moreover, this effect is "dose-dependent," both in terms of the s allele (one copy or two) and in terms of the frequency and severity of the abuse.[8] Thus, the most vulnerable to depression are individuals with the s allele/s allele (s/s) genotype, and the least vulnerable are those with the l allele/l allele (l/l) genotype, with s/l individuals having intermediate risk. This finding is all the more extraordinary because this polymorphism has been shown to be functional: s/s and s/l individuals exhibit reduced SERT binding sites in PET imaging studies compared with l/l individuals. Note that individuals with the l/l genotype are immune to the depressogenic effects of early life trauma, representing a disease-resistant haplotype. This original observation by Caspi and colleagues[8] has now been replicated by most subsequent studies.

Another allele, the Lg, or Goldman polymorphism, which is similar functionally to the l allele, has recently been discovered. It confers some protection against depression and may account for some of the variance in the studies to date. Some studies that focused exclusively on stressful life events have found no evidence that 5-HTTLPR moderates the relationship between stressful life events and depression. This difference is likely explained in part by the wide variety of stressors and stress assessment methods included in these studies and the age of the individual at the time of the abuse/neglect. There is robust evidence that the 5-HTTLPR polymorphism moderates the relationship between childhood abuse or maltreatment and depression. A recent metaanalysis conducted by Karg and colleagues[59] confirms these findings.

Other genes involved in CRF and HPA axis regulation have been implicated in vulnerability to depression associated with early life stress. One of the authors' studies investigated several single-nucleotide polymorphisms (SNPs) in the CRF1 receptor gene (CRHR 1) and their role in moderating adult depression in individuals who experience early life stress in the form of child abuse. The CRHR 1 plays a key role in the regulation of the HPA axis in response to stress. It mediates the effect of CRF on the pituitary to release ACTH, which in turn stimulates the production of cortisol. In addition, CRF activity at the CRHR 1 in extrahypothalamic regions produces symptoms of anxiety and depression. The authors' study found that several SNPs and two haplotypes (TAT and TCA) formed by these SNPs mediated the interaction between early adverse events and risk for depression. The study revealed that the TAT and TCA haplotypes had a protective effect on the severity of adult depressive symptoms among individuals who had moderate to severe childhood abuse. These results were validated in two distinct ethnically different populations (a predominantly African American group of lower socioeconomic status and a group of mostly white women of higher socioeconomic status). The genotypes and haplotypes that constitute variants of CRHR 1 may serve as potential predictors of both risk and resilience for adult depression in men and women with a history of child abuse.[60]

A recent study by Polanczyk and colleagues[61] attempted to answer the question of how adverse experiences in childhood can result in depression that emerges years later during adulthood. Their theory focused on the effects of emotional arousal and memory consolidation and the potential role played by CRHR 1. The amygdala, which contains a significant number of CRHR 1 receptors, plays a crucial role in the consolidation of memories of emotionally charged experiences. Previous findings suggest that negative and ruminative memories play a role in the development of depression in some patients. The authors argued that individuals who have two copies of the TAT protective haplotype CRHR 1 gene may end up having impaired activation of fear memory consolidation processes, resulting in relatively unemotional processing of memories of adverse childhood experiences. This impaired activation, leading to a nonemotional cognitive processing of emotionally charged events, may protect these individuals from depression in later years. These findings suggest a possible mechanism for the protective effects of CRHR 1 gene variants on the development of adult depression following childhood maltreatment. Obviously, subsequent studies need to replicate these findings and explore other potential mechanisms for this interaction.

The FKBP5 gene, coding with FK506-binding protein 51(FKBP5), a co-chaperone regulating glucocorticoid receptor (GR) sensitivity, is also implicated in HPA axis regulation. Its mechanism of action involves cortisol induction of FKDP5 expression and, in turn, FKBP5 binding to the GR, reducing its affinity for cortisol. Several SNPs within the FKBP5 gene have been identified, including one that increases FKBP5 protein expression, namely the high-induction allele T. A recent study demonstrated that this SNP was associated with an altered cortisol response to stress. T allele homozygotes had a significantly slower recovery of stress-induced cortisol response and higher anxiety during recovery.[62] Appel and colleagues[63] demonstrated that individuals carrying the TT genotype who had had severe physical abuse (and severe sexual and emotional abuse) were at significantly higher risk for major depression in adulthood. Interestingly, individuals with a history of childhood neglect did not show a similar interaction.[63] This finding is of considerable interest and begs further study. Research on this gene has also led to an interesting treatment finding: depressed patients carrying the TT genotype showed a significantly faster response to a variety of antidepressants of different classes than CT or CC genotypes.[64]

In a different study, Binder and colleagues[65] identified four SNPs of the FKBP5 gene that interact with severity of childhood abuse to predict adult PTSD symptoms.

These variations in the FKBP5 gene potentially serve as predictors of both risk and resilience for adult PTSD among survivors of early sexual and physical abuse.[65]

Additionally, Ressler and colleagues[66] examined a more complex G×G×E interaction of CRHR1 and 5-HTTLPR polymorphisms and measures of childhood abuse on risk for adult depression. This study demonstrated that there is an interaction between 5-HTTLPR and CRHR1 variants and childhood abuse that predicts adult depression. Individuals carrying the risk alleles in both genes (5-HTTLRP s/s or s/l and zero copies of CRHR1 TCA protective allele) exhibited clinically significant depressive symptoms at less severe levels of childhood abuse than individuals with no or only one of the risk alleles. The protective CRHR1 allele was overrepresented in a subgroup of individuals with a history of childhood abuse but no lifetime major depression. Moreover, the protective effects of the CRHR1 TCA haplotype were only observed in individuals carrying the 5-HTTLRP l/l genotype (therefore in the absence of the s allele). However, sufficiently severe levels of childhood abuse seem to overcome any amount of genetic "protection."[66]

Another study examining G×G×E interactions found a significant three-way interaction between a brain-derived neurotrophic factor (BDNF) gene polymorphism with the 5-HTTLPR gene and a history of early life trauma in predicting depression.[67] Children who had both the BDNF gene Val66Met polymorphism and the s/s 5-HTTLPR genotype had the highest depression scores, but only in the maltreated subgroup. A significant four-way interaction also emerged in this study: social support was found to moderate risk for depressive symptoms in children with childhood maltreatment carrying both vulnerable phenotypes. This finding obviously has significant therapeutic implications.

In summary, the association between the stress of childhood trauma and depression is mediated by a number of neurobiological pathways (CRF and HPA axis dysregulation, immune system dysregulation) and moderated by complex genetic mechanisms.

EPIGENETICS

The field of epigenetics (the study of heritable changes in gene expression or cellular phenotype caused by mechanisms other than changes in the underlying DNA sequence) has contributed further to an understanding of developmental changes occurring in early life in response to childhood adversity. A number of molecular mechanisms leading to structural genetic modifications are involved in the regulation of gene expression.

DNA methylation is the best-characterized epigenetic modification. It seems that promoter-specific DNA methylation is correlated with gene silencing, but gene body (nonpromoter) DNA methylation correlates with increased gene activity. Using postmortem brain tissue from suicide victims, McGowan and colleagues[68] found evidence of methylation of the promoter region of the GR gene in the hippocampus of those with a history of childhood abuse. No such methylation pattern was found in suicide victims without childhood abuse. In this case, the methylation likely silenced the GR gene, resulting in decreased GR expression and potentially, increased stress response.

Demethylation may be able to reverse the changes in gene expression associated with the methylation process. Weaver and colleagues[69] showed that methionine, a dietary modulator of methylation, was able to reverse both the DNA methylation pattern of the GR promoter and stress responses in rats that experienced early maternal deprivation, indicating that epigenetic effects of early life stress may be reversible.

Histone modifications and noncoding RNA-mediated regulation of gene expression are two other important epigenetic mechanisms implicated in the developmental changes caused by early life stress. A number of animal studies have demonstrated that interfering with early mother-infant interactions, both prenatally and postnatally, can lead to developmental changes caused by epigenetic modifications. However, there is evidence that the postnatal handling of offspring exposed to prenatal stress can offset many of the detrimental effects of stress, suggesting that a positive postnatal experience may potentially reverse stress-induced epigenetic modifications.[70] Clearly, the combination of genetic and environmental influences, mediated in part by epigenetic changes at critical periods of development, determine whether an individual will be vulnerable or resilient to developing subsequent stress-related disorders.

IMPLICATIONS FOR PREVENTION AND TREATMENT

In this section the authors discuss genetic, neurobiological, and psychological factors that characterize individuals with early life trauma who seem resilient to stress[71] as compared with those who develop subsequent depression. These resilient individuals may carry protective SNPs that moderate environmental stress, including protective polymorphisms in the 5-HTTLPR, CRHR1, FKBP5, and BDNF genes. Additionally, a number of psychosocial factors have been associated with resilience, including positive emotions/optimism, cognitive flexibility, an active coping style, and social support.

Specifically, positive affectivity has been shown to decrease autonomic activity and promote adaptive coping.[72] Cognitive flexibility, the ability to reframe and find positive meaning in an adverse event, seems to result in decreased activation of the amygdala and increased activation of the medial prefrontal cortex.[73] Individuals who use active coping strategies exhibit low levels of denial and avoidance and a high ability to problem-solve, which has been linked to improved capacity to handle stress. Active coping may decrease the risk of developing fear-conditioned associations to a traumatic event and later on, decreased intensity of traumatic memories on reexposure to traumatic stimuli.[74] Finally, the availability of and openness to social support have been shown to promote resilience to a variety of health outcomes.[75] Social support promotes resilience among individuals exposed to childhood sexual abuse.[76] In human studies, low social support has been associated with neuroendocrine changes indicative of heightened reactivity to stress, such as increased blood pressure and pulse.[77]

The authors have highlighted a variety of factors that seem to characterize individuals who show resilience to stress and adversity. They now discuss the implications of these findings in the prevention and treatment of depression.

There are few predictors of treatment response in depression, but childhood trauma has clearly emerged as one. Early life adversity has been associated with lower rates of response and remission, higher rates of relapse, and a more chronic course of depression. However, to date few randomized controlled studies have specifically addressed the impact of early life trauma on treatment response in depression. Uher,[78] in a recent review, briefly discusses four adult and four adolescent treatment studies of depression. All studies concluded that a history of childhood maltreatment predicted poor treatment outcome (treatment modalities in these studies included use of antidepressants, psychotherapy, or a combination). One curious finding that emerged from the adolescent studies was that cognitive behavior therapy (CBT) was associated with poorer outcomes in this particular population compared with antidepressants. Larger studies need to be conducted in the future to corroborate this finding.[78]

Only one study to date has reported differential effectiveness of treatment modalities in depressed individuals with a history of childhood abuse. Nemeroff and colleagues[79] reanalyzed data from a large multicenter treatment trial of chronically depressed patients, comparing the efficacy of an antidepressant, nefazodone, psychotherapy (cognitive-behavioral analysis system of psychotherapy), or the combination, by subdividing the patients according to a history of childhood trauma. The likelihood of achieving remission in depressed patients with an early life adverse event was twice as high with psychotherapy when compared with antidepressant treatment and three times as high specifically for those with parental loss. Combination treatment was no better than psychotherapy alone. This differential response to treatments suggests that there may be variable neurobiological pathways leading to depression and psychotherapy and pharmacotherapy affect these pathways in different ways.[80] This study has significant implications for the treatment of chronic depression in individuals with early life trauma. Further studies are needed to compare the effectiveness of other forms of psychotherapy and pharmacotherapy and to identify the critical elements of response in both modalities.

Overall, it seems that patients with early life trauma and depression present a multitude of psychological and biological characteristics that render treatment problematic. Psychologically these patients are characterized by lack of trust, poor or volatile relationships, frequent isolation, poor self-image, insecure attachment, cognitive distortion, and emotional dysregulation. This psychological profile is the mirror image of what the authors see in individuals with psychological resilience.

TREATMENT APPROACHES FOR INDIVIDUALS WITH EARLY LIFE TRAUMA AND DEPRESSION
Psychotherapy

In the past 30 years, more than 150 controlled and comparative studies have examined the efficacy of psychological treatments of depression (these studies included CBT, interpersonal therapy, psychodynamic psychotherapy, supportive psychotherapy, and others). In general, evidence that one type of psychotherapy for depression was more effective than another is lacking.

To date, however, no clear psychotherapeutic approach to depression in individuals with early life trauma has been established. Some forms of group therapy have been effective in symptom reduction in survivors of childhood trauma. Emotion-focused therapy, a 20-week individual psychotherapy focusing on better emotional regulation and improved interpersonal relationships, seems effective in the treatment of adults who had childhood trauma.[81] The few studies that are available, however, do not exclusively address the treatment of depression but more generally, improvement in multiple domains of psychopathology.

Fava and Tomba[82] have developed Well-Being Therapy, a short-term (8–12 sessions) individual psychotherapy that is structured and focused on current problems and states and has a large educational component. This form of therapy, based on Ryff's[83] cognitive model of psychological well-being, focuses on specific psychological domains including environmental mastery, personal growth, purpose in life, autonomy, self-acceptance, and positive relations with others. The difference between Well-Being Therapy and standard CBT is one of focus. Whereas traditional CBT tends to address areas of psychological distress, Well-Being Therapy primarily addresses instances of emotional well-being. Even though this form of treatment has been validated in a number of randomized control studies, it has not been studied in patients with an acute and severe episode of depression. It currently seems to benefit patients who have partially responded to other forms of treatment but who continue to experience residual symptoms. This form of psychotherapy that focuses on positive emotions nonetheless raises interesting questions for future research on the effectiveness of positive psychology, such as the following:

- What are the essential therapeutic elements in a positive psychological approach when treating depression associated with childhood trauma?
- Can a positive emotional approach more effectively lead to recovery and resilience?
- Are there epigenetic effects of positive emotions and cognitions on reversing the negative sequelae of trauma?

Psychodynamic psychotherapy is another treatment modality that warrants serious discussion and consideration in this population. Given its emphasis on conflict, meaning, developmental arrests, attachment and relationships, and multiple symptomatic domains and its focus on the therapeutic alliance and the inevitable disruptions that occur in the context of transference and countertransference, this form of treatment may be particularly effective in this population. Unfortunately, no controlled randomized outcome studies that evaluate the effectiveness of this treatment for this population are available. A recent meta-analysis by Abbass and colleagues[84] indicated that short-term psychodynamic psychotherapy may be effective in patients with depression and comorbid personality disorder. Several new studies are currently under way examining the effectiveness of mentalization in the treatment of depression, but so far the results have been mixed.[85] A recent pilot study examined the effectiveness of dynamic interpersonal therapy (DIT), a brief psychodynamic intervention, as a treatment for depression. This small study of 16 patients found that DIT was associated with a significant reduction of depressive symptoms, but larger randomized controlled studies are needed.[86]

Beutel and colleagues[87] recently reported that psychodynamic psychotherapy effectively regulated the amygdala-hippocampal hyperactivation and the prefrontal deactivation in patients with panic disorder. A recent Finnish study compared short-term psychodynamic psychotherapy and fluoxetine using PET scans to measure CNS 5-HT1A receptors. The 5-HT1A receptor system has been implicated in the pathophysiology of depression. Both treatments were equally effective, but the psychotherapy group had a significant increase in the 5-HT1A receptor density compared with the medication group. The mechanism of action of psychodynamic psychotherapy on this change in the serotonin system is unknown.[88] These findings, however, add weight to the hypothesis that psychotherapy could lead to changes in gene expression.

Similarly, Lehto and colleagues[89] measured changes in midbrain SERT availability in depressed patients who received psychodynamic psychotherapy. After 12 months of therapy, midbrain SERT densities significantly increased in patients with atypical but not classical depression.[89] Future studies are needed to confirm these findings. These neuroimaging studies suggest that psychodynamic psychotherapy is differentially effective compared with antidepressants in the treatment of patients with depression and a history of childhood maltreatment.

Pharmacotherapy

Several laboratory animal studies have demonstrated that SSRI antidepressants can reverse certain of the neurobiological effects brought on by trauma.[90] For instance, 3 weeks of treatment with paroxetine, an SSRI, of adult rats that had experienced maternal deprivation reduced their abnormally high CNS CRF mRNA expression as well as serum ACTH and corticosterone concentrations. These neuroendocrine changes reverted to abnormal on discontinuation of the SSRI.[91]

It seems now that normalization of neuroendocrine system dysregulation is necessary in order to achieve remission from depression. Electro-convulsive therapy and fluoxetine, an SSRI, significantly reduce CSF CRF concentrations in treatment-responsive patients. To date, however, there have been few studies investigating the neuroendocrine effects and efficacy of antidepressants specifically in individuals with depression and a history of childhood trauma.

Klein and colleagues[92] studied patients with chronic major depressive disorder enrolled in a 12-week open-label trial of algorithm-guided pharmacotherapy. Among completers, 32% of patients with a history of clinically significant childhood abuse achieved remission compared with 44% of patients without such a history. Variables predicting a lower probability of remission included a history of maternal overcontrol, paternal abuse, paternal indifference, and sexual abuse. These findings indicate that depressed patients with a history of childhood adversity are less responsive to pharmacotherapy.[92]

It is reasonable to think that by reducing the HPA axis activation and toning down the limbic system and the immune system, antidepressants could play a complementary and synergistic role to psychotherapy in the treatment of depression with childhood adversity. In fact, DeRubeis and colleagues[93] studied the neuromechanisms affected either by CBT or antidepressants in the course of treatment of depression. Their findings indicate that CBT primarily increases prefrontal function and therefore cognitive control, whereas antidepressants act on the amygdala, which is actively involved in the processing of negative emotions.[93]

SUMMARY

In summary, depressed patients with a history of childhood trauma may have a distinct depression endophenotype characterized by a specific neurobiology and risk genotype that may be responsive to different treatment strategies than depressed patients without childhood adversity. Based on current findings, treatment strategies should be multimodal and include the following[94]:

1. Psychotherapy that addresses a number of domains, such as emotional regulation, cognitive reframing, careful exploration of past traumatic events, attachment, and interpersonal relationships in a safe and trusting therapeutic environment.
2. The therapy should likely be longer term in order to effectively impact those domains.
3. Pharmacotherapy that will be effective in quieting the body's hyperresponsiveness to stress and reverse epigenetic modifications induced by trauma and stress.
4. Environmental interventions that provide a support network (maternal care, a positive family environment, the support of a close friend) have all been shown to attenuate the impact of childhood abuse.

In addition, there is great potential in the identification of genomic biomarkers to help guide us in the identification of traumatized individuals who are susceptible to depression. These indices may also help identify those for whom the immediate provision of treatment may have a preventive effect and may someday guide us in the development of novel pharmacologic approaches.

REFERENCES

1. Kessler RC, Berglund P, Demler O, et al; National Comorbidity Survey Replication. The epidemiology of major depressive disorder: results from the National Comorbidity Survey Replication (NCS-R). JAMA 2003;289:3095–105.
2. Evans DL, Charney DS, Lewis L, et al. Mood disorders in the medically ill: scientific review and recommendations. Biol Psychiatry 2005;58:175–89.
3. Trivedi MH, Rush AJ, Wisniewski SR, et al. STAR*D Study Team: evaluation of outcomes with citalopram for depression using measurement-based care in STAR-D: implications for clinical practice. Am J Psychiatry 2006;163:2840.
4. Sullivan PF, Neale MC, Kendler KS. Genetic epidemiology of major depression: review and meta-analysis. Am J Psychiatry 2000;157:1552–62.
5. Mann JJ, Malone KM, Psych MR, et al. Attempted suicide characteristics and cerebrospinal fluid amine metabolites in depressed inpatients. Neuropsychopharmacology 1996;15:576–86.
6. Drevets WC, Frank E, Price JC, et al. PET imaging of serotonin 1A receptor binding in depression. Biol Psychiatry 1999;46:1375–87.
7. Charney DS. Monoamine dysfunction and the pathophysiology and treatment of depression. J Clin Psychiatry 1998;59(Suppl 14):11–4.
8. Caspi A, Sugden K, Moffitt TE, et al. Influence of life stress on depression: moderation by a polymorphism in the 5-HTT gene. Science 2003;301:386–9.
9. Ressler KJ, Nemeroff CB. Role of norepinephrine in the pathophysiology of neuropsychiatric disorders. CNS Spectr 2001;6:663–6, 670.
10. Nemeroff CB, Entsuah R, Benattia I, et al. Comprehensive pooled analysis of remission (COMPARE) with venlafaxine vs SSRIs. Biol Psychiatry 2008;63:424–34.
11. Dunlop BW, Nemeroff CB. The role of dopamine in the pathophysiology of depression. Arch Gen Psychiatry 2007;64:327–37.
12. Meyer JH, Kruger S, Wilson AA, et al. Lower dopamine transporter binding potential in striatum during depression. Neuroreport 2001;12:4121–5.
13. Nestler EJ, Carlezon WA Jr. The mesolimbic dopamine reward circuit in depression. Biol Psychiatry 2006;59:1151–9.
14. Vythilingam M, Heim C, Newport J, et al. Childhood trauma associated with smaller hippocampal volume in women with major depression. Am J Psychiatry 2002;159: 2072–80.
15. Mayberg HS, Liotti M, Brannan SK, et al. Reciprocal limbic-cortical function and negative mood: converging PET findings in depression and normal sadness. Am J Psychiatry 1999;156:675–82.
16. Drevets WC. Prefrontal cortical-amygdalar metabolism in major depression. Ann NY Acad Sci 1999;877:614–37.
17. Sachar EJ, Hellman L, Fukushima DK, et al. Cortisol production in depressive illness: a clinical and biochemical clarification. Arch Gen Psychiatry 1970;23: 289–98.
18. Evans DL, Burnett GB, Nemeroff CB. The dexamethasone suppression test in the clinical setting. Am J Psychiatry 1983;140:586–9.
19. Ising M, Kunzel HE, Binder EB, et al. The combined dexamethasone/CRH test as a potential surrogate marker in depression. Progr Neuropsychopharmacol Biol Psychiatry 2005;29:1085–93.
20. Nemeroff CB, Widerlov E, Bissette G, et al. Elevated concentrations of CSF corticotropin-releasing factor-like immunoreactivity in depressed patients. Science 1984; 226:1342–4.

21. Merali Z, Du L, Hrdina P, et al. Dysregulation in the suicide brain: mRNA expression of corticotropin-releasing hormone receptors and GABAA receptor subunits in frontal cortical brain region. J Neurosci 2004;24:1478–85.

22. Nemeroff CB, Bissette G, Akil H, et al. Neuropeptide concentrations in the cerebrospinal fluid of depressed patients treated with electroconvulsive therapy: corticotrophin-releasing factor, β-endorphin and somatostatin. Br J Psychiatry 1991;158:59–63.

23. Heinrichs SC, Menzaghi F, Merlo Pich E, et al. The role of CRF in behavioral aspects of stress. Ann NY Acad Sci 1995;771:92–104.

24. Heim C, Shugart M, Craighead WE, et al. Neurobiological and psychiatric consequences of child abuse and neglect. Dev Psychobiol 2010;52:671–90.

25. Heim C, Newport DJ, Heit S, et al. Pituitary-adrenal and autonomic responses to stress in women after sexual and physical abuse in childhood. JAMA 2000;284:592–7.

26. Heim C, Mletzko T, Purselle D, et al. The dexamethasone/corticotropin-releasing factor test in men with major depression: role of childhood trauma. Biol Psychiatry 2008;63:398–405.

27. Currier MB, Nemeroff CB. Inflammation and mood disorders: proinflammatory cytokines and the pathogenesis of depression. Anti-Inflammatory & Anti-Allergy Agents in Medicinal Chemistry 2010:9,212–20.

28. Anisman H, Merali Z, Poutler MS, et al. Cytokines as a precipitant of depressive illness: animal and human studies. Curr Pharm Des 2005;11:963–72.

29. Schiepers OJ, Wichers MC, Maes M. Cytokines and major depression. Prog Neuropsychopharm Biol Psychiatr 2005;29:201–17.

30. Lanquillon S, Kreig JC, Benning-Abu-Shach U, et al. Cytokine production and treatment response in major depressive disorder. Neuropsychopharmacol 2000;29:370–79.

31. Mohr DC, Goodkin DE, Islar J, et al. Treatment of depression is associated with suppression of nonspecific and antigen-specific T(H)1 receptors in multiple sclerosis. Arch Neurol 2001;58:1081–6.

32. Anisman J, Ravindran AV, Griffiths J, et al. Interleukin-I beta production in dysthymia before and after pharmacotherapy. Biol Psychiatry 1999;8:141–74.

33. Chrousos GP. The hypothalamic-pituitary-adrenal-axis and immune-mediated inflammation. N Engl J Med 1995;332:1351–62.

34. Ramamorthy S, Ramamorthy JD, Prasad PD, et al. Regulation of the human serotonin transporter by interleukin-1 beta. Biochem Biophys Res Commun 1995;216:560–7.

35. Bell C, Abrams J, Nutt D. Tryptophan depletion and its implications in psychiatry. Br J Psychiatry 2001;178:399–405.

36. Shuto H, Kataoka Y, Horikawa, T et al. Repeated interferon-alpha administration inhibits dopaminergic neural activity in the mouse brain. Brain Res 1997;747:348–51.

37. McNally L, Bhagwagar Z, Hannestad J. Inflammation, glutamate and glia in depression: a literature review. CNS Spectr 2008;13:501–10.

38. Rudisch B, Nemeroff CB. Epidemiology of comorbid coronary artery disease and depression. Biol Psychiatry 2003;54:227–40.

39. Muller N, Schwarz MJ, Dehning S, et al. The cyclo-oxygenase-2 inhibitor celecoxib has therapeutic effects in major depression: results of a double-blind, randomized, placebo-controlled add-on pilot study to reboxetine. Mol Psychiatry 2006;11:680–4.

40. Tyring S, Gottleib A, Papp K, et al. Etanercept and clinical outcomes, fatigue and depression in psoriasis: double-blind placebo-controlled randomized phase III trial. Lancet 2006;367:29–35.

41. Kiecolt-Glaser JK, Loving TJ, Stowell JR, et al. Hostile marital interactions, proinflammatory cytokine production and wound healing. Arch Gen Psychiatr 2005;62:266–72.

42. Pace TW, Metzko TC, Alagbe O, et al. Increased stress-induced inflammatory response in male patients with major depression and increased early life stress. Am J Psychiatr 2006;163:1630–3.

43. Danese A, Pariate CM, Caspi A, et al. Childhood maltreatment predicts adult inflammation in a life-course study. Proc Natl Acad Sci USA 2007;104:1319–24.

44. Gorey KM, Leslie DR. The prevalence of child sexual abuse: integrative review adjustment for potential response and measurement biases. Child Abuse Negl 1997;21:391–8.

45. Holmes WC, Slap GB. Sexual abuse of boys: definition, prevalence, correlates, sequelae, and management. JAMA 1998;280:1855–62.

46. Horowitz LA, Putman FW, Noll JG, et al. Factors affecting utilization of treatment services by sexually abused girls. Child Abuse Negl 1997;21:35–48.

47. McCauley J, Kern DE, Kolodner K, et al. Clinical characteristics of women with a history of childhood abuse: unhealed wounds. JAMA 1997;277:1362–68.

48. Mullen PE, Martin JL, Anderson JC, et al.The long–term impact of the physical, emotional, and sexual abuse of children: A community study. Child Abuse Negl 1996;20:7–21.

49. Young EA, Abelson JL, Curtin GC, et al. Child adversity and vulnerability to mood and anxiety disorders. Depress Anxiety 1997;5:66–72.

50. Zlotnick C, Ryan CE, Miller IW, et al. Childhood abuse and recovery from major depression. Child Abuse Negl 1995;19:1513–6.

51. Bremner JD, Southwick SM, Johnson DR. Childhood physical abuse and combat related posttraumatic stress disorder in Vietnam veterans. Am J Psychiatry 1993;150: 235–39.

52. Portegijs PJ, Jeuke FM, van der Horst FG, et al. A troubled youth: relations with somatization, depression and anxiety in adulthood. Fam Prac 1996;13:1–11.

53. Stein MB, Walker JR, Anderson G, et al. Childhood physical and sexual abuse in patients with anxiety disorders and in a community sample. Am J Psychiatry 1996; 153:275–7.

54. Heim C, Newport J, Mletzko T, et al. The link between childhood trauma and depression: insights from HPA axis studies in humans. Psychoneuroendocrinology 2008;33:693–710.

55. Kaplan MJ, Klinetob NA. Childhood emotional trauma and chronic posttraumatic stress disorder in adult outpatients with treatment resistant depression. J Nerv Ment Dis 2000;188:596–601.

56. Lara ME, Klein DN, Kasch KL. Psychosocial predictors of the short-term course and outcome of major depression: a longitudinal study of a nonclinical sample with recent onset episodes. J Abnorm Psychol 2000;109:644–50.

57. McGloin JM, Widom CS. Resilience among abused and neglected children grown up. Dev Psychopathol 2001;13(4):1021–38.

58. Collishaw S, Pickles A, Messer J, et al. Resilience to adult psychopathology following childhood maltreatment: evidence from a community sample. Child Abuse Negl 2007;31:211–29.

59. Karg K, Burmeister M, Shedden K, et al. The Serotonin transporter promoter variant (5-HTTLPR), stress, and depression meta-analysis revisited. Arch Gen Psychiatry 2011;68(5):444–54.

60. Bradley RG, Binder EB, Epstein M, et al. Influence of child abuse on adult depression: moderation by the corticotropin-releasing hormone receptor gene. Arch Gen Psych 2008;65:190–200.
61. Polanczyk G, Caspi A, Williams B, et al. Protective effect of CRHR1 gene variants on the development of adult depression following childhood maltreatment: replication and extension. Arch Gene Psych 2009;66:978–85.
62. Ising M, Depping AM, Siebertz A, et al. Polymorphisms in the FKBP5 gene region modulate recovery from psychosocial stress in healthy controls. Eur J Neurosci 2008;28:389–98.
63. Appel K, Schwahn C, Mahler J, et al. Moderation of adult depression by a polymorphism in the FKBP5 gene and childhood physical abuse in the general population. Neuropsychopharmacology 2011;36:1982–91.
64. Binder EB, Salyakina D, Lichtner P, et al. Polymorphisms in FKBP5 are associated with increased recurrence of depressive episodes and rapid response to antidepressant treatment. Nat Genet 2004;36:1319–25.
65. Binder EB, Bradley RG, Liu W, et al. Association of FKBP5 polymorphisms and childhood abuse with risk of posttraumatic stress disorder symptoms in adults. JAMA 2008;299(11):1–15.
66. Ressler KJ, Bradley B, Mercer K, et al. Polymorphisms in CRHR1 and the serotonin transporter loci: gene x gene x environment interactions on depressive symptoms. Am J Med Genet B Neuropsychiatr Genet 2009;153B:812–24.
67. Kaufman H, Yang BZ, Douglas-Palumberi H, et al. Brain-derived neurotrophic factor-5-HTTLPR gene interactions and environmental modifiers of depression in children. Biol Psychiatry 2006;59(8):673–80.
68. McGowan PO, Sasaki A, D'Alesso AC, et al. Epigenetic regulation of the glucocorticoid receptor in human brain associates with childhood abuse. Nat Neurosci 2009; 12:342–48.
69. Weaver IC, Champagne FA, Brown SE, et al. Reversal of maternal programming of stress responses in adult offspring through methyl supplementation: altering epigenetic marking later in life. J Neurosci 2005;25:11045–54.
70. Dudley KJ, Li X, Kobor MS, et al. Epigenetic mechanisms mediating vulnerability and resilience to psychiatric disorders. Neurosci Behav Rev 2011;35:1544–51.
71. Charney DS, Psychobiological mechanisms of resilience and vulnerability: implications for successful adaptation to extreme stress. Am J Psychiatry 2004;161:195–216.
72. Folkman S, Moskowitz JT. Positive affect and the other side of coping. Am Psychol 2000;55:647–54.
73. Ochsner KN, Bunge SA, Gross JJ, et al. Rethinking feelings; an fMRI study of the cognitive regulation of emotion. J Cogn Neurosci 2002;14:1215–29.
74. Southwick S, Vythilingam M, Charney D. The psychobiology of depression and resilience to stress: implications for prevention and treatment. Annu Rev Clin Psychol 2005;1:255–91.
75. Berkman LF. The role of social relations in health promotion. Psychosom Med 1995;57:245–54.
76. Jonzon E, Lindblad F. Adult female victims of child sexual abuse: multitype maltreatment and disclosure characteristics related to subjective health. J Interpers Violence 2005;20:651–66.
77. Uchino BN, Cacioppo JT, Kiecolt-Glaser JK. The relationship between social support and physiological processes: a review with emphasis on underlying mechanisms and implications for health. Psychol Bull 1996;119:488–531.

78. Uher R. Genes, environment, and individual differences in responding to treatment for depression. Harv Rev Psychiatry 2011;19(3):109–24.
79. Nemeroff CB, Heim CM, Thase ME, et al. Differential responses to psychotherapy versus pharmacotherapy in patients with chronic forms of major depression and childhood trauma. Proc Natl Acad Sci USA 2003;100:14293–6.
80. Mayberg HS. Modulating dysfunctional limbic-cortical circuits in depression: towards development of brain-based algorithms for diagnosis and optimised treatment. Br Med Bull 2003;65:193–207.
81. Paivo SC, Neuwenhuis JA. Efficacy of emotion focused therapy for adult survivors of child abuse: a preliminary study. J Trauma Stress 2001;14:115–33.
82. Fava GA, Tomba E. Increasing psychological well-being and resilience by psychotherapeutic methods. J Pers 2009;77:1903–34.
83. Ryff CD. Happiness is everything, or is it: explorations on the meaning of psychological well-being. J Pers Soc Psychol 1989;6:1069–81.
84. Abbass A, Town J, Driessen E. The efficacy of short-term psychodynamic psychotherapy for depressive disorders with comorbid personality disorder. Psychiatry 2011;74(1):58–71.
85. Taubner S, Kessler H, Buchheim A, et al. The role of mentalization in the psychoanalytic treatment of chronic depression. Psychiatry 2011;74(1):49–57.
86. Lemma A, Target M, Fonagy P. The development of a brief psychodynamic intervention (dynamic interpersonal therapy) and its application to depression: a pilot study. Psychiatry 2011;74(1):41–8.
87. Beutel ME, Stark R, Pan H, et al. Changes of brain activation pre- post short-term psychodynamic inpatient psychotherapy: an fMRI study of panic disorder patients. Psychiatry Res 2010;184:96–104.
88. Karlsson H, Hirvonen J, Kajander J, et al. Research Letter: psychotherapy increases brain serotonin 5 HT1A receptors in patients with major depressive disorder. Psychol Med 2010;40:523–28.
89. Lehto SM, Tolmunen T, Joensuu M, et al. Changes in midbrain serotonin transporter availability in atypically depressed subjects after one year of psychotherapy. Prog Neuropsychopharmacol Biol Psychiatry 2008;32:229–37.
90. Gutman D, Nemeroff CB. Neurobiology of early life stress: rodent studies. Semin Clin Neuropsychiatry 2002;7:89–95.
91. Huot RL, Thrivikraman KV, Meaney MJ, et al. Development of adult ethanol preference and anxiety as a consequence of neonatal maternal separation in Long Evans rats and reversal with antidepressant treatment. Psychopharmacology (Berlin) 2001;158:366–73.
92. Klein D, Arnow B, Barkin J, et al. Early adversity in chronic depression: clinical correlates and response to pharmacotherapy. Depress Anxiety 2009;26:701–10.
93. DeRubeis RJ, Siegle GJ, Hollon SD. Cognitive therapy versus medication for depression: treatment outcomes and neural mechanisms. Nat Rev Neurosci 2008;9:788–96.
94. Craighead WE, Nemeroff CB. The impact of early trauma on response to psychotherapy. Clin Neurosci Res 2005;4:405–11.

The Varieties of Depressive Experience: Diagnosing Mood Disorders

S. Nassir Ghaemi, MD[a],*, Paul A. Vöhringer, MD[a,b],
Derick E. Vergne, MD[a]

KEYWORDS

- Depression • Diagnosis • Mood disorder • Phenomenology
- Psychopathology • Jaspers

"Depression" is not simply depression. There are many varieties, with manic and anxiety symptoms being prominent aspects. To understand depression, we need to understand much beyond depression.

It is not enough to say simply, "the patient meets criteria for major depressive disorder" (MDD); there are thousands of ways to meet criteria for MDD. And it is not even clear that meeting criteria for MDD is scientifically very meaningful. MDD represents an extremely broad spectrum of depressive conditions, and the first step is to carefully describe the clinical symptoms. Unfortunately, although the *Diagnostic and Statistical Manual of Mental Disorders, Third Edition,* (DSM-III) was meant to enhance the science of nosology, it has lead to the "death of phenomenology".[1] The supposedly temporary description of diagnostic criteria has led to a reification of those criteria such that clinicians and researchers do not carefully assess patients' actual symptoms but only whether they meet DSM-defined criteria. This American phenomenon has infected many countries.

The careful study of the phenomenology of psychiatric conditions is absolutely necessary before one can even begin to discuss diagnoses. This tradition of attention to psychopathology is strongest in Germany, and specifically in Heidelberg, where Karl Jaspers and Kurt Schneider established this approach. In that effort, the authors believe the iconic duo of Freud and Kraepelin is missing a third part: Karl Jaspers.

This work was partly supported by grant number 5R01MH78060-5 from the National Institute of Mental Health (S.N.G.) and a scholarship from the National Commission for Scientific and Technological Research (CONICYT) of the government of Chile (P.A.V.).

Disclosures: Ghaemi, Research grant (Pfizer), Research consulting (Sunovion). No other disclosures for coauthors.

^a Mood Disorders Program, Department of Psychiatry, Tufts Medical Center, Tufts University School of Medicine, 800 Washington Street #1007, Boston, MA 02111, USA
^b Hospital Clinico, Facultad de Medicina, Universidad de Chile, Santiago, Chile
* Corresponding author.
E-mail address: nghaemi@tuftsmedicalcenter.org

Psychiatr Clin N Am 35 (2012) 73–86
doi:10.1016/j.psc.2011.11.008
0193-953X/12/$ – see front matter © 2012 Elsevier Inc. All rights reserved.

psych.theclinics.com

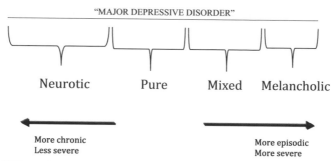

Fig. 1. The MDD spectrum.

Study of the *General Psychopathology* by Jaspers would be excellent training for psychiatrists who want to understand nosology.[2,3] What follows is a psychopathologic analysis of MDD.

HETEROGENEITY OF DEPRESSION
The MDD Spectrum: Melancholic, Neurotic, Mixed, and Pure Depression

The authors believe MDD represents four distinct and different kinds of depression: melancholic, neurotic, mixed, and pure types (**Fig. 1**), which are described in this article.

To appreciate this heterogeneity, some historical comments are needed. As a single unified construct, MDD has less and less scientific validity, yet it persists largely unchanged through each successive revision of DSM. In the authors' view, MDD is extremely broad, encompassing many more conditions than even the broadest notions of the bipolar spectrum, yet whereas the broad bipolar spectrum is passionately attacked by many, MDD is treated as a straightforward entity.

MDD was a political compromise in DSM-III, grafted onto science, as documented in a recent history based on the minutes of the DSM-III committees.[4] The original concept was to replace the broad and amorphous psychoanalytic concept of neurosis with more discrete, scientifically sound diagnoses of severe depression and specific anxiety conditions (phobias, panic attacks, obsessive-compulsive disorder, [OCD]). This laudable impulse was impeded by the political process of DSM revision. The scientific work was based largely on the efforts of the neo-Kraepelinian Washington University of St Louis researchers and their collaborators. That group wanted to propose a diagnosis of major unipolar depression, with criteria set up so as to exclude all mild depressive conditions and with the term *unipolar* used to indicate distinct episodes rather than the mild chronic symptoms of neurosis. Similarly, mild anxiety syndromes would be deleted from DSM-III and replaced with specific severe conditions like OCD. This proposal was met with resistance by the American Psychiatric Association's leadership and general assembly, most of whom were psychoanalytic practitioners. The most common diagnosis in psychoanalytic practice was neurotic depression, which meant mild depression and anxiety—both symptoms specifically excluded from the Washington University nosology. The head of the DSM-III revision, Robert Spitzer, trying to negotiate between the two groups, proposed that the research-based severe condition be called major depression, and the psychoanalytically-useful milder condition be called minor depression. The psychoanalytic groups objected that a "minor" diagnosis might receive minor insurance reimbursement, so the term *minor depression* was dropped, but *major* was retained, with the milder depressive criteria initially meant for minor depression folded into the "major" diagnosis.[4] Similarly, for the anxiety conditions, Spitzer created a new term, *generalized anxiety disorder* (GAD), to include the mild nonspecific anxiety symptoms that had been excluded initially based on the neo-Kraepelinian research studies. In the end, the majority of GAD criteria overlapped with MDD criteria. Many of the more chronic mild depressive symptoms were subsumed in a new category of dysthymia.

Given this origin of our current diagnoses of MDD and GAD, perhaps it is not surprising that twin studies show complete genetic correlation between the two diagnostic constructs.[5] In other words, there is no genetic (nor probably biological) distinction to be made between MDD and GAD. This similarity may have to do with the fact that both diagnoses were constructed for professional reasons rather than on scientific grounds. This historical background provides evidence for the fact that MDD frequently overlaps with the diagnoses of dysthymia and GAD. There is no deep biological reason for this "comorbidity"; it is the result of how these definitions were constructed.

Even the pragmatic claim that MDD is useful in orienting clinical practice has been put into doubt by our best studies of antidepressants, such as the disappointing long-term results of the STAR*D study.[6,7] No biological class of drugs can work effectively in a very heterogeneously defined illness.

If this conclusion is correct, the authors believe that the broad and heterogenous concept of MDD—the untouchable third rail of psychiatry—needs to be questioned.

Neurotic Depression

The spectrum of MDD includes, therefore, this mixture of mild depressive and anxiety symptoms that we now call MDD with comorbidity of dysthymia and GAD, but that used to be called, more simply, neurotic depression.

Neurotic depression patients have less severe depression and more prominent anxiety symptoms, as well as a high degree of sensitivity to psychosocial stressors, than is usual in recurrent unipolar depression, and they are likely to follow a chronic, not clearly episodic, course.[8]

The concept of neurotic depression is not vague. One of the authors (S.N.G.) has published, following the work of Sir Martin Roth, specific diagnostic criteria that can be used to validate this diagnosis in research studies, as well as to guide clinicians in reliably identifying it in clinical practice (**Box 1**).[7] The authors view neurotic depression psychopathologically—descriptively, not psychoanalytically. They make no conjectures about unconscious emotional causes. The key feature, as in Kraepelin's tradition, is *course*: neurotic depression is chronic; nonneurotic depressive conditions are episodic.

The chronicity of neurotic depression does not imply severity; in fact, the reverse is the case: these patients have mild to moderate depressive symptoms in general. Chronicity does not mean that there are never episodes. Patients with neurotic depression are especially prone to episodes because of their moderately depressed baseline; this is why even a slight psychosocial stressor can tip them over the threshold of an official DSM major depressive episode. But they tip just as easily back below that threshold to their moderately depressed baseline. In other words, they experience DSM major depressive episodes frequently but briefly and in immediate relation to psychosocial stressors.

The main problem for such patients is not these brief full depressive episodes; it is the chronic moderate depressive baseline. In this group, as the much-debated recent antidepressant metaanalyses show, antidepressants are least effective compared with placebo (mild depression).[9] STAR*D also showed lower antidepressant response in MDD with anxiety (consistent with neurotic depression or mixed depression, see following) versus nonanxious MDD (consistent with pure depression or melancholia).[10]

> **Box 1**
> **Modified Roth diagnostic criteria for neurotic depression**
>
> A. Depressed mood leading to severe subjective distress or marked functional impairment.
>
> B. Meeting 2 to 4 of the following criteria: Sleep decreased or increased, decreased interest in usual activities, decreased self-esteem, decreased energy, decreased concentration, decreased or increased appetite, suicidal ideation, but not meeting DSM-V criteria for a major depressive episode (ie subsyndromal major depressive episode symptoms).
>
> C. Prolonged or frequent worries or anxiety nearly daily for most of each day or sustained or frequently recurring multiple somatic symptoms (eg, gastrointestinal distress, headaches, paresthesias) with no secondary medical cause.
>
> D. Criteria A to C present over at least 6 months, during the majority of early every day.
>
> E. Mood or other symptoms apparently reactive to adverse or favorable changes in circumstances or everyday events.
>
> F. Absence of severe psychomotor retardation, guilt, anger, agitation, or psychotic features.
>
> G. DSM-IV major depressive episode criteria are not met during more than half of the duration of features A to G.
>
> *Adapted and expanded from* Roth S, Kerr T. The concept of neurotic depression: a plea for reinstatement. In: Pichot P, Rein W, editors. The clinical approach in psychiatry. Paris (France): Synthelabo; 1994. *From* Ghaemi SN. Why antidepressants are not antidepressants: STEP-BD, STAR*D, and the return of neurotic depression. Bipolar Disord 2008;10:957–68; with permission.

In the authors' view, that depressive baseline reflects temperament, which one might call dysthymia, but not illness—not a separate disease.

Historically, this concept fell into disrepute after the decline of psychoanalytic assumptions; indeed, if by neurotic one means anxious or depressive symptoms caused by unconscious emotional drives or defenses, then the term is suffused with psychoanalytic assumptions. But most psychiatrists in most of Europe never used the term *neurosis* this way. Outside of psychoanalytic circles, the term *neurotic* meant, descriptively, mildly depressed and anxious without any presumption as to cause. There was no inherent connotation of unconscious or conscious or biological or psychological causation. The term was one of pure descriptive psychopathology: mild symptoms of anxiety or depression. Severe depression was termed *melancholia*. And mania, of course, was a different set of symptoms. With these nonpsychoanalytic uses in mind, the authors agree with the stand of Sir Martin Roth in the famous British debates with Aubrey Lewis over the nosology of depression.[11] Roth held that the demise of neurotic depression, as a result of the conflict between psychoanalysts and neo-Kraepelinians, was regrettable.[12] Neurotic depression—as a pure construct of chronic mild depression and anxiety—was clinically sound and scientifically valid and distinguishable from melancholic episodes.

It is the authors' view that research since those debates of the 1970s has tended to support Roth's position that there are many subtypes of depression, one of which is neurotic depression, as opposed to Lewis's view (assumed by DSM-III onward) that all depressive conditions are essentially similar (hence the one broad diagnosis of MDD).

Melancholia

The type of depression termed *melancholia* is severe and generally unassociated with anxiety, unlike neurotic depression. Patients are severely psychomotor-retarded, with marked anhedonia. The cardinal feature of melancholia is complete absence of mood reactivity: patients are not labile (unlike mixed depression, see following), and they are generally unresponsive to psychosocial stressors (unlike neurotic depression); bad events cannot make them feel worse because they cannot feel any worse; good events do not cheer them up at all.[13] Melancholic depression is episodic, not chronic, and more common in bipolar disorder than unipolar depression.[14]

This depression is severe and dangerous; suicide risk is high. These episodes are lengthy, often lasting a few months at minimum, and up to a year. Rapid treatment, whether with antidepressants or electroconvulsive therapy, is essential. These treatments have proved effective, as seen in the recent debated metaanalyses, in which antidepressants were clearly more effective than placebo in severe depression,[9] which the authors see as a reflection of melancholia. In this group, however, modern antidepressants (like serotonin reuptake inhibitors) are relatively ineffective compared with traditional antidepressants (like tricyclic agents).[15]

Melancholia is unmistakable: it is the severe depression one sees in the psychiatric literature going back to the mid 19th century at least, and probably earlier, much the same as is seen today.[16]

Mixed Depression

The current broad *Diagnostic and Statistical Manual of Mental Disorders, Fourth Edition* (DSM-IV) definition of MDD entails, conversely, a narrow definition of mania, and especially of the acute mixed episode (requiring that full mania criteria be met at the same time as full depression criteria). Patients can thus be diagnosable with MDD with one, two, or three manic symptoms (along with a major depressive episode), because that presentation is still below the high threshold set for the DSM-IV mixed episode. Some data indicate that up to one-half of subjects with MDD have one to three manic symptoms,[17] which has been termed *mixed depression*.[18] Studies showing benefit with neuroleptics in MDD and bipolar depression may reflect the long-known efficacy of such agents for mixed states.[19] Lack of benefit with antidepressants may also reflect this lack of attention to mixed depression in the broad MDD diagnosis: research on depressive mixed states in bipolar depression, published from the STEP-BD database, found no benefit with antidepressants,[20] which is consistent with the older literature on lack of benefit with antidepressants in mixed episodes in general.[21]

A major proponent of the concept of mixed depression is Athanasios Koukopoulos, who has also supplied specific diagnostic criteria (**Box 2**), which can be validated or refuted in research studies, and which can be used to reliably identify these patients in clinical practice. The definition provided by Koukopoulos emphasizes irritability, agitation, and mood lability as the core features of mixed depression. Those patients with depression who have these other features are mixed, in this investigator's approach; patients may also have anxiety as with neurotic depression, but their symptoms are episodic and severe, unlike those with neurotic depression. Melancholia, in contrast, does not involve marked irritability, and lability and agitation are absent by definition.

Mixed depression is more common in bipolar disorder than MDD but it is frequently present in MDD as well, perhaps arguing against the whole distinction between bipolar and unipolar illnesses, hallowed in DSM-III. Indeed, in the Kraepelinian definition of manic-depressive insanity, there was no relevance to polarity: it did not matter if mood episodes were depressive or manic; what mattered was that mood episodes occurred at all and were recurrent.[21] Thus, 100 depressive episodes (without any mania, ever) was manic-depressive illness; 10 manic episodes were the same illness. One reason, in the authors' view, that Kraepelin may have ignored

> **Box 2**
> **Modified Koukopoulos diagnostic criteria for mixed depression**
>
> The presence of DSM-IV–defined acute major depressive episode, for 2 weeks or longer, with three or more of the following criteria:
>
> A. Absence of psychomotor retardation
>
> B. Talkativeness
>
> C. Psychic agitation or inner tension
>
> D. Distinct description of suffering and or frequent spells of weeping
>
> E. Flight of ideas
>
> F. Marked irritability or unprovoked rage
>
> G. Marked mood lability or marked mood reactivity
>
> *Adapted from* Koukopoulos A, Sani G, Koukopoulos AE, et al. Melancholia agitata and mixed depression. Acta Psychiatr Scand Suppl 2007;(433):50–7; with permission.

polarity was that, by having a broad concept of mixed states, Kraepelin concluded that poles did not exist. Most mood episodes, in Kraepelin's view (influenced by Weygandt) were mixed, and thus not specifically at one pole or the other.[22] Pure depressive and pure manic episodes, in contrast, were less common. This approach is partly confirmed by recent studies that indicate that the majority of mood episodes in persons with mood disorders (MDD or bipolar) are in fact mixed, broadly defined, rather than purely depressive (melancholic) or purely manic (euphoric).[23–25]

The DSM-5 draft proposal incorporates some of these ideas about mixed depression, but in a different way than proposed by Koukopoulos. As is typical with DSM revisions, there is concern about specificity (in delineating mixed depression from nonmixed depression). Because in the DSM view irritability and agitation are nonspecific and occur in other kinds of depression, those core symptoms of mixed depression are not counted in the proposed DSM-5 definition of MDD with an added mixed specifier. Rather, the proposed definition would require the presence of at least three manic symptoms occurring simultaneously with a fully syndromal episode of depression: namely, elevated mood, decreased need for sleep, goal-directed activity, increased energy and visible hyperactivity, grandiosity, accelerated speech, and racing thoughts. Symptoms that are characteristic of both depression and mania are not included in the new mixed specifier, specifically distractibility, irritability, agitation, insomnia, and indecisiveness.

Whereas the DSM-5 changes are an important step toward recognizing the common occurrence of mixed manic and depressive symptoms, it would seem to be problematic to exclude, on conceptual grounds, specifically those symptoms that most commonly occur when manic and depressive symptoms happen together. This exclusion would be akin to excluding auditory hallucinations from the diagnosis of schizophrenia because they also commonly occur in mania, or excluding headache from the diagnosis of meningitis because it also happens in migraine.

Pure Depression

We are left with a final category, one that is not uncommon but that essentially reflects the absence of the others. Some depressed patients still have some mood reactivity and some interests as opposed to complete anhedonia; they are somewhat functional and might still even work, as opposed to being completely debilitated and severely psychomotor-retarded. These patients may meet DSM-defined clinical depression criteria but have no manic symptoms at all and have little or no anxiety. Their illness is usually episodic with normal euthymia between episodes, as opposed to mild to moderate chronic depression. They are not melancholic, mixed, or neurotic, but they are clinically depressed.

This group would be said to have pure (or vanilla) depression. This diagnosis is similar to what has been called typical depression. The authors prefer not to use the word *typical*, because it immediately conjures the contrast of atypical depression which, although commonly used in the past decades, does not seem to the authors to represent a valid depressive subtype. Usually what has been meant by atypical depression vacillates among the other depressive subtypes provided previously. Often, one refers to the presence of marked mood reactivity and anxiety: that kind of atypical depression is better understood as neurotic depression. Sometimes, atypical refers to increased sleep and increased appetite; although often claimed, the consistent occurrence of such features together has not been consistently empirically validated. In the authors' experience, many patients will have increased sleep but decreased appetite or decreased sleep and increased appetite. It has been suggested that increased sleep and appetite are more common in anergic bipolar depression, but that picture is no different than the severely psychomotor-retarded, mood nonreactive syndrome of melancholia, which indeed is more common in bipolar than unipolar depression.[14] So in that sense, atypical depression seems to reflect melancholia.

The authors' view is that the nonspecificity of atypical features in psychopathology is reason to drop the term and instead clearly define whether we are describing neurotic, melancholic, or mixed depression. In those patients who are none of the above, we are faced with moderately severe, episodic pure (vanilla) depression.

Because the prior reliance on the heterogeneous, unitary MDD concept has driven most psychopharmacology studies, it is not known whether antidepressants would be especially more effective in such episodic pure depressive patients than they are in mixed or neurotic depression. The authors' hypothesis is that this is the group in whom modern antidepressants like serotonin reuptake inhibitors are most effective.

MISUNDERSTANDING OF PSYCHOPATHOLOGY

There are many misconceptions about psychopathology that complicate the diagnosis of depression. In this section, two important problems are pointed out: lack of attention to the phenomenology of insight in mood disorders and simplistic approaches to attribution of psychosocial causation.

Insight

A key underappreciated aspect of the psychopathology of depression is the phenomenon of insight. Insight reflects awareness in the self that something is wrong, that one might have an illness of depression, or have mania, or be out of touch with reality in some way (psychosis). Lack of insight, or the inability to understand and conceptualize illness as a reality, is perhaps the greatest hurdle in psychiatric practice.[26] This aspect is one of the biggest challenges when facing disorders such as mania, psychosis, delusions, or even chronic substance abuse or dependence.

Current practice for severe depressive illnesses generally involves short-term hospitalizations, on the order of 1 week or less. In such settings, patients are discharged when control of symptoms has been achieved, but insight, which requires much more time to improve, is often still lacking. This lack of insight then leads to medication noncompliance and rehospitalization: the revolving door phenomenon.

Another aspect of the relevance of insight is that about one-half of patients with mania do not have insight,[27] whereas most patients with depression have insight.[28] Thus, in the large group of depressive illnesses that are bipolar, misdiagnosis commonly occurs as unipolar or MDD because patients report depressive, but deny manic, symptoms. This underdiagnosis of bipolar disorder in depressive populations remains an endemic problem, despite claims to the contrary.[29]

Split-Brain Psychiatry: Why Psychosocial Events May Not Matter

Many clinicians, both novice and experienced, make the common error of attributing depression to psychosocial events: the patient is depressed because X happened. This viewpoint has been used to launch a generalized critique of the medicalization of sadness.[30]

The assumptions behind this view were long ago described by Aristotle, who famously taught as follows: there are different types of causes; some causes set the chain of effects in motion (the first cause); some have their impact later in the chain such that they produce the effect immediately (the efficient cause). One of the greatest errors in understanding depression is to mistake first and efficient causes. The first cause in depression is genetics and early life environment; without these biological susceptibilities, later efficient causes could never produce a clinical depressive episode. The efficient causes are the immediate life events that trigger a clinical depression at that time—the divorce, job loss, or death that precedes this episode of depression. The first cause is necessary for later depression, although not sufficient; it usually is not enough to lead to the actual depressive episodes of adult life. The efficient causes are not necessary—they occur without depression in other people, and even in the same person do not invariably produce depression—but they sometimes are sufficient: in some persons they can lead to depression whenever they occur. So, first causes are necessary but usually not sufficient; efficient causes are often sufficient, but not necessary. One usually needs both, and neither alone is the single cause of depression.

Besides this logical rationale for why efficient causes should be deemphasized, there is a strong biological rationale based on split-brain studies in neurology[31] conducted in refractory epilepsies treated with corpus callosotomy. In right-handed patients after split-brain surgery, the split between language and vision can be tested. If an image is shown to the right hemisphere (in the left visual field) of, for example, a woman talking on a phone, the experimenter who asks the patient, "What do you see?" will get an answer; a wrong answer, but an answer nonetheless:

"I see a friend," the subject might say.

"What is the friend doing?"

"Cooking dinner."

Then with a phone nearby, the experimenter can ask the subject, "Show me what you saw." The subject will pick up the phone. The split-brain epilepsy patient knows what is seen by the right hemisphere, but cannot speak it. What is most interesting is that the patient does not say, "I do not know," or "I am unsure," or some such. Even when prompted before the experiment by the researcher saying, "Now remember, you have had split-brain surgery for your seizures, keep that in mind when you answer my questions," patients rarely say that they do not know what they saw or why they feel as they do about what they saw. That is the way our brains operate: Our brains are rationalizing machines; we are designed to come up with plausible explanations for what we experience.

Reasons are always provided; they are not infrequently incorrect. Aristotle's final cause looms behind.

A good example of this kind of assumption is found in a recent study of German psychologists to whom researchers gave two vignettes, one of a person with severe depression and another of a person with mania.[32] The cases were set up so as to clearly meet DSM-IV definitions of a major depressive episode or a manic episode. The psychologists were asked to diagnose the cases as major depression, mania, or neither. Ninety-five percent of them correctly diagnosed the case of DSM-IV–defined major depression; only 38% of the psychologists diagnosed the case of mania correctly (53% saw it as depression). The researchers put in a wrinkle: half of the vignettes for the case of mania stated that the man in the case (who had happy mood, decreased need for sleep, increased activity level, increased talkativeness, and impulsive behavior) had just started a new relationship with a girlfriend; the other half of the vignettes for the case of mania said nothing about an external trigger for the symptoms. In the girlfriend case, the correct diagnosis of mania dropped to 23%; in the nongirlfirend case it rose to 60%. Having a girlfriend or not is irrelevant to determining whether a person is experiencing a manic episode; yet most of us naturally think this way.

MODELS OF DEPRESSION

How one diagnoses depressive conditions is strongly influenced by one's conceptual model of what depression is all about. The most common conceptual approach these days is the biopsychosocial model; psychoanalytic and behavioral theories are also popular. The following sections show the limitations of these approaches and the importance of two neglected, separate (but related) alternatives: method-based psychiatry and the existential tradition.

Freud and Cognitive-Behavioral Therapy

Freudian theory and cognitive-behavioral therapy (CBT) are the two standard schools of thought in current psychology. The authors do not deny the utility of both psychoanalytic and CBT-based approaches to some kinds of depression, but they do deny the utility of their use in most or all kinds of depression.

Psychoanalytic theories are based on the concept of inwardly directed aggression, and CBT approaches on such approaches as learned helplessness models or social deprivation paradigms. The psychoanalytic view was developed by Freud in *Mourning and Melancholia* largely as a response to the planned presentation of views by Freud's erratic pupil, Victor Tausk, on manic-depressive illness.[33] Freud's theory of depression followed the practice of psychoanalytic therapy rather than vice versa. A theory had to be developed to explain the practice. The learned helplessness and social deprivation models, on the other hand, grew out of the experimental psychology literature and were later used in CBT and interpersonal treatment approaches.

The authors do not discuss these approaches in detail here, because they are so frequently discussed in the literature. Suffice it to say that they have their limits.

The Biopsychosocial Model

One response to the limitations of any pure theory, such as psychoanalytic or CBT approaches, is to combine them. This response is the basic idea behind the biopsychosocial (BPS) model: more is better. This view, although ecumenical, is empty.

Many clinicians seem to use the BPS model in a rote manner, never really defining what they mean. One of the authors (S.N.G.) has examined this matter in detail and studied the discussions of the BPS model in the works of its originators, Roy Grinker and George Engel, and in recent articles and books that attempt to describe and promote it.[34] The authors' conclusion is that, at bottom, the BPS model reflects, and translates into, eclecticism.

Engel claimed, "*All three levels*, biological, psychological, and social, must be taken into account *in every health care task*" (italics added).[35] No single illness or patient or condition can be reduced to any one aspect. They are all, more or less equally, relevant in all cases at all times. This claim, as stated, is trivial, and if advanced untrivially, takes us far beyond the BPS model.

Beyond the formal definition given previously, there is another ultimate, rarely explicit, rationale for the BPS model: eclecticism. Grinker[36] forthrightly argued for a "struggle for eclecticism" as opposed to psychoanalytic dogmatism. Yet where Grinker was sober and limited in his goals, Engel was expansive. Grinker identified the key: BPS advocates really seek eclectic freedom, the ability to "individualize treatment to the patient," which has come to mean, in practice, being allowed to do whatever one wants to do. This eclectic freedom borders on anarchy: one can emphasize the "bio" if one wishes, or the "psycho" (which is usually psychoanalytic among many BPS advocates), or the "social." But there is no rationale as to why one heads in one direction or the other; it is like going to a restaurant and getting a set of ingredients rather than a plate of food[37]; one can put them all together any way one likes. This freedom results in the ultimate paradox: being free to do whatever one chooses, one enacts one's own dogmas (conscious or unconscious). Eclecticism becomes a new dogmatism.

Supporters of the BPS model may claim that the authors set up the model here as a straw man. This is not so; all of the claims discussed previously are based on primary sources in the writings of Engel and Grinker, which one of the authors (S.N.G.) has documented in book-length form.[34] These views may seem controversial to some only because many proponents of the BPS model these days seem not to have studied the many papers written by Grinker and Engel in the 1960s and 1970s. Both claimed these ideas were relevant to all phases of psychiatry: not just teaching, but also practice, and even research. If this eclecticism seems extreme to some who would still wish to support the BPS model, then, like Marxists who disavow Marx, they would need to explain how and why their views differ from those of Engel and Grinker and also why such revisions should still be seen as related to the original BPS model that became so popular in the 1980s.

Outside of the historical question of what Engel and Grinker thought and what BPS advocates now think, the authors believe there remains this major conceptual problem for those who support the BPS model: how do they avoid mere eclecticism, with all its limitations? This question is not a matter simply for theorizing. For 3 decades the BPS approach has ruled psychiatry in teaching and practice. As the authors discuss in detail elsewhere,[34] it has proved to be eclecticism in reality.

Alternatives to the BPS Model

Are these approaches the only alternatives? Biomedical reductionism (the medical model) versus the BPS model; eclecticism versus dogmatism. The BPS approach only shines when opposed to straw men. But there are alternatives to both the BPS model and any specific theory. One alternative is what the authors call method-based psychiatry, derived from the work of Karl Jaspers; another is the existential approach to psychiatry and psychology. Both can be related to what has been called the medical humanist model, as developed by William Osler.[38]

Jaspers,[2,3] who realized that theories rose and fell with their methods, saw two major methods in psychiatry: the objective/empiric versus the subjective/interpretive. Methodology determined the strengths, and weaknesses, of theories. Rather than advocating one or the other method, Jaspers called for methodologic consciousness:

we need to be aware of what methods we use, their strengths and limitations, and why we use them. Dogmatists hold that one method is sufficient, BPS eclectics that methods should always be combined, Jaspers that (depending on the condition) sometimes one, sometimes another, method is best. Jaspers' nondogmatic, noneclectic approach was a method-based psychiatry.[39]

Osler (reinterpreting Hippocrates) argued that the physician's role was to treat disease in the body (biomedical reductionism) while attending to the human being—the person—who has the disease. Osler applied the medical model humanistically. Where disease is present, one treats the body; where disease is ameliorable but not curable, one still treats, with attention to risks; and where no disease exists (some patients have symptoms, but no disease; eg, cough, rather than pneumonia) one attends to the human being as a person. This approach (which captures the Hippocratic aim to cure sometimes, to heal often, to console always) has all the strengths and none of the weaknesses of the BPS model.[40]

Applied to depression, the BPS model often results in simplistic, vague, eclectic treatment. All patients are presumed to have some biological aspect to their depression, so all get antidepressants. All are presumed to have psychosocial aspects, so all get psychotherapies. Combined treatment is better than either alone; the more the better. Some studies support this approach in certain circumstances[41]; others do not in other circumstances.[42] But the generic opinion that everyone should get everything[43] is not scientifically sound.

What would the alternative medical humanist method-based approach be? All patients are human beings, whether or not they have diseases of the body. So they should all be seen first as humans with stories and feelings about their diseases (if they have diseases). So if a patient has severe recurrent unipolar depression as a disease, that disease should be treated, taking a biological approach primarily (as with medications); some attention should also be given to how that human being feels about having that disease (although this need not entail formal psychotherapy). If a patient has, neurotic depression, which may reflect a personality trait in interaction with life stresses, then the disease-oriented biological approach would not be most appropriate (medications would be foregone or used only short-term), and the main focus would be on the person himself or herself (psychotherapy would be the prime focus of treatment). The method-based approach requires us to identify what *kind* of depression is present, and then to tailor one's method of practice to that *type* of depression. One size does not fit all.

The Existential Tradition

The authors' critique of the biopsychosocial approach to depression is not meant to imply that all depression is purely biomedical. This is a false straw-man dichotomy. Indeed, the authors believe most people who are attracted to the BPS model are attracted not because they like it but because they hate biomedical reductionism. The authors tried to show earlier that one can agree with the premises while drawing a different conclusion: other alternatives to biomedical reductionism exist. One of these alternatives is *biological existentialism*.[44] This idea, found in the work of Karl Jaspers and William Osler, has to do with realizing that some people have diseases, and when they do, those diseases can be understood reductionistically and biologically. But some people, if not most, do not have diseases; they suffer from being human beings. Their suffering is the same as everyone else's: being unhappy because of the limits and traumas of life. This experience is the existential aspect of all human suffering, and specifically of depression. One needs to have a humanistic awareness rooted in literature—not science, not even psychology—to appreciate these aspects of existential depression.[45]

In some persons, depression is not a disease; there is no melancholia, no mania, and no temperament trait of neuroticism. Generally, such existential depression is not severe. Nor is it always motivated by external events. Grief after the death of a loved one or after a traumatic event can trigger such existential unhappiness. But it can be in some people that, to a mild degree, there is a certain unhappiness that resides deep in the mind.

This unhappiness is not another subtype of MDD; it is normal sadness, a realistic assessment of human existence, of the reality of living and dying and illness and loss. It may be that this mild existential depression lies behind the psychological research identifying some uniquely positive aspects to depression: increased realism and empathy.

It has been repeatedly shown that depressed people are more realistic than the nondepressed in several experiments that measure sense of control: depressive realism.[46] Depressive patients with self-reported depression scores correctly attributed errors to themselves as opposed to when errors were experimentally manipulated outside. In contrast, normal subjects reported more control over experimental tasks than they really possessed. Realism may partly reflect increased insight of depression, and its converse may be decreased insight in mania, as described previously.[28] Depressive realism may also be reflected in existential despair,[47] an awareness of the unchanging limits of human existence, especially illness and death.

The authors have proposed that if depressive realism is a valid phenomenon, then it would support the application of existential psychotherapy methods to those with depression.[48]

A similar conclusion might be drawn from research on empathy in mood disorders; although few such studies exist, empathy seems to be increased in depressed patients compared with other psychiatric diagnoses and normal controls.[49] Because empathy is a core treatment modality of existential psychotherapy,[2] the enhancement of empathy in depression raises another interesting link between depression and existential psychotherapy.

The tradition of existential psychotherapy has numerous offshoots; here the authors focus on Jaspers' tradition wherein the emphasis was on empathy, on understanding the first-person experience of the patient, on seeing the treatment as an encounter between two human beings, each of which would change in the process.[3] This existential approach would seem to apply well to mild depression in which enhanced realism and empathy would allow for fruitful interactions between psychotherapist and patient.

Existential psychotherapy models may be especially useful in existential depression, and even, perhaps, in neurotic depression, when trying to address long-term personality-based perspectives on existence.

SUMMARY

Biopsychosocial eclecticism has led, the authors believe, to a simplistic acceptance of a unitary view of MDD with little scientific solidity. The authors propose a return to careful psychopathology as the basis of all nosology, which has led to identifying four main types of depressive illness, and a method-based, existential approach to understanding depression.

REFERENCES

1. Andreasen NC. DSM and the death of phenomenology in America: an example of unintended consequences. Schizophr Bull 2007:33(1):108–12.

2. Jaspers K. General psychopathology. Baltimore (MD): Johns Hopkins University Press; 1998.

3. Ghaemi SN. The concepts of psychiatry. Baltimore (MD): Johns Hopkins University Press; 2007.

4. Shorter E. Before Prozac: the troubled history of mood disorders in psychiatry. New York: Oxford University Press; 2009.

5. Kendler KS, Neale MC, Kessler RC. Major depression and generalized anxiety disorder: same genes, (partly) different environment? Arch Gen Psychiatry 1992;49:716–22.

6. Rush AJ, Trivedi MH, Wisniewski SR, et al. Acute and longer-term outcomes in depressed outpatients requiring one or several treatment steps: a STAR*D report. Am J Psychiatry 2006;163(11):1905–17.

7. Ghaemi SN. Why antidepressants are not antidepressants: STEP-BD, STAR*D, and the return of neurotic depression. Bipolar Disord 2008;10(8):957–68.

8. Rodriguez BF, Bruce SE, Pagano ME, et al. Relationships among psychosocial functioning, diagnostic comorbidity, and the recurrence of generalized anxiety disorder, panic disorder, and major depression. J Anxiety Disord 2005;19(7):752–66.

9. Kirsch I, Deacon BJ, Huedo-Medina TB, et al. Initial severity and antidepressant benefits: a meta-analysis of data submitted to the Food and Drug Administration. PLoS Med 2008;5(2):e45.

10. Fava M, Rush AJ, Alpert JE, et al. Difference in treatment outcome in outpatients with anxious versus nonanxious depression: a STAR*D report. Am J Psychiatry 2008; 165(3):342–51.

11. Shorter E. The doctrine of the two depressions in historical perspective. Acta Psychiatr Scand Suppl 2007;(433):5–13.

12. Roth S, Kerr, T. The concept of neurotic depression: a plea for reinstatement. In: Pichot P, Rein W, editors. The clinical approach in psychiatry. Paris (France): Synthelabo; 1994. p. 339–68.

13. Parker G, Fink M, Shorter E, et al. Issues for DSM-5: whither melancholia? The case for its classification as a distinct mood disorder. Am J Psychiatry 2010;167(7):745–7.

14. Parker G, Roy K, Wilhelm K, et al. The nature of bipolar depression: implications for the definition of melancholia. J Affect Disord 2000;59(3):217–24.

15. Parker G. 'New' and 'old' antidepressants: all equal in the eyes of the lore? Br J Psychiatry 2001;179:95–6.

16. Shorter E. A History of psychiatry. New York: John Wiley and Sons; 1997.

17. Angst J, Azorin JM, Bowden CL, et al. Prevalence and characteristics of undiagnosed bipolar disorders in patients with a major depressive episode: the BRIDGE study. Arch Gen Psychiatry 2011;68(8):791–8.

18. Koukopoulos A, Albert MJ, Sani G, et al. Mixed depressive states: nosologic and therapeutic issues. Int Rev Psychiatry 2005;17(1):21–37.

19. Robertson MM, Trimble MR. Major tranquillisers used as antidepressants. A review. J Affect Disord 1982;4(3):173–93.

20. Goldberg JF, Perlis RH, Ghaemi SN, et al. Adjunctive antidepressant use and symptomatic recovery among bipolar depressed patients with concomitant manic symptoms: findings from the STEP-BD. Am J Psychiatry 2007;164(9):1348–55.

21. Goodwin F, Jamison K. Manic depressive illness. 2nd edition. New York: Oxford University Press; 2007.

22. Salvatore P, Baldessarini RJ, Centorrino F, et al. Weygandt's on the mixed states of manic-depressive insanity: a translation and commentary on its significance in the evolution of the concept of bipolar disorder. Harv Rev Psychiatry 2002;10(5):255–75.

23. Calugi S, Litta A, Rucci P, et al. Does psychomotor retardation define a clinically relevant phenotype of unipolar depression? J Affect Disord;129(1–3):296–300.

24. Cassano GB, Rucci P, Frank E, et al. The mood spectrum in unipolar and bipolar disorder: arguments for a unitary approach. Am J Psychiatry 2004;161(7):1264–9.

25. Koukopoulos A, Sani G, Koukopoulos AE, et al. Melancholia agitata and mixed depression. Acta Psychiatr Scand Suppl 2007;(433):50–7.

26. David AS. Insight and psychosis. Br J Psychiatry 1990;156:798–808.

27. Ghaemi SN, Stoll AL, Pope HG. Lack of insight in bipolar disorder: the acute manic episode. J Nerv Ment Dis 1995;183:464–7.

28. Ghaemi SN, Rosenquist KR. Insight in mood disorders: an empirical and conceptual review. In: Amador X, David A, editors. Insight and psychosis. Oxford (UK): Oxford University Press: 2004. p. 101–18.

29. Smith DJ, Ghaemi SN. Is underdiagnosis the main pitfall when diagnosing bipolar disorder? Yes. BMJ 2010;340:c854.

30. Horwitz A, Wakefield J. The loss of sadness. New York: Oxford University Press; 2007.

31. Gazzaniga MS. The mind's past. Berkeley (CA): University of California Press; 1998.

32. Bruchmuller K, Meyer TD, Diagnostically irrelevant information can affect the likelihood of a diagnosis of bipolar disorder. J Affect Disord 2009;116(1–2):148–51.

33. Roazen P. Brother animal: the story of Freud and Tausk. New York: Knopf; 1969.

34. Ghaemi SN. The rise and fall of the biopsychosocial model: reconciling art and science in psychiatry. Baltimore (MD): Johns Hopkins University Press; 2009.

35. Engel GL. The biopsychosocial model and the education of health professionals. Ann N Y Acad Sci 1978;310:169–87.

36. Grinker RR Sr. A Struggle for eclecticism. Am J Psychiatry 1964;121:451–7.

37. McHugh P, Slavney P, Perspectives of psychiatry. 2nd edition. Baltimore (MD): Johns Hopkins University Press; 1998.

38. Osler W. Aequanimitas. 3rd edition. Philadelphia: The Blakiston Company; 1932.

39. Ghaemi SN. The rise and fall of the biopsychosocial model. Br J Psychiatry 2009; 195(1):3–4.

40. Ghaemi SN. Toward a Hippocratic psychopharmacology. Can J Psychiatry 2008; 53(3):189–96.

41. Thase ME, Friedman ES, Fasiczka AL, et al. Treatment of men with major depression: a comparison of sequential cohorts treated with either cognitive-behavioral therapy or newer generation antidepressants. J Clin Psychiatry 2000;61(7):466–72.

42. Frank E, Kupfer DJ, Wagner EF, et al. Efficacy of interpersonal psychotherapy as a maintenance treatment of recurrent depression: contributing factors. Arch Gen Psychiatry 1991;48:1053–9.

43. Gabbard GO, Kay J. The fate of integrated treatment: whatever happened to the biopsychosocial psychiatrist? Am J Psychiatry 2001;158(12):1956–63.

44. Ghaemi SN. On the nature of mental disease: the psychiatric humanism of Karl Jaspers. Existenz 2008;3(2).

45. Mendelowitz E. Meditations on Oedipus: Becker's Kafka, Nietzsche's metamorphosis. Journal of Humanistic Psychology 2006;46:385–431.

46. Alloy LB. Abramson LY. Depressive realism: four theoretical perspectives. In: Alloy LB, editor. Cognitive processes in depression. New York: Guilford Press;1988. p. 223–65.

47. Havens LL. Ghaemi SN. Existential despair and bipolar disorder: the therapeutic alliance as a mood stabilizer. Am J Psychother 2005;59(2):137–47.

48. Ghaemi SN. Feeling and time: the phenomenology of mood disorders, depressive realism, and existential psychotherapy. Schizophr Bull 2007;33(1):122–30.

49. Galvez JF, Thommi S, Ghaemi SN. Positive aspects of mental illness: a review in bipolar disorder. J Affect Disord 2010;128(3)185–90.

Treatment Selection in Depression: The Role of Clinical Judgment

Elena Tomba, PhD[a], Giovanni A. Fava, MD[a,b],*

KEYWORDS

- Depressive disorder • Clinical judgment
- Antidepressive agents • Psychotherapy • Clinimetrics

Key Points

- Clinical judgment should guide the selection of treatment options in depression
- Pharmacotherapy remains the treatment of choice of the acute episode, but it is unlikely to entail solution to complex array of symptoms that are associated with depression
- Sequential strategies addressing residual symptomatology (particularly cognitive-behavioral therapy following pharmacotherapy) appear to be a promising strategy of integration of different options
- Treatment of depression may be conceptualized as integrated treatment of the various components of symptomatology, lifestyle and social adjustment

---

Selection of treatment according to evidence-based medicine relies primarily on randomized controlled trials and meta-analyses. However, this evidence applies to the "average" patient and ignores the fact that customary clinical taxonomy does not include patterns of symptoms, severity of illness, effects of comorbid conditions, timing of phenomena, rate of progression of illness, responses to previous treatments, and other clinical distinctions that demarcate major prognostic and therapeutic differences among patients who otherwise seem to be deceptively similar because they share the same diagnosis.[1,2]

Indeed, the American Psychiatric Guideline for the treatment of patients with major depressive disorder states that "the ultimate recommendation regarding a particular clinical procedure or treatment plan must be made by the psychiatrist in light of the

---

The authors have nothing to disclose.

[a] Department of Psychology, University of Bologna, Viale Berti Pichat 5, 40127 Bologna, Italy
[b] Department of Psychiatry, State University of New York at Buffalo, 462 Grider Street, Buffalo, NY 14215, USA
* Corresponding author. Department of Psychology, University of Bologna, Viale Berti Pichat 5, 40127 Bologna, Italy.
E-mail address: giovanniandrea.fava@unibo.it

Psychiatr Clin N Am 35 (2012) 87–98
doi:10.1016/j.psc.2011.11.003
0193-953X/12/$ – see front matter © 2012 Elsevier Inc. All rights reserved.

psych.theclinics.com

clinical data, the psychiatric evaluation, and the diagnostic and treatment options available. Such recommendations should incorporate the patient's personal and socio-cultural preferences and values in order to enhance the therapeutic alliance, adherence to treatment, and treatment outcomes."[3(p9)] This is what actually occurs in clinical practice, but it is often dismissed as an expression of highly subjective clinical evaluation. The average depressed patient appears to express stronger preferences for psychotherapy than for antidepressant medications,[4] a finding that is of considerable clinical import given that treatment preference is a potent moderator of response to therapy.[5] Patients receiving their preferred treatment (whether pharmacotherapy or psychotherapy) respond significantly better than those who do not receive their preferred therapy.[6]

There has been considerable improvement in the accuracy of clinical judgment in psychiatry, particularly to the extent that it is guided by clinimetrics, the science of clinical measurement.[2] In psychiatry, as in other fields of medicine, there is also increasing awareness of a need for augmenting practice guidelines with patient-specific recommendations that take into account individual variables and history, as well as previous treatment responses.[7,8]

Rather than focusing on behavioral variables, personalized medicine has generally advocated for a focus on biological markers that may predictive of treatment response.[9] It is also possible, however, to outline treatment options as filtered by clinical judgment according to the clinimetric perspective[2] and not simply by comparing treatment options for the average patient in the treatment of the acute episode of depression and in prevention of relapse. This article examines how clinimetrics can guide clinical judgment, particularly in relation to decisions about whether and when to recommend psychotherapy and when to recommend antidepressant medications. It does not discuss specific distinctions within pharmacotherapies and psychotherapies or clinical situations such as treatment resistant depression, which are dealt with elsewhere.

PATIENT EVALUATION OVERVIEW

A number of assessment strategies may supplement the information provided by a diagnostic interview.[10]

Staging

Box 1 outlines the staging method according to the basic steps of development of unipolar depression, ranging from prodroma177l to the residual and chronic forms, in a longitudinal view of development of disturbances.[11] **Box 2** examines previous history of treatment resistance.[2]

Macroanalysis

The majority of patients with depression do not quantify for one, but for several Axis I and Axis II disorders.[12] The method of macroanalysis[2,13] establishes a relationship between co-occurring syndromes and problems on the basis of where treatment should begin in the first place (**Fig. 1**). Macroanalysis starts from the assumption that, in most cases, there are functional relationships with other more or less clearly defined problem areas, and that the targets of treatment may vary during the course of disturbances. For instance, a patient may present with a major depressive disorder, agoraphobia, marital crisis (as a result of obsessional traits that create areas of conflict with his or her spouse), and obsessive ruminations (which lead to a chronic state of indecision). In terms of macroanalysis, the clinician, after a thorough interview

---

Box 1
Stages of development of major depressive disorder

1. Prodromal phase (anxiety, irritable mood, anhedonia, sleep disorders)

   a. No depressive symptoms

   b. Minor depression

2. Major depressive episode

3. Residual phase

   a. No depressive symptoms

   b. Dysthymia

4. a. Recurrent depression

   b. Double depression

5. Chronic major depressive episode (lasting at least 2 years without interruptions)

---

with the patient, could place into a hierarchy the syndromes and symptoms of comorbidity by considering the patient's needs. The clinician could thus give priority to pharmacotherapy of major depressive disorder, leaving to post-therapy assessment the determination of the relationship of agoraphobia to marital crisis and obsessional ruminations. Will they wane as anxious epiphenomena or will they persist, despite some degree of improvement? Should, in this latter case, further treatment be necessary? If the clinical decision of tackling one syndrome may be taken during the initial assessment, the subsequent steps of macroanalysis require a reassessment after the first line of treatment has terminated (**Fig. 2**). The hierarchical organization that is chosen may depend on a variety of factors (urgency, availability of treatment tools, chronological appearance of symptoms), including the patient's preferences and priorities. Macroanalysis is not only a tool for the therapist, but can also be used to inform the patient about the relationship between different problem areas and motivate the patient for change.

Microanalysis

Macroanalysis can be supplemented by microanalysis, a detailed analysis of specific symptoms that can be performed by additional interviewing or by a specific observer or self-rated rating scales, such as the Clinical Interview for Depression[14] in relation

---

Box 2
Staging of levels of treatment resistance in unipolar depression

Stage 0: No history of failure to respond to therapeutic trial of antidepressant drugs

Stage 1: Failure of at least one adequate therapeutic trial of antidepressant drugs

Stage 2: Failure of at least two adequate trials of antidepressant drugs

Stage 3: Failure of three or more adequate therapeutic trials of antidepressant drugs

Stage 4: Failure of three or more adequate trials including at least one concerned with augmentation/combination with psychotherapy

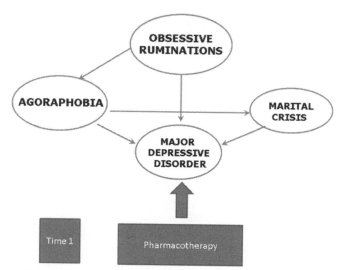

Fig. 1. Macroanalysis before first-line of treatment. A patient presents with major depressive disorder, obsessive ruminations about health anxiety, agoraphobia, and marital crisis. At time 1, the therapist could give priority to prescribing antidepressant drug therapy.

to variables such as reactivity to environmental stimuli or intensity of phobic fears.[15] Biomarkers, such as brain structural and functional measures,[16] genomic evaluations,[16,17] neuroendocrine investigations,[16] and polysomnography[18] could be conceptualized as biological forms of microanalysis. If the predictive value of markers

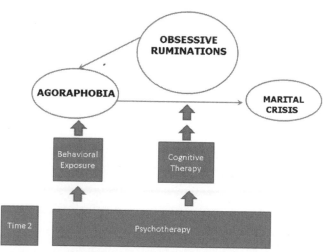

Fig. 2. Macroanalysis after first-line of treatment. At time 2, the therapist decides to intervene on residual comorbidity (avoidance agoraphobia and obsessive ruminations) using homework exposure in the first sessions and cognitive restructuring afterwards to emphasize the negative effects respectively of excessive social withdrawal and ruminations that lead to communicative difficulties with the partner.

such as the serotonin transporter gene-linked polymorphic region (5-HTTLPR) in the uncharacterized patient appears to be disappointing or controversial,[17] their use in the setting of macroanalysis may be more rewarding. It is like a primary care physician prescribing specific tests on clinical suspicion instead of as a general screening battery.

Repeated Assessment

There is increasing evidence that a single cross-sectional evaluation may not be sufficient for disclosing symptomatology that is related to the depressive episode (eg, anxiety) or bipolar trends.[2]

ACUTE PHASE

When the clinician is confronted with the presence of a major depressive disorder, pharmacotherapy or psychotherapy may be pursued. Even though the two types of treatment are roughly equivalent for the average case,[3,19] there are important distinctions when clinical judgment is applied to the specific patient, as outlined in detail later. Further, one course of treatment is unlikely to yield full recovery from the acute episode in the majority of cases. Residual symptoms are the rule in 80% to 90% of patients.[10,11] Both first-line and second-line treatments should be planned, even in case of successful response to the initial treatment.

First-Line Treatment

Antidepressant drugs offer a number of advantages in specific clinical situations:

- There are readily available.
- They can be administered by nonpsychiatric physicians without specialized training.
- They act in a few weeks.
- The magnitude of benefit of antidepressant medication compared with placebo increases with severity of depressive symptoms[20]; antidepressants are thus the treatment of choice in severe and melancholic depression.

There are also disadvantages:

- Side effects of drugs.
- Potential interactions with medical conditions.[21,22]
- Previous unsuccessful trials with medications (see **Box 2**). From a clinical viewpoint, it is quite different to treat a patient pharmacologically who displayed positive responses to previous therapeutic trials (stage 0) and a patient who failed to respond to various adequate trials (stage 4). In the former case the patient is likely to respond to the same treatment that was effective before, whereas in the latter situation the evidence clearly indicates that the more trials are performed, the more resistant and intolerant to new drug treatments the patient becomes.[11]

If a patient has experienced loss of therapeutic effect during antidepressant treatment (**Box 3**), a new antidepressant is more likely to yield the same result,[23,24] probably due to a mechanism of oppositional tolerance.[24] Continued pharmacologic treatment may recruit processes that oppose the initial acute effect of a drug, leading to loss of clinical effect and even paradoxical responses. When drug treatment ends, these processes may operate unopposed, at least for some time, triggering extended withdrawal phenomena, inducing resistance to the same treatment and

> **Box 3**
> **Staging of loss of therapeutic effects during continuation or maintenance antidepressant treatment**
>
> Stage 0: No loss of therapeutic effect
>
> Stage 1: Loss of therapeutic effects after adequate response in a therapeutic trial
>
> Stage 2: Loss of therapeutic effects after adequate response in two therapeutic trials
>
> Stage 3: Loss of therapeutic effects after adequate responses in three or more therapeutic trials

increasing vulnerability to relapse.[24] A recent meta-analysis on the risk of relapse after antidepressant discontinuation[25] provides support to the oppositional model of tolerance.[24]

Evidence-based psychotherapy (particularly cognitive behavioral treatment and interpersonal therapy) has a few advantages in the treatment of the acute phase episode:

- It has fewer side effects, particularly in the setting of medical disease.[26]
- It does not seem to induce phenomena of resistance.[27]
- It may yield better long-term prognosis.[19]

There are also disadvantages:

- Patients need motivation for psychotherapy.[4–6]
- Competent psychotherapists may not be available.[28]
- Remission from depression tends to be slower than with pharmacotherapy.[19]

Combined treatment (pharmacotherapy and psychotherapy) may offer slight advantages compared to each of the treatments alone in the average case of depression.[29] The benefits are, however, clear cut in chronic forms of mood disorders and double depression.[30]

Second-Line Treatment

Frequently outcomes of initial treatment will require implementation of second-line treatments. First-line treatments are unlikely to ameliorate disturbances that precede the onset of the depressive episode, requiring additional treatments. Further, repeat assessments may expose problematic areas that were not revealed in the first macro-analysis (see **Fig. 2**). Even when first-line treatment is successful, residual symptoms are the rule.[10,11] Some residual symptoms of depression may progress to become prodromal symptoms of relapse.[11] This has led to the development of a sequential strategy based on the use of pharmacotherapy in the acute phase of depression and cognitive behavioral therapy in its residual phase[10] (**Box 4**).

While psychotherapy of residual symptoms is performed, there are two options as to pharmacotherapy. One consists of continuation of drug treatment during the residual phase. The other involves tapering and discontinuation of antidepressant drugs during psychotherapy. Because this latter variant was found to entail significant benefits compared to continuation treatment in a recent meta-analysis,[31] it is the model presented here (see **Box 4**). In a particularly successful randomized controlled trial,[32] cognitive–behavior therapy of residual symptoms was supplemented by lifestyle modification[33] (eg, physical exercise, appropriate rest, limiting exposure to chronic life stress situations) and well-being therapy.[34] The addition of a well-being

---

Box 4
Steps for implementing the sequential approach in recurrent depression

1. Careful assessment of patient 3 months after starting antidepressant drug treatment, with special reference to residual symptoms

2. Cognitive behavioral treatment for residual symptoms, including cognitive restructuring or homework exposure

3. Tapering of antidepressant drug treatment at the slowest possible pace., such as 25 mg of a tricyclic drug every other week

4. Addition of well-being enhancing therapy (well-being therapy) and lifestyle modification

5. Discontinuation of antidepressant drugs

6. Careful assessment of patient 1 month after drug discontinuation

---

promoting strategy was based on research suggesting that psychological well-being stimulates resilience and confers a protective effect[34] against further depressive episodes.

In this model, psychotherapy addresses only problems and symptoms that were unaffected by drug treatment. Second-line psychotherapy can thus be briefer and more targeted than psychotherapy applied in the initial phase. It still requires motivation and availability of competent therapists, however. An alternative approach is to provide additional pharmacotherapeutic strategies that may address symptoms such as fatigue or insomnia.[5] A potential disadvantage to adding medications is the potential induction of oppositional tolerance.[24] For instance, many patients who did not respond to initial treatment in the STAR* D trial and underwent the various phases of treatment, including augmentation/combination, were characterized by refractory states with low remission, high relapse, and high intolerance rates.[11] Probably the most important insight that was gained from the STAR*D approach, essentially based on switching/augmentation/combination pharmacologic strategies, is that only a small minority of patients survived continuing care without relapsing or dropping out.[11,35]

PREVENTION OF RECURRENCE

The chronic and recurrent nature of major depressive disorder is gaining increasing attention.[36] Approximately 8 of 10 people experiencing a major depressive disorder will have one or more further episodes during their lifetime, that is, a recurrent major depressive disorder. In some patients, the episodes become increasingly frequent. This latter course appears to be the more prevalent, both in psychiatric and primary care settings.[36] Partial remission between episodes, rather than full recovery, appears to be the rule, and it is associated with residual disability.[11]

There are two advantages in keeping antidepressant drug treatment indefinitely:

- There is a reduction in the likelihood of relapse.[37,38]
- It is a simple procedure that does not require additional time investment.

The disadvantages, however, are many:

- The prophylactic effects of antidepressants decrease with the number of episodes[38]; this means that drug treatment is less helpful in the patients who need more protection.

- Duration of drug treatment does not affect long-term prognosis once the drug is discontinued.[39]
- Loss of clinical effect during long-term antidepressant treatment is a common and vexing problem[24] (see **Box 2**). Dose increase is likely to yield only a transient response, and loss of response may also trigger subsequent refractoriness.
- With second-generation antidepressants, long-term side effects (such as weight gain, sexual dysfunction, bleeding, risk of fracture and osteoporosis) may emerge and are unlikely to disappear with time.[40,41]

Intermittent Drug Treatment

The treatment of recurrence of depression can also be managed by treatment of the new episode with the same or other antidepressant and discontinuation with remission ensues. The appearance of prodromal symptoms generally precedes the full syndrome by weeks or months.[11] An early intervention on relapse was found to significantly shorten the length of depressive episode.[42] As a result, relatively frequent follow-up visits and education of patients and their family members to recognize the patient's characteristic prodromal symptoms (which appear to be similar across episodes of the same patient) may potentially increase the efficacy of this approach.[26]

There are the following advantages:

- In several naturalistic studies, patients who took antidepressants intermittently had a better outcome than those who took them regularly.[24] It cannot be excluded, however, that those who had the most severe symptoms were the ones who needed to take the drug continuously.
- There are periods free of drugs and side effects.
- Some patients would discontinue antidepressant drug treatment regardless of the physician's advice to continue treatment.[43] It is a common clinical experience that sometimes patients choose the most unfavorable time for stopping the drug without consulting the physician. Planned drug discontinuation may promote adherence.

There are also a few disadvantages:

- Drug discontinuation may elicit the phenomenon of resistance. Patients may not respond on subsequent trials, though they had a good response to that medication at the time it was discontinued.[24]
- Discontinuation syndromes are frequent, particularly with selective serotonin reuptake inhibitors (SSRIs), and despite slow tapering.[44]
- There should be a close monitoring of the patient's clinical status.

Sequential Treatment

The use of the sequential combination of drug treatment of the acute episode of depression, followed by psychotherapy in the residual phase, has been tested in a number of controlled trials.[5]

The following advantages were detected:

- There is a significant reduction in relapse rates,[31] which particularly applies to recurrent depression.[5]
- It is an intensive intervention divided in two phases and not a maintenance strategy that requires unspecified added costs.

- It may allow discontinuation of drug treatment.[31]

Its disadvantages are as follows:

- Patients should be motivated for psychotherapy, which may be difficult when drug treatment has overcome the most bothersome symptoms (patients may perceive an improvement in their clinical status yielded by drug treatment as an indication of full recovery, neglecting areas that are still problematic; the physician may collude with the patient in this illusion of wellness).
- Competent psychotherapists should be available and there should be close coordination with administration of drug treatment.

CLINICAL JUDGMENT

In clinical practice, psychiatrists weigh factors such as the progression of disease, the overall severity of the disorder, the patient's social support and adaptation, resilience and reaction to stressful life circumstances, and response to previous treatment.[2] The customary clinical taxonomy in psychiatry (*Diagnostic and Statistical Manual* [DSM]) does not include patterns of symptoms, severity of illness, effects of comorbid conditions, timing of phenomena, rate of progression of illness, responses to previous treatments, and other clinical distinctions that demarcate major prognostic and therapeutic differences among patients. Though these factors are likely to affect significantly how patients respond to various psychotherapeutic and pharmacologic treatments, depressed patients may be treated as deceptively similar because they share the same psychiatric diagnosis.

Several assessment strategies that reflect clinical judgment are nonetheless available: the use of diagnostic transfer stations instead of diagnostic endpoints using repeated assessments (when making a diagnosis, thoughtful clinicians seldom leap from a clinical manifestation to a diagnostic endpoint; the clinical reasoning goes through a series of "transfer stations," where potential connections between presenting symptoms and pathophysiologic process are drawn); subtyping versus integration of different diagnostic categories; staging; and macro- and microanalysis, broadening of clinical information (encompassing psychological well-being and subclinical symptomatology).[2]

SUMMARY

The selection of treatment in depression should be filtered by clinical judgment, taking into consideration a number of clinical variables, such as characteristics and severity of depressive episode, co-occurring symptomatology and problems (not necessarily syndromes), medical comorbidities, and patient's history with particular reference to treatment of previous episodes, if they occurred. Such information should be placed within what is actually available in the specific treatment setting and should be integrated with the patient's preferences.

In clinical practice, on the one end, clinical decisions may be affected by irrational factors (eg, exposure to massive doses of pharmaceutical propaganda or familiarity with a specific psychotherapy or medication). On the other end, psychiatrists often use sophisticated forms of clinical judgment that are suitable for clinical challenges but are not addressed by current research strategies.[2] There is increasing awareness of the need of differentiating depression according to specific subtypes,[45,46] yet clear-cut indications for these subdivisions are still missing. The role of biomarkers, despite many promising research strategies, is still far from offering reliable clinical guidance.[16–18] In the meanwhile, there are important indications that come from clinical research. Treatment of depression may be conceptualized as integrated treatment of the various components of symptomatology, lifestyle, and social adjustment. An integrated treatment model, discussed in detail elsewhere,[2,8,10] is realistic and practical, and not just idealistic. It may be frustrating to those who like oversimplified biological models; however, approaches that integrate clinimetrics, patient priorities, lifestyle issues, and clinical judgment are more in keeping with the complexity of clinical situations and the challenge of depression treatment.

REFERENCES

1. Feinstein AR, Horwitz RI. Problems in the "evidence" of the "evidence-based medicine." Am J Med 1997;103:529–35.
2. Fava GA, Rafanelli C, Tomba E. The clinical approach process in psychiatry: a clinimetric approach. J Clin Psychiatry 2011. DOI: 10.40881JCP.10r06444.
3. Work Group on Major Depressive Disorder. Practice guideline for the treatment of patients with major depressive disorder. 3rd edition. Am J Psychiatry 2010;167 (October Suppl):1–118.
4. Raue PJ, Schulberg HC, Heo M, et al. Patients' depression treatment preferences and initiation, adherence and outcome: a randomized primary care study. Psychiatr Serv 2009;60:337–43.
5. Kocsis JH, Leon AC, Markowitz JC, et al. Patient preference as a moderator of outcome for chronic forms of major depressive disorder treated with nefazodone, cognitive behavioral analysis system of psychotherapy, or their combination. J Clin Psychiatry 2009;70:354–61.
6. Mergl R, Henkel V, Allgaier AK, et al. Are treatment preferences relevant in response to serotonergic antidepressants and cognitive behavioral therapy in depressed primary patients? Psychother Psychosom 2010;79:131–5.
7. Owens DK. Improving practice guidelines with patient-specific recommendations. Ann Intern Med 2011;154:683–4.
8. Tomba E. Nowhere patients. Psychother Psychosom 2012;81:69–72.
9. Bartova L, Berger A, Pezawas L. Is there a personalized medicine for mood disorders? Eur Arch Psychiatry Clin Neurosci 2010;260(Suppl 2):S121–S126.
10. Fava GA, Tomba E. New modalities of assessment and treatment planning in depression: the sequential approach. CNS Drugs 2010;24:453–65.
11. Fava GA, Tomba E, Grandi S. The road to recovery from depression. Psychother Psychosom 2007;76:260–5.
12. Zimmerman M, Chelminski I, McDermut W. Major depressive disorder and Axis I diagnostic comorbidity. J Clin Psychiatry 2002;63:187–93.
13. Emmelkamp PMG, Bouman TK, Scholing A. Anxiety disorders. Chichester (UK): John Wiley; 1993. p. 55–67.
14. Guidi J, Fava GA, Bech P, et al. The clinical interview for depression. Psychother Psychosom 2011;80:10–27.
15. Fava GA, Rafanelli C, Tomba E, et al. Sequential combination of cognitive behavioural treatment and well-being therapy in cyclothymic disorder. Psychother Psychosom 2011;80:136–43.
16. Leuchther AF, Cook IA, Hamilton SP, et al. Biomarkers to predict antidepressant response. Curr Psychiatry Rep 2010;12:553–62.
17. Taylor MJ, Sen S, Bhagwagar Z. Antidepressant response and the serotonin transporter gene-linked polymorphic region. Biol Psychiatry 2010;68:536–43.
18. Schulthorpe KD, Douglass AB. Sleep pathologies in depression and the clinical utility of polysomnography. Can J Psychiatry 2010;55:413–21.

19. Spielmans GI, Berman MI, Usitalo AN. Psychotherapy versus second generation antidepressants in the treatment of depression. J Nerv Ment Dis 2011;199:142–9.
20. Fournier JC, de Rubeis RS, Hollon SD, et al. Antidepressant drug effects and depression severity. JAMA 2010;303:47–53.
21. Looper KJ. Potential medical and surgical complications of serotonergic antidepressant medications. Psychosomatics 2007;48:1–9.
22. Niewstraten C, Labiris NR, Holbrook A. Systematic overview of drug interactions with antidepressant medications. Can J Psychiatry 2006;51:300–16.
23. Fabbri S, Fava GA, Rafanelli C, et al. Family intervention approach to loss of clinical effect during long-term antidepressant treatment. J Clin Psychiatry 2007;68: 1348–51.
24. Fava GA, Offidani E. The mechanisms of tolerance in antidepressant action. Prog Neuro- Psychopharmacol Biol Psychiatry 2011;35:1593–602.
25. Andrews PW, Kornstein SG, Haberstadt LJ, et al. Blue again: perturbational effects of antidepressants suggest monoaminergic homeostasis in major depression. Front Psychol 2011;2:159.
26. van Straten A, Geraedts A, Verdonck-de Leeuw I, et al. Psychological treatment of depressive symptoms in patients with medical disorders. J Psychosom Res 2010;69: 23–32.
27. Leykin Y, Amsterdam JD, deRubeis RJ, et al. Progressive resistance to a selective serotonin reuptake inhibitor but not to cognitive therapy in the treatment of major depression. J Consult Clin Psychol 2007;75:267–76.
28. Kuyken W, Tsivrikos D. Therapist competence, comorbidity and cognitive behavioral therapy for depression. Psychother Psychosom 2009;78:42–8.
29. Cuijpers P, van Straten A, Hollon SD, et al. The contribution of active medication to combined treatments of psychotherapy and pharmacotherapy for adult depression. Acta Psychiatr Scand 2010;121:415–23.
30. Keller MB, McCullough JP, Klein DN, et al. A comparison of nefazodone, the cognitive behavioral-analysis system of psychotherapy, and their combination for the treatment of chronic depression. N Engl J Med 2000;342:1462–70.
31. Guidi J, Fava GA, Fava M, et al. Efficacy of sequential integration of psychotherapy and pharmacotherapy in major depressive disorder. Psychol Med 2011;41:321–31.
32. Fava GA, Ruini C, Rafanelli C, et al. Six year outcome of cognitive behavior therapy for prevention of recurrent depression. Am J Psychiatry 2004;161:1872–6.
33. Tomba E. Assessment of lifestyle in relation to health. Adv Psychosom Med 2012;32: 72–96.
34. Fava GA, Tomba E. Increasing psychological well-being and resilience by psycho-therapeutic methods. J Personality 2009;77:1903–34.
35. Pigott HE, Leventhal AM, Alter GS, et al. Efficacy and effectiveness of antidepressants: current status of research. Psychother Psychosom 2010;79:267–79.
36. Judd LL. The clinical course of unipolar major depressive disorders. Arch Gen Psychiatry 1997;54:989–91.
37. Geddes JR, Carney SM, Davies C, et al. Relapse prevention with antidepressant drug treatment in depressive disorders: a systematic review. Lancet 2003;361:653–61.
38. Kaymaz N, Van Os J, Loonen AJM, et al. Evidence that patients with single versus recurrent episodes are differentially sensitive to treatment discontinuation. J Clin Psychiatry 2008;69:1423–36.
39. Viguera AC, Baldessarini RJ, Friedberg J. Discontinuing antidepressant treatment in major depression. Harvard Rev Psychiatry 1998;5:293–306.
40. Moret C, Isaac M, Briley M. Problems associated with long-term treatment with selective serotonin reuptake inhibitors. J Psychopharmacol 2009;23:967–74.

41. Fava GA. Statistical alchemy for drug treatment of generalized anxiety disorder. Psychother Psychosom 2011;80:261–3.

42. Kupfer DJ, Frank E, Perel JM. The advantage of early treatment intervention in recurrent depression. Arch Gen Psychiatry 1989;46:771–5.

43. Simon GE, von Korff M, Heiligenstein JH, et al. Initial antidepressant choice in primary care. JAMA 1996;275:1897–902.

44. Fava GA, Bernardi M, Tomba E, et al. Effects of gradual discontinuation of selective serotonin reuptake inhibitors in panic disorder with agoraphobia. Int J Neuropsychopharmacol 2007;10:835–8.

45. Lichtenberg P, Belmaker RH. Subtyping major depressive disorder. Psychother Psychosom 2010;79:131–5.

46. Bech P. Struggle for subtypes in primary and secondary depression and their mode-specific treatment or healing. Psychother Psychosom 2010;79:331–8.

Cognitive Behavioral Therapy for Depression

Donna M. Sudak, MD

KEYWORDS

- Cognitive–behavioral therapy • Depression
- Behavioral activation • Cognitive restructuring • Suicide

Cognitive–behavioral therapy (CBT) for depression is one of the best researched treatments in all of medicine.[1] As developed by Aaron T. Beck in the 1970s,[2] CBT for depression employs the highly potent strategies of behavioral activation and the relapse-preventing interventions of belief change and cognitive restructuring. As this article discusses, CBT is also substantially more durable than medication in patients who respond to treatment. Because not all patients with depression respond to medication, and many continue to have residual symptoms that interfere with their quality of life and incur a risk for relapse, CBT can play a major role in the treatment of this significant, often deadly public health problem.

EVIDENCE FOR THE USE OF CBT FOR MAJOR DEPRESSION

CBT is an effective treatment for acute major depression, with efficacy greater than or equal to that of medication in mild, moderate, and severe episodes of major depression.[3] In addition, when CBT is employed either with or without medication, treatment is more durable than with medication alone.[4] There is a nearly 50% reduction in relapse rates as compared to medication in patients who receive CBT alone and remit.[5] This trend was recently confirmed in a meta-analytic study that determined that patients who respond to acute phase CBT treatment alone for acute depression have a 61% chance of complete recovery relative to patients treated with medication alone, who have a 39% chance of complete recovery.[6]

The most evidence about the efficacy of CBT relative to other forms of psychotherapy for depression compares CBT and interpersonal therapy (IPT). The first large-scale comparison between these two forms of treatment, the National Institute of Mental Health Treatment of Depression Collaborative Research Program (NIMH TDCRP), reported a superior result for IPT in patients with severe depression,[7] and a less robust response for CBT relative to pharmacotherapy. Many subsequent studies[8] and reanalysis of the data from the TDCRP[9] have found that CBT for severe

The author has nothing to disclose.
Department of Psychiatry, Drexel University College of Medicine, PO Box 45358, Philadelphia, PA 19124, USA
E-mail address: donna.sudak@drexelmed.edu

Psychiatr Clin N Am 35 (2012) 99–110
doi:10.1016/j.psc.2011.10.001
0193-953X/12/$ – see front matter © 2012 Elsevier Inc. All rights reserved.

depression is equally as effective as medication. A recent large-scale study[10] comparing CBT and IPT showed that both were equally effective in treating outpatients with depression, but that patients with more severe depression had a significantly better response with CBT.

EVIDENCE FOR THE USE OF CBT COMBINED WITH MEDICATION FOR MAJOR DEPRESSION

Many of the early studies of CBT were conducted to evaluate the superiority of medication or therapy. The studies that included a comparison of the combination to either treatment showed a nonsignificant trend for a superior result when treatment is combined compared to either treatment alone.[11] Comparing CBT or medication for depression relative to the combination is a challenge because each individual treatment is quite effective relative to placebo. This means a large sample of patients must be studied to show a statistical advantage for the combination. Several authors[12,13] responded to this methodologic difficulty by performing statistical manipulations of existing data, showing that a significantly greater number of depressed patients will respond when a combination of treatments is given: one additional responder for each five patients treated with the combination in the data from 685 patients analyzed in the Friedman study and a significant advantage with a number needed to treat of 7.14 in the Cuijpers review of 16 studies (852 patients). Further, when we combine antidepressant medication and CBT no deleterious effects occur. A large study of chronically depressed patients that employed a form of CBT (cognitive–behavioral analysis system of psychotherapy) with and without medication[14] also resulted in a superior outcome for patients treated with the combination relative to either treatment alone. In addition, this study provided data that can guide decision making regarding what treatment to offer particular patients (see "Patient Selection").

An additional benefit of combined CBT and medication treatment is that patients receiving antidepressant medication remain in treatment longer and take medication more regularly when therapy is added.[15] Nonadherence to antidepressant medication is a substantial problem, with rates of nonadherence reported to be as high as 50% to 83% of patients.[16]

Finally, there is a significant body of work investigating the sequential application of medications and CBT in patients who have either acute or chronic depression. These studies have employed a variety of CBT applications (group and individual, treatment of varying lengths) prescribed after initial successful treatment with medication. A review of these studies[17] indicates a statistically significant increase in durability in patients who receive the combination regardless of whether antidepressant medication is continued. Many of these studies have been reviewed in a recent publication about the use of medication with CBT.[18]

THEORETICAL BASIS SUPPORTING CBT FOR DEPRESSION

One premise that underlies the practice of CBT is the cognitive–biological–social model.[19] This model states that a large number of influences—biological, genetic, temperamental, social, and developmental—can interact in the brain and influence information processing. Thus, biological predisposition, learned behavioral patterns, and interpersonal and social stressors are all potential contributory and maintenance factors to depressive illness. Next the model incorporates the fact that all humans organize experiences internally to make sense of the world efficiently and to guide behavior. Beck's theory of depression[16] states that in a negative mood state this information processing is highly negatively biased and frequently inaccurate. Depression, for example, is assumed to begin when a particular life stress interacts with a particular depressive diathesis—a set of beliefs and thinking biases. When these beliefs are activated it influences the patient's information processing, leading to selective attention to negative experiences and possibilities.[20] Such faulty information processing leads to the negative thinking, withdrawal, and inactivity typical of depression. Negative thinking further influences mood, behavior, and physiology so that the patient's social and interpersonal functioning deteriorates. These behavioral changes lead to more negative thoughts and interpersonal and social consequences that frequently confirm the patient's negative view of the world. The "cognitive triad"—negative thoughts about the self, others, and the future—as described by Beck[21] produces an ongoing and relentless cycle with hopelessness and suicidal ideation an understandable endpoint. Therapy interventions target this triad both with cognitive restructuring and behavioral experiments, with the goal of modifying this negative information processing system with rational and objective data.

In addition, learning theory provides a substantial theoretical underpinning in CBT. Patients learn particular ways to evaluate themselves, others, and their experiences that may perpetuate problems by influencing information processing and retrieval. For example, patients may develop ideas about personal vulnerability ("Bad things are likely to happen to me") through which all experiences are filtered, with selective attention to negative outcomes and discounting positive experience.

Skill deficits are considered to be additional risk factors for the initiation and maintenance of depression. For example, someone who has the experience early in life that people will be harsh and critical of any efforts he makes may develop a belief that he is incompetent, and that the safest action is to not try new things. This strategy can cause the accumulation of multiple skill deficits over time. A vicious circle of low expectations, lack of effort, little reinforcement, and low mood ensues. Therefore skill deficits are assessed and remediated when present in the treatment.

Learning theory significantly influences the structure of treatment as well. Patients are taught the tools of treatment with a rationale: that they will continue to use these tools in the future because these strategies will prevent relapse. CBT typically entails the use of "homework"—irrespective of what practicing skills outside of session are called in therapy. This modification occurs because many patients have a negative view of the concept of "homework." Patients are assigned tasks to complete outside of sessions because the key to learning new skills is practice, and repeated practice is required before new skills are automatic and generalized. Data support patients' participation in homework as a predictor of recovery and treatment durability. Patients who continue to use CBT skills outside of the session are less likely to relapse.[22]

A particular modification of CBT in depression is that the therapist is sensitive to the memory deficits and slowed thinking typical of depressed patients and therefore customizes interventions to ensure that the patient retains material from the session. For example, therapy with depressed patients includes frequent verbal and written summaries of important points discovered in the session. Assignments are written down and given to the patient at the end of the hour. Homework is tailored so that small assignments are given at the start of treatment to make it likely to be successful. The therapist carefully discusses obstacles to homework completion and attends to the patient's thoughts and beliefs about the assignment before the patient leaves the session.

Finally, predictors of positive outcome in CBT for depression other than homework completion have been determined. First, careful therapist adherence to the specific techniques and procedures of CBT is more important to a good outcome than the therapeutic alliance itself.[23,24] Patients who have a dramatic session-to-session improvement in rating scales for depression (so called "sudden gains") are also more likely to have long-term remission of depression.[25] Although the reason for such a correlation is unclear, one could speculate that patients who dramatically improve resonate with the model and would continue to apply treatment strategies in the future.

CBT IN CLINICAL PRACTICE

Core strategies of CBT are designed to exploit patient strengths and capabilities and to teach new skills. The therapeutic alliance is active and collaborative. In essence the therapist functions as a teacher and coach, and works together with the patient. At the start of treatment the therapist and patient jointly set goals to accomplish in therapy. Goal setting is particularly important in depression because it increases motivation and helps the patient to direct his or her efforts to change behaviors that are most likely to help his or her mood (ie, sleep, appetite, activity). The therapist and patient work together to help the patient accomplish the goals that are determined to be a focus of treatment and to increase more objective and functional thinking.

Educating the patient is another important early focus in treatment. Patients are taught about depression as an illness and about the model and rationale for the procedures of CBT. Tools employed to facilitate learning include reviewing knowledge acquired from session to session ("bridging") and summarizing key points within and at the end of the session. Socratic questions and behavioral experiments are essential ingredients used as treatment progresses because patients are much more likely to believe information that they discover on their own.

Planning treatment is another feature of CBT for depression. Therapy is structured carefully and sensitively to maximize the efficiency of treatment and minimize the patient's anxiety. The therapist is responsible for keeping therapy goal focused and on track. Elements common to most sessions include jointly setting an agenda, identifying specific problems to discuss in the session, and then directly working to solve them. In addition, the therapist frequently summarizes the important points made in the session and directly asks for feedback from the patient about his understanding of the session and his reactions to it. This increases the patient's engagement and corrects any misconceptions that could occur. Treatment plans are individualized according to the patient's conceptualization. A patient with severe anergia and anhedonia, for example, will require significant amounts of behavioral activation (see "Behavioral Activation") early in treatment before instituting cognitive modification. Patients who are highly hopeless and suicidal will require direct methods to modify this thinking and engage in treatment at the start (see "Hopelessness and Suicidal Ideation"). Patients with interpersonal "emergencies" (eg, school or work performance that could lead to dismissal) may require direct problem-solving and interpersonal intervention early in treatment to mitigate significant life problems that would complicate treatment. In general, patients begin with interventions designed to remedy behavioral deficits and to normalize activities of daily living.

Subsequent sessions teach patients to identify "automatic thoughts"—thoughts that occur rapidly in response to particular situations and that are associated with a negative mood shift or undesirable behaviors (see "Cognitive Interventions"). The patient is then instructed to use inductive reasoning to examine these thoughts and generate more accurate or functional alternatives. Finally, common themes suggested by patterns of automatic thoughts and an understanding of the patient's specific developmental and interpersonal life experiences help the therapist and patient jointly conceptualize the particular rules and beliefs that generate the patient's vulnerability to depressed mood in the presence of particular activating events.

Behavioral experiments and experiential techniques are added to inductive reasoning to evaluate and modify these ideas. Belief change has been shown to convey a particular advantage in increasing the durability of treatment response.[23,26]

Behavioral Activation

Behavioral activation is an essential element of CBT for moderate to severe depression. Behavioral activation employed alone is as effective as CBT or pharmacotherapy for acute depression[27] and may be more helpful than standard CBT in patients with substantial Axis II comorbidity who can obtain only brief courses of psychotherapy.[28] Lewinsohn originally described and researched the use of behavioral methods as a treatment for depression.[29] The foundation for these interventions is the idea that behavior that makes sense to a depressed person (ie, inactivity, social withdrawal) causes low levels of positive reinforcement in that person's life. Behavioral interventions counter the tendency to avoid and withdraw that is common to depression. The goal is both to increase the patient's sense of self-efficacy and to address urgent needs such as sleep, eating, and self-care that may have been neglected during the depressive episode.

The first step in this intervention involves teaching the patient to self-monitor to assess current activity levels. The therapist and patient jointly identify activities previously valued by the patient that the patient has decreased and any activities of daily living that the patient is avoiding. If patients cannot identify any activities that are of interest, the Pleasant Events Schedule[30] may be employed to help the patient remember previous activities that were pleasurable or to provide affordable and accessible new activities that may increase enjoyment. Identified activities are assigned to attempt at specific times of the day, particularly those times that are associated with increased symptoms of depression. Activity thus occurs according to a plan, instead of the patient waiting for motivation and energy to occur. Then patients are asked to observe changes that occur in their mood state when they engage in planned activities. This experiment tests faulty predictions the patient makes about success or failure and assesses the outcome of action on the patient's mood. In addition to assigning pleasurable activities, the therapist may help the patient to make step-by-step plans for activities that appear to be too overwhelming and help the patient to plan, troubleshoot, and execute such activities (eg, graded task assignment).

Behavioral activation is also an excellent tool to employ in primary care when patients are depressed, with or without adjunctive pharmacologic treatment. In this setting it is important to make certain that the task identified is important to the patient and that the amount of activity prescribed not too overwhelming. The more specific an assignment is, the more likely it will be done, and written reminders of what the patient will attempt to do are crucial: a prescription for a specific activity, with whom, when, and the rationale for the activity is ideal. It is also of key importance for the physician to ask about the assignment at the next visit or the patient will not place sufficient value on completing tasks.

Practitioners familiar with longer inpatient admissions for major depression have seen behavioral activation at work, as inpatient programs force patients to be up and about and participate in daily activities. In an outpatient setting, including primary care settings, providers must be persistent and not discouraged by the inertia depressed patients experience. Consistent, creative troubleshooting of obstacles, both real and perceived, is the key to success.

Another benefit of behavioral activation is that patterns of thought the patient has that are associated with withdrawal and avoidance (eg, "It's no use," "I don't have the energy," "I will feel worse if I try and I fail") become evident when the patient is instructed to engage in activity. These thoughts can be evaluated and tested by increasing activity. Behavioral activation also targets skill deficits that put the patient at risk for difficulties in social interactions (eg, lack of assertive communication or poor social skills). Such training ensures that future social interactions may be more rewarding and satisfying and enhance mood.

Cognitive Interventions

After patients engage in behavioral activation the therapist continues to work with the patient to accomplish the goals of treatment, and the specific focus shifts to identify, examine, and generate more logical and functional ways of thinking about personal experiences, as cognitive changes are associated with patient improvement.[31] Several mechanisms can produce changes in thinking in CBT. Behavioral change may change cognitive processes at a number of levels, as patients draw new conclusions from actual life experiences.

Targets of CBT sessions are automatic thoughts, cognitive errors, and misattributions, which are identified and then examined to generate more accurate and functional ideas, rules, and conclusions. The process of identifying automatic thoughts—the thoughts just below the surface of conscious awareness—is often easier when the patient is taught to look for them by first identifying mood shifts. Mood changes are easily recognized because one function of human emotion is to get one to pay attention. At the time of a mood shift the patient is taught to ask "What was going through my mind?"[32] Other clinical tools that are used to help patients identify automatic thoughts include lists of cognitive distortions[32] and various types of thought change records[32,33] that help the patient learn to recognize such thoughts and their relationship to mood and behavior.

After the patient can identify automatic thoughts easily, the next step is to use logical analysis to see if the thought is true, partly true, or untrue. Particular attention is paid to evaluating the evidence supporting or refuting thoughts, getting perspective by looking at potential alternative responses (eg, asking the patient if he or she would say such a thing to a friend in such a circumstance), or asking what investigation the patient could conduct to determine if the thought in question is true. As the patient begins to see that thoughts can be changed, and that when believable and more accurate alternatives are substituted he or she feels and functions better, the model for treatment is reinforced. The patient is instructed to practice evaluating negative thinking in typical problematic situations outside the session.

One important treatment consideration is what to do if the automatic thought or belief that the patient has is actually true. Therapists cannot always know in advance whether or not this is the case. Patients contending with difficult life events may work with therapists to identify whether their thoughts about such events represent problems to be solved or whether they have ascribed any faulty meaning to difficult life circumstances. For example, the parent of a child with cancer may believe something he or she did caused the cancer to occur—such a thought would magnify suffering in an already painful time. In such a situation therapy would focus on grieving, active coping, and accurate evaluation of responsibility.

Once the patient is capable of changing automatic thoughts with some proficiency, the therapist can shift the therapeutic focus to uncovering the rules, assumptions, and beliefs that make the patient more vulnerable life events and negative thinking. Uncovering misattributions and the meaning underlying commonly occurring automatic thoughts can help the patient understand the foundation for the thinking he has. This process is reserved for later sessions because such meanings and core beliefs can be extremely painful to uncover. The therapist and patient share the specific conceptualization of the patient's development of such beliefs about the world, the self, and others to facilitate the patient's self-knowledge and increase motivation for change.

Changing beliefs and assumptions is a more challenging process than changing automatic thoughts. When patients are reluctant to change, examining the advantages and disadvantages of changing beliefs or identifying possible and attainable other ways to believe is a first step. Many patients have difficulty with relinquishing ideas that seem protective or that are so fundamental to their identity. A number of methods have been identified to help patients change beliefs. These include the cognitive continuum,[33] historical tests of beliefs,[32] and behaving "as if" the belief is true.[34] Trial-based cognitive therapy is a newer tool that focuses on activating positive beliefs in session with promising results.[35] Patients with Axis II difficulties may require assistance to generate positive and more functional beliefs; often their life experiences have been so depriving and their enduring interpersonal dysfunction is so severe that they cannot develop alternative ideas about themselves or others without the therapist's help. Finally, the patient is taught that strengthening new beliefs will require collecting supportive data for some time, and homework entails completing logs that collect supportive evidence day by day.

Termination

Termination in CBT for depression is somewhat different from termination in other therapeutic approaches. The therapist has consistently provided written materials and summarized the patient's learning throughout treatment and the initial process of termination involves reviewing what the patient has learned. Then the patient and therapist predict and provide solutions for those situations that may be a problem for the patient in the future (relapse prevention). "Booster sessions"—therapy sessions that are scheduled at gradually longer intervals—ensure the durability of what the patient has learned. Booster sessions are not designed for "getting the news." Rather, the patient is instructed to prepare by identifying problems that have occurred in the interval and specifying which tools used from therapy he used. This material is reviewed in the session with a goal to consolidate learning and troubleshoot the patient's use of skills.

Hopelessness and Suicidal Ideation

Hopelessness is an important treatment target in CBT for depression. Hopelessness is a strong predictor of suicidal ideation, suicidal intention, and suicide completion.[36,37] Because patients with severe depression frequently manifest hopelessness early in treatment, the therapist must intervene to actively counter the patient's hopeless thinking before the patient knows the tools used in CBT that evaluate and modify irrational negative thinking. This does not mean that the therapist tells the patient not to think that things are hopeless; instead, the therapist guides the patient in the session to examine evidence about whether his or her situation is actually hopeless, highlighting perhaps the positive evidence the patient discards or omits because of the pervasive nature of the mood state. The therapist also modifies automatic thoughts "on the spot" with hopeless patients, particularly if patients ask rhetorical questions (eg, "what's the use?"). The patient is asked to answer such questions seriously and the therapist uses Socratic questions to guide the patient to more rational conclusions.

The process of CBT may combat hopelessness as well. The therapist's collaboration with the patient and the ability to educate the patient about depression and about the relationship between thinking, mood, and behavior is a powerful tool to instill hope. Providing a specific plan to help the patient that is backed by a solid rationale and empirical evidence for efficacy is a potent agent to boost morale; setting goals provides tangible guideposts to improve function.

Of particular importance in any treatment for depression is how the treatment manages suicidal ideation. Patients who are suicidal and treated with CBT can derive specific benefits regarding suicidal behavior in and of itself, independent of the diagnosis of the patient. Several studies have shown that CBT applied specifically to patients with suicidal behavior can decrease the frequency of such behavior in the future, compared to treatment as usual.[38,39] The therapist's activity and accurate optimism about the effectiveness of CBT for depression is a powerful force on its own to combat suicidal thinking and despair. In addition, specific strategies of CBT when applied to suicidal thinking, whether or not such thinking is related to depression, have been shown to be useful in deterring suicide attempts.[38] First, therapists identify the patient's strengths and help the patient to access memories of effective prior coping. The goal of this intervention is to increase the flexibility of the patient's thinking and to generate options to deal with life problems other than suicide. Another important procedure is to identify specific reasons for living and remain engaged in life.[40] Hopelessness and suicidal thinking are monitored from session to session and are made the primary agenda item if they are present. The therapist and patient make specific, detailed, written plans for activities outside of sessions that include what to do if the patient begins to feel worse. These are often in the form of coping cards, written cards that have "bullet points" containing the essence of solutions developed in the session. In a clinical situation, when hopeless and suicidal thoughts have been successfully restructured in a session, the new way of thinking, plus a plan for action to counter such thoughts, and a crisis plan if these strategies are ineffective are given to the patient to read and use on a regular basis.

PATIENT SELECTION

Cost-effective and efficient treatment would be easier to deliver if one had a "crystal ball" that helped to determine which patient would respond to which treatment for depression. Data derived from research to guide treatment selection are scarce. Patient preference is an obvious factor to consider, as is cost and availability. Trends do exist that should inform our choices until better information is available. For example, in the Keller study,[14] patients with prominent symptoms of anxiety[41] or insomnia[42] had much better outcomes if they received combined treatment relative to psychotherapy alone. Patients in the same study who had a history of childhood abuse did not do as well if they received pharmacotherapy alone.[43]

Fournier and colleagues[44] looked at predictors of response to CBT relative to medication and determined that marriage, unemployment, and history of a recent stressful life event predicted a better response to CBT relative to medication. Likewise, Leykin and colleagues[45] found that the greater the number of prior exposures to antidepressants, the less likely the response to medication compared to CBT. Severity of depression[46] increases the likelihood of response to medication given without therapy, but durability and the question of residual symptoms may still make CBT a desirable choice in such patients. Finally, the presence of significant Axis II psychopathology means that medication[47] or behavioral activation[28] is each likely to be more effective than CBT for depression delivered in a time-limited format.

When patients have comorbid Axis II difficulties and have interest and resources to be in CBT in a longer format, the therapist modifies treatment to pay closer attention to establishing and strengthening the relationship with the patient, and may spend more time with solving interpersonal problems with the patient. Such patients also must understand the conceptualization the therapist develops and the role that long-held beliefs and strategies play in the problems they have had throughout their lives. The therapist often provides other, more functional perspectives and interpersonal strategies in this case, rather than expect the patient to discover these by inductive reasoning.

In addition to the aforementioned research findings, other clinical features may make CBT more or less applicable in a particular patient. Because CBT requires that the patient learns new skills, patients who are cognitively impaired are less good candidates for CBT. Patients who cannot form interpersonal relationships may also require modifications of "standard" CBT to allow for time to learn that the therapist can be trusted and to agree to participate in treatment. Patients who "resonate" with the model and who can easily express and identify thoughts and emotions, and who do not blame others for their difficulties are ideal candidates for CBT (and likely for any other form of psychotherapy). Skillful CBT practitioners can modify standard treatment by attending to a patient's affect and feedback, and engage with patients who are more challenging so that this evidence-based therapy can be implemented in more difficult patients.

SUMMARY

CBT is a valuable treatment for mild, moderate, and severe forms of major depression. It is equally effective and more durable than medication alone, and the combination of medication and CBT may increase the response rate and extend durability when CBT is employed after pharmacotherapy is successful. Therapist competence has been shown to influence outcomes in CBT for depression.[48] Practitioners who wish to learn more about CBT may access a wide variety of educational materials: basic texts,[32,49,50] course offerings at major scientific meetings, and local and national training centers are available. The Academy of Cognitive Therapy website (www.academyofct.org) provides detailed information about obtaining training and certification in CBT.

REFERENCES

1. Butler AC, Chapman JE, Forman EM, et al. The empirical status of cognitive-behavioral therapy: a review of meta-analyses. Clin Psychol Rev 2006;26:17–31.
2. Beck AT. Cognitive therapy: nature and relation to behavior therapy. Behav Ther 1970;1:184–200.
3. Dreissen E, Hollon SD. Cognitive behavioral therapy for mood disorders: efficacy, moderators and mediators. Psychiatr Clin North Am 2010;33(3):537–55.
4. Hollon SD, DeRubeis RJ, Shelton RC, et al. Prevention of relapse following cognitive therapy versus medications in the treatment of moderate to severe depression. Arch Gen Psychiatry 2005;62:417–22.
5. Hollon SD, Stewart MO, Strunk D. Enduring effects for cognitive behavioral therapy in the treatment of depression and anxiety. Annu Rev Psychol 2006;57:285–315.
6. Vittengl JR, Clark LA, Dunn TW, et al. Reducing relapse and recurrence in unipolar depression: a comparative meta-analysis of cognitive-behavioral therapy's effects. J Consult Clin Psychol 2007;75(3):475–88.
7. Elkin I, Shea MT, Watkins JT, et al. National Institute of Mental Health Treatment of Depression Collaborative Research Program: general effectiveness of treatments. Arch Gen Psychiatry 1989;46:971–82.
8. DeRubeis RJ, Hollon SD, Amsterdam JD, et al. Cognitive therapy vs medications in the treatment of moderate to severe depression. Arch Gen Psychiatry 2005;62(4): 409–16.

9. DeRubeis RJ, Gelfand LA, Tang TZ, et al. Medications versus cognitive behavior therapy for severely depressed outpatients: mega-analysis of four randomized comparisons. Am J Psychiatry 1999;156:1007–13.

10. Luty SE, Carter JD, McKenzie JM, et al. Randomised controlled trial of interpersonal psychotherapy and cognitive-behavioural therapy for depression. Br J Psychiatry 2007;190:496–502.

11. Hollon SD, Jarrett RB, Nierenberg AA, et al. Psychotherapy and medication in the treatment of adult and geriatric depression: which monotherapy or combined treatment. J Clin Psychiatry 2005;66:465–8.

12. Friedman ES, Wright JH, Jarrett RB, et al. Combining cognitive therapy and medication for mood disorders. Psychiatr Ann 2006;36(5):320–8.

13. Cuijpers P, VanStraten A, Hollon SD, et al. The contribution of active medication to combined treatments of psychotherapy and pharmacotherapy for adult depression: a meta-analysis. Acta Psychiatr Scand 2010;121(6):415–23.

14. Keller MB, McCullough JP, Klein DN, et al. A comparison of nefazodone, the cognitive behavioral-analysis system of psychotherapy, and their combination for the treatment of chronic depression. N Engl J Med 2000;342:1462–70.

15. Pampallona S, Bollini P, Tibaldi G, et al. Combined pharmacotherapy and psychological therapy for depression. Arch Gen Psychiatry 2004;61:714–9.

16. Aikens JE, Nease DE, Klinkman MS. Explaining patient's beliefs about the necessity and harmfulness of antidepressants. Ann Fam Med 2008;6:23–9.

17. Paykel ES. Cognitive therapy in relapse prevention for depression. Int J Neuro-Psychopharmacol 2007;10:131–6.

18. Sudak DM. Combined treatment for major depression. In: Combining CBT and medication: an evidence-based approach. Hoboken (NJ): John Wiley & Sons; 2011. p. 55–80.

19. Wright JH. Integrating cognitive behavioral therapy and pharmacotherapy. In: Leahy, RL, editor. Contemporary cognitive therapy: Theory, research, and practice. New York: Guilford; 2004. p. 341–66.

20. Beck AT. The evolution of the cognitive model of depression and its neurobiological correlates. Am J Psychiatry 2008;165:969–77.

21. Beck AT. Depression: Clinical, experimental, and theoretical aspects. New York: Harper and Row; 1967.

22. Strunk DN, DeRubeis RJ, Chiu AW, et al. Patients' competence and performance of cognitive therapy skills: relation to the reduction of relapse risk following treatment for depression. J Consult Clin Psychol 2007;75(4):523–30.

23. DeRubeis RJ, Feeley M. Determinants of change in cognitive therapy of depression. Cogn Ther Res 1990;14:469–82.

24. Feeley M, DeRubeis RJ, Gelfand LA. The temporal relation of adherence and alliance to symptom change in cognitive therapy for depression. J Consult Clin Psychol 1999;67(4):451–89.

25. Tang TZ, DeRubeis RJ. Sudden gains and critical sessions in cognitive-behavioral therapy for depression. J Consul Clin Psychol 1999;67(6):894–904.

26. Hollon SD, Evans MD, DeRubeis RJ. Cognitive mediation of relapse prevention following treatment for depression: implications of differential risk. In: Ingram RE, editor. Psychological aspects of depression. New York: Plenum; 1990. p. 117–36.

27. Dimidjian S, Hollon SD, Dobson S, et al. Randomized trial of behavioral activation, cognitive therapy, and antidepressant medication in the acute treatment of adults with major depression. J Consult Clin Psychol 2006;74(4):658–70.

28. Coffman SJ, Martell CR, Dimidjian S, et al. Extreme nonresponse in cognitive therapy: can behavioral activation succeed where cognitive therapy fails? J Consult Clin Psychol 2007;75(4):531–41.

29. Lewinsohn PM. A behavioral approach to depression. In: Friedman RM, Katz MM, editors. The psychology of depression: contemporary theory and research. New York: John Wiley & Sons; 1974. p. 157–85.

30. MacPhillamy DJ, Lewinsohn PM. The pleasant events schedule: studies on reliability, validity, and scale intercorrelation. J Consult Clin Psychol 1982;50(3):363–80.

31. Garratt G, Ingram RE. Cognitive processes in cognitive therapy: evaluation of the mechanisms of change in the treatment of depression. Clin Psychol Sci Pract 2007;14(3):224–39.

32. Beck JS. Cognitive therapy: basics and beyond. New York: Guilford; 1990.

33. Greenberger D, Padesky CA. Mind over mood. New York: Guilford; 1995.

34. Dobson KS. Cognitive therapy for depression. In: Whisman MA, editor. Adapting cognitive therapy for depression. New York: Guilford Press; 2008. p. 3–35.

35. deOliveira IR. Trial-based thought record (TBTR): Preliminary data on a strategy to deal with core beliefs by combining sentence reversion and the use of an analogy to a trial. Rev Brasil Psiquiatr 2008;30:12–8.

36. Beck AT, Kovacs M, Weissman A. Hopelessness and suicidal behavior – an overview. JAMA 1975;234:1146–9.

37. Beck AT, Steer RA, Kovacs M, et al. Hopelessness and eventual suicide: a 10-year prospective study of patients hospitalized with suicidal ideation. Am J Psychiatry 1985;142:559–62.

38. Brown G, Have TT, Henriques GR, et al. Cognitive therapy for the prevention of suicide attempts: a randomized controlled trial. JAMA 2005;294:563–70.

39. Tarrier N, Taylor K, Gooding P. Cognitive-behavioral interventions to reduce suicidal behavior: a systemic review and meta-analysis. Behav Modif 2008;32(1):77–108.

40. Wright JS, Sudak DM, Turkington D, et al. Treating hopelessness and suicidality. In: High yield cognitive-behavior therapy for brief sessions: an illustrated guide. Washington, DC: APPI Press; 2010. p. 145–66.

41. Ninan PT, Rush AJ, Crits-Christoph P, et al. Symptomatic and syndromal anxiety in chronic forms of major depression: effect of nefazodone, cognitive behavioral analysis system of psychotherapy, and their combination. J Clin Psychiatry 2002;63(5):434–41.

42. Thase ME, Rush J, Mamber R, et al. Differential effects of nefazodone and cognitive behavioral analysis system of psychotherapy on insomnia associated with chronic forms of major depression. J Clin Psychiatry 2002;63(6):493–500.

43. Nemeroff CB, Heim CM, Thase ME, et al. Differential responses to psychotherapy versus pharmacotherapy in patients with chronic forms of major depression and childhood trauma. Proc Natl Acad Sci USA 2003;100 (24):14293–6.

44. Fournier JC, DeRubeis RJ, Shelton RC, et al. Prediction of response to medications and cognitive therapy in the treatment of moderate to severe depression. J Consult Clin Psychol 2009;77(4):775–87.

45. Leykin Y, Amsterdam J, DeRubeis R, et al. Progressive resistance to a selective serotonin reuptake inhibitor but not to cognitive therapy in the treatment of major depression. J Consult Clin Psychol 2007;75(2):267–76.

46. Fournier JC, DeRubeis RJ, Hollon SD, et al. Antidepressant drug effects and depression severity: a patient-level meta-analysis. JAMA 2010;303(1):47–53.

47. Fournier JC, DeRubeis RJ, Shelton RC, et al. Antidepressant medications vs. cognitive therapy in people with or without personality disorder. Br J Psychiatry 2008;192: 124–9.

48. Strunk DR, Brotman MA, DeRubeis RJ, et al. Therapist competence in cognitive therapy for depression: predicting subsequent symptom change. J Consult Clin Psychol 2010;78:429–37.
49. Sudak DM. Cognitive behavior therapy for clinicians. Philadelphia: Lippincott Williams & Wilkins; 2006.
50. Wright JH, Basco MR, Thase ME. Learning cognitive-behavior therapy: an illustrated guide. Washington, DC: American Psychiatric Publishing; 2006.

Psychodynamic Treatment of Depression

Patrick Luyten, PhD[a,b,*], Sidney J. Blatt, PhD[c]

KEYWORDS

- Depression • Mood disorder • Psychoanalytic
- Psychodynamic • Treatment • Efficacy • Effectiveness

Key Points: SUMMARY OF KEY FINDINGS CONCERNING PSYCHODYNAMIC TREATMENT OF DEPRESSION

○ Psychodynamic treatments for depression are readily accepted by many depressed patients as a viable treatment

○ Brief psychodynamic treatment

- Is superior to control conditions, is equally effective as other active psychological treatments, and treatment effects are often maintained in the long run

- Is as effective as pharmacotherapy in the acute treatment of mild to moderate depression, and either alone or in combination with medication is associated with better long-term outcome compared with pharmacotherapy alone

○ Longer-term psychoanalytic treatment and psychoanalysis

- May be indicated in patients with complex, chronic psychological disorders characterized by mood problems, often with comorbid anxiety and personality problems.

- May be more effective in the long run compared with brief treatment for depression, although more research is needed in this context.

○ Evidence suggests that psychoanalytic treatment is also effective in children and adolescents

---

Over the last 2 decades, there has been a remarkable increase in research into psychodynamic treatments (PT) for depression.[1–4] This article reviews the key theoretical assumptions of PT for depression and summarizes findings concerning

---

The authors have nothing to disclose.

ª Department of Psychology, University of Leuven, Tiensestraat 102 PO Box 3722, 3000 Leuven, Belgium

ᵇ Research Department of Clinical, Educational and Health Psychology, University College, London, UK

ᶜ Departments of Psychiatry and Psychology, Yale University, New Haven, CT, USA

* Corresponding author. Department of Psychology, University of Leuven, Tiensestraat 102 PO Box 3722, 3000 Leuven, Belgium.

E-mail address: patrick.luyten@psy.kuleuven.be

Psychiatr Clin N Am 35 (2012) 111–129
doi:10.1016/j.psc.2012.01.001
0193-953X/12/$ – see front matter © 2012 Elsevier Inc. All rights reserved.

psych.theclinics.com

the efficacy and effectiveness of these interventions alone and in combination with pharmacotherapy in adults, children, and adolescents. Issues of suitability and acceptability are also discussed as well insights into the mutative factors in these treatments. We close this article with a summary and implications for future research and treatment guidelines.

SPECIFICITY OF THE PSYCHODYNAMIC APPROACH: COMMON AND SPECIFIC FACTORS IN PSYCHODYNAMIC TREATMENTS OF DEPRESSION

Meta-analyses have identified very few, if any, differences in the efficacy of bona fide psychotherapies for a number of conditions, including depression.[5,6] This may be because the effects of these treatments are only in part related to specific techniques. Other factors may account for a larger portion of the variance in treatment outcome; it has been estimated that only 15% is predicted by specific techniques, 30% by common factors (eg, providing support), 15% by expectancy and placebo effects, and 35% to 40% by extratherapeutic effects (eg, spontaneous remission, positive events or changes).[7] Moreover, it has been difficult to find differences among treatments because most studies have focused on symptom remission in brief, highly structured, and manualized interventions. Furthermore, most randomized, controlled trials (RCTs) have only had power to investigate noninferiority compared with other active treatments and thus may be unable to detect meaningful differences between treatments. Research focusing on outcomes broader than symptom remission, as well as long-term effects, may be more promising as discussed below.

Psychodynamic Specific Features

Notwithstanding the many common features of treatments for depression (such as provision of hope, support, and a theoretical framework concerning the origins of and potential cure for the disorder), studies do show important differences between psychodynamic and other treatments. For instance, relative to cognitive–behavioral therapists, psychodynamic therapists tend to have a stronger emphasis on[8]:

1. Affect and emotional expression
2. Exploration of patients' tendency to avoid topics (ie, defenses)
3. Identification of recurring patterns in behavior, feelings, experiences, and relationships
4. The past and its influence on the present
5. Interpersonal experiences
6. The therapeutic relationship
7. Exploration of wishes, dreams, and fantasies.

These findings are largely congruent with work done in the United Kingdom in the context of the Improving Access to Psychological Therapies initiative. This demonstrates that although psychodynamic competencies overlap to some extent with those of other treatments (such as the ability to engage the client and establish a positive therapeutic alliance), there are a number of competencies specific to psychodynamic therapy (such as the ability to work with transference and countertransference and to recognize and work with defenses).[9] The focus on competencies has also led to the development of dynamic interpersonal therapy, a promising novel psychodynamic treatment for depression that integrates features of a number of current empirically supported PT of depression. Dynamic interpersonal therapy is currently being evaluated in an RCT.[2]

Aside from these specific techniques and competencies, a number of general assumptions, rooted in psychodynamic theory,[10] further define the specificity of the psychodynamic approach to the treatment of depression.

Psychodynamic Approaches Focus on the Patient's Internal World

First, perhaps more so than any other treatment, PT focus on the patient's internal world, that is, representations or cognitive affective schemas of self and others that influence our perceptions, thoughts, feelings and actions, including an emphasis on the role of unconscious motivation and intentionality. The emphasis in psychodynamic approaches to depression is on how (unconscious) motivational factors lead the patient to (mis)perceive and (mis)interpret external reality and experiences and to create, unwillingly, problems that maintain depressive symptoms, particularly in interpersonal relationships. For instance, highly dependent individuals may unconsciously avoid any manifest expression of aggression in close relationships for fear of abandonment, although they may feel very frustrated and dissatisfied. Likewise, because of their high standards and competitiveness, highly self-critical individuals may unconsciously and unwittingly elicit criticism and dislike by others, reinforcing their belief that that nobody really likes or loves them.[11] Of course, these tendencies are likely to be influenced by social–environmental factors (eg, growing up in a family characterized by low parental warmth or working in a competitive work environment) and by biological factors, some of which are discussed below.

Yet, psychoanalytic approaches to depression emphasize the need to understand the subjective experience of the disorder. As we discuss in more detail below, a focus on the phenomenology of depression has not only allowed researchers from different theoretical strands to delineate different types of depressive experiences. This has also facilitated research into neurobiological and social factors related to depression[12–14] and led to an awareness of the role of distortions in mentalization, that is, the ability to reflect on the self and others in terms of mental states, both as a cause and a consequence of depression. These distortions may not only influence the course but also the treatment of this disorder.[2,13]

Psychodynamic Approaches Take a Developmental Perspective

Second, psychodynamic approaches have always emphasized the importance of a developmental perspective in conceptualizing and treating depression, and recent research has provided dramatic support for these assumptions. For instance, the emphasis in contemporary models of depression concerning the impact of early adversity on the programming of the main human stress system and the existence of critical time windows in development, when biological/psychological systems are especially sensitive to environmental experiences, are congruent with assumptions about the role of early developmental factors in the causation of depression.[15–17] Psychoanalytic treatment approaches more specifically emphasize the role of insight into the past in changing attitudes and feelings in the present, offering the possibility of a "new beginning."[18] Moreover, even in brief PT of depression that focus less on the past, developmental antecedents of behavior, thoughts, feelings, and attitudes are always taken into account.[2]

Psychodynamic Approaches are Person Centered

Finally, psychodynamic approaches of depression are more *person* than *disorder* centered. The view, supported by empirical research,[19,20] is that depression is not categorically distinct from subclinical depression and from normality and that depression is not a discrete disorder, distinct from other Axis I and Axis II disorders. Depression is first and foremost considered to be a basic affect that signals a discrepancy between a wished-for state and an actual state of the self; it is not necessarily considered something pathologic. It is seen as a primordial, probably for evolutionary reasons prewired, signal affect or a basic "building block" of the individual's internal affective world. From a psychoanalytic perspective, both normal and disrupted development involve ongoing attempts by the individual, throughout the life span, to find an optimal balance between biological givens and the demands of the environment.[11] Depression is, thus, not conceptualized in terms of a static end state, but as reflecting continuing attempts of the individual, however maladaptive, to find a (better) balance between endowment and experience.[21] Together with anxiety and aggression, depression is seen as a basic emotional response of the individual, in particular to feelings of loss of a wished-for state. Depression, anxiety, and aggression are, thus, inextricably linked. This also explains the high comorbidity of depression and anxiety and the largely artificial distinction between these 2 disorders in psychiatric classification.[22] Viewing depression as a basic affect suggests there is no qualitative but only quantitative distinction between normal and "pathological" mood, with depression situated on a continuum ranging from mild dysphoria to clinical depression, a view supported by taxometric studies.[23]

Person- and disorder-centered approaches should be seen as complementary. Studies clearly show that most patients seek help from psychoanalytically trained therapists primarily for (chronic) mood problems, often in combination with anxiety and personality problems.[24,25] In response, a substantial empirical tradition focusing on depression and its treatment has emerged within the psychoanalytic tradition.

THEORETICAL PERSPECTIVES
Historical Developments

Freud aptly described depression as a psychic wound or hemorrhage ("innere Verblutung"), a kind of "hole in the psyche" ("ein Loch im psychischen") that drains all energy of the individual.[26] From a psychoanalytic perspective, the core features of depression indeed refer to a problem related to desire, that is, the relationship of the individual to his wishes, ideals, and ambitions[27,28] or "wished-for state."[29] The depressed patient's complaints can be seen as indicative of a continuous and often very painful confrontation resulting from the gap between his ideals and ambitions, his wished-for state of the self and the actual state of the self. This may lead to feelings of helpless or hopelessness,[30] possibly explaining the typical feelings of anhormia (lack of drive) and anhedonia observed in depressed individuals. Yet, this state is also often accompanied by anxiety (anxious or agitated depression), and aggression toward the self or others. In Kleinian[31] and attachment-based[32] approaches, aggression toward the self and others (eg, because of self-criticism or disappointment) is seen as playing a prominent role in depression. Moreover, feelings of pain and exhaustion also typically color the clinical picture, as is also expressed in the high co-occurrence and comorbidity between depression, pain, and fatigue syndromes.[33] By contrast, in (hypo)manic states, which are almost the opposite of depression in terms of symptoms, the individual appears to be at one with his ego ideal.[34] Although these observations are still relevant clinically, traditional psychoanalytic theories of depression were often overspecified, lacked theoretical precision, and were too broad to be empirically tested.

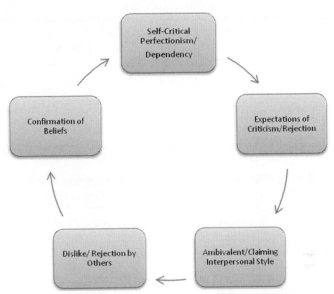

Fig. 1. Treatment focus: dysfunctional transactional styles associated with personality-related vulnerability for depression.

Personality and the Dynamics of Depression

In the early 1970s, Blatt[35] provided a view of depression that has been the basis for almost 40 years of empirical research and most contemporary psychodynamic approaches to depression.[11,14,20,36,37] Congruent with earlier psychoanalytic theorizing, he argued that in the phenomenologic experience of depression, 2 central issues can be identified: one relating to loneliness, feelings of neglect, and abandonment, the other to self-worth, responsibility, and guilt. As a result of this distinction, investigators from both the psychodynamic and cognitive–behavioral tradition have focused on 2 independent personality dimensions in depression,[35,38,39] an interpersonal dimension, reflecting high levels of dependency, and a self-critical dimension that involves extensive preoccupation with self-definition and autonomy. Beck,[38] from a cognitive-behavioral perspective, similarly distinguished sociotropy and autonomy, personality dimensions that, in the extreme, confer vulnerability for depression.

Considerable evidence indicates that the dependency and self-critical personality dimensions are associated with differences in the onset, course, and clinical expression of depression,[14,20,35] basic personality style,[11] relational and attachment style,[21,40] and current and early life experiences.[41,42] Perhaps most importantly, as discussed in the final section of this article, these 2 dimensions are also related to treatment response across different therapeutic modalities.[43]

Evidence also indicates that high levels of dependency and self-criticism are associated both with increased stress sensitivity and the generation of stress, particularly through so-called dysfunctional interpersonal transactional styles,[20,44,45] which often are the central focus in PT of depression (**Fig. 1**). These findings are particularly relevant given that stress and adversity play a major role in the causation of depression.[46,47]

Individuals with high levels of dependency or self-criticism tend to behave in ways that elicit particular responses from others. These reactions often confirm the individual's fear of rejection and abandonment or of disapproval, thereby creating a vicious cycle. For example, high levels of dependency have been associated with annoyance and resentment in others, eventually leading to rejection and abandonment, thereby confirming fears associated with high levels of dependency. Similarly, high levels of self-criticism are associated with ambivalence toward others because of fear of criticism and disapproval. Accordingly, others perceive these individuals as cold, competitive, and distant, confirming the highly self-critical individual's belief that others do not like and disapprove of them.

Attachment, Mentalization, and the Neurobiology of Depression

Attachment

Blatt's and Beck's models are conceptually and empirically linked to attachment theory,[20] fostering dialogue between psychoanalytic, developmental psychopathology, and neuroscience approaches to depression.[13,48] Contemporary research suggests that 2 dimensions, avoidance and anxiety, underlie attachment styles[49,50] and that these are conceptually related to Blatt's concepts of self-definition and relatedness, respectively. The attachment avoidance dimension refers to "discomfort with closeness and with discomfort depending on others"[49] and is typically associated with the use of attachment deactivation strategies. In times of distress, automatic unconscious strategies are activated that involve denying attachment needs and asserting one's own autonomy, independence, and strength. The attachment anxiety dimension, in contrast, involves "fear of rejection and abandonment."[49] In times of stress, the attachment system becomes hyperactivated leading to frantic attempts to find security, support, and relief, often expressed in demanding or clingy behavior.

Evidence from various strands of research support the key role of attachment in depression.[13] Vulnerability to depression is related to both attachment hyperactivation and deactivation strategies.[51,52] Insecure attachment has been shown to be prospectively related to recurrent depression and is associated with more depressive episodes and residual symptoms, longer use of antidepressants, greater impairments in social functioning,[53] and suicide.[54] As noted, early adversity, and disruptive attachment experiences in particular, play a central role in the causation of depression.[46] This may explain, at least in part, the role of increased responsivity to both daily and major life stressors in the causation and course of depression.[46,55] Furthermore, both animal[56–58] and human[59–61] research suggests that the neuropeptide oxytocin (and potentially also vasopressin), which is involved in neural systems underlying attachment,[56,62] plays a key role in stress regulation. This hormone is involved in affiliative behavior (eg, pair bonding, maternal care, and sexual behavior), social memory, and social support[63] and has stress-reducing and anxiolytic effects,[56] again indicating the close relationship between attachment history, depression, and anxiety.[48]

The emphasis on attachment in depression is further reinforced by findings on the role of impairments in social cognition, and mentalizing in particular, in depression.[2,64]

Mentalization

Mentalizing refers to the imaginative mental activity involving interpretation of the self and others in terms of mental states, such as feelings, desires, wishes, and goals. It enables us to navigate the social world and is typically acquired in the context of (early) attachment relationships. Impairments in mentalizing have been associated with depression, and they may, in part, underlie the interpersonal problems typically associated with this disorder (for a detailed review, see Luyten and coworkers[13]).

As well as having a causative role, it is likely that impairments in mentalizing also result from depression. Depressed mood impairs the capacity of an individual to reflect on both the self and others, and when he or she does mentalize, it is likely to be distorted. As a result, modes of thinking that antedate full mentalizing re-emerge that help understand the phenomenologic experience of depression. For example, in the psychic equivalence mode, psychological and physical pain and emotional and physical exhaustion are equated, possibly explaining the high comorbidity of pain, fatigue, and depression.[65,66] Psychological experiences are felt as too real; psychological pain means bodily pain, and criticism by others is felt as a physical attack on the integrity of the self. Findings on the common neural circuits underlying psychological and physical pain show that these experiences are closely intertwined; rejection literally hurts.[67] In the pretend mode, thoughts and feelings are severed from reality, which is typically expressed in overly detailed, highly cognitive, or affectively overwhelming narratives, often characterized by rumination, self-blame, or the relentless blaming of others. In the teleological mode, only observable behavior or material causes can be real. The patient can only feel loved if there is also a physical expression of love, which may lead to frantic attempts to elicit care and love from attachment figures, including the therapist (eg, demanding longer or more sessions or asking to be hugged or touched, which may lead to boundary violations). In this mode, suicidal thoughts and gestures often lead others, including professionals, to similarly revert to a teleological mode in an attempt to demonstrate love, care, and concern.

EFFICACY AND EFFECTIVENESS OF PSYCHODYNAMIC THERAPY FOR DEPRESSION

Over the last decades, a range of brief and long-term psychodynamically based treatments for depression have been empirically evaluated in children, adolescents, and adults. Although some of these treatments have been based on generic psychodynamic treatment principles,[68–73] others have been more explicitly rooted in extant psychodynamic findings concerning depression.[2,74] These treatments differ to the extent that they emphasize supportive and expressive techniques (although they all include elements of both) and whether their primary focus is interpersonal or intrapsychic. Despite these differences, as noted, these treatments have in common a focus on recurring patterns in feelings and relationships with the aim to increase the patient's insight into these patterns, so that he or she can change them.[8] Several recent reviews and meta-analyses have addressed their efficacy and effectiveness.[4,75,76] Below we critically review the findings.

Efficacy and Effectiveness of Psychodynamic Treatment Alone

A recent meta-analysis of 23 studies with a total of 1365 patients found that brief psychoanalytic therapy (BPT) for depression was associated with large symptom reductions (Cohen's $d = 1.34$) that were maintained at 1-year follow-up.[4] BPT was found superior to control conditions ($d = 0.69$). After treatment, BPT was slightly less effective than other psychotherapies ($d = 0.30$), yet these differences disappeared at 3- and 12-month follow-up ($d = 0.05$ and $d = 0.29$, respectively). Moreover, individual BPT ($d = 1.43$) was more effective compared with group BPT ($d = 0.83$) and was as effective as other individual psychotherapies after treatment ($d = 0.19$) and at 3- and 12-month follow-up ($d = 0.05$ and $d = 0.31$, respectively; all nonsignificant). These results are surprisingly good, given that in early trials, BPT was often included as a control condition.

The use of BPT as a control may also explain, in part, why some previous reviews found BPT to be inferior to other therapies, including cognitive behavioral treatment (CBT). In the meta-analysis by Gloaguen and colleagues,[77] for example, Wampold and coworkers[5] found that once non–bona fide therapies were removed, superiority of CBT over other therapies could no longer be demonstrated. A recent meta-analysis of RCTs comparing the efficacy of BPT to CBT in major depressive disorder, similarly found no differences in changes in depressive and general psychiatric symptoms nor social functioning.[78]

Specific types of depression and BPT

Reviews and meta-analyses focusing on specific types of depression and related conditions similarly support the efficacy and effectiveness of BPT. Abbass and colleagues[79] recently presented a meta-analysis of BPT in patients with depression and comorbid personality disorder, showing moderate to large effect sizes that were maintained at treatment follow-up. These findings are important, as estimates of comorbidity between major depression and personality disorder typically range between 35% and 65%.[80] Maina and colleagues[81] compared the efficacy of BPT, brief supportive therapy (ST), and a wait-list condition (WL) in the treatment of minor depressive disorder. Both BPT and ST were superior to the WL at treatment termination, and BPT was superior to ST at 6-month follow-up. In one RCT focusing on pathologic grief, it was found that group BPT was superior to a WL control group.[82] In a second RCT of this group, there was a patient–treatment interaction; patients with high quality of object relationships showed greater improvement with regard to grief symptoms in insight-oriented BPT, whereas those with low-level object relations showed greater gains in supportive BPT.[83] These findings are congruent with those from studies showing that patients with lower levels of personality organization may benefit more from treatments with a greater emphasis on supportive interventions.[84] Yet, for general symptoms, insight-oriented BPT was superior regardless of level of object relations.

Although BPT is highly effective for a considerable subgroup of patients suffering from depressive disorders, a substantial proportion do not improve, as is the case with other brief treatment.[85] Recent studies suggest that only about 50% of depressed patients show a response to brief treatment and that relapse figures can be as high as 75%.[19,20,85,86] A recent follow-up study found that 42% of patients treated with BPT for depression had a recurrence within a 5-year time span, which is similar to findings in follow-up studies of other brief psychological treatments, such as CBT.[87]

Long-term perspective in depression treatment

Current treatment guidelines, therefore, emphasize the role of a long-term perspective in the management of depression, stressing continuation and maintenance treatment, with a focus on relapse prevention.[85] In this context, studies concerning longer-term psychoanalytic treatment (LTPT) are highly relevant, as LTPT focuses on patients suffering from chronic mood problems, which often result from a combination of depression, anxiety, and significant personality and relational problems. Studies by Knekt and colleagues[88,89] are particularly pertinent in this context. They conducted an RCT comparing BPT, LTPT, and solution-focused therapy in 326 patients with depressive and anxiety disorders. During the first year, BPT was superior to LTPT, during the second year there were no differences between these treatments, and at 3-year follow-up LTPT outperformed both BPT and solution-focused therapy, with no differences between the latter 2 treatments. These findings are consistent with the assumption that LTPT is characterized by a slower rate of change compared with brief treatment (probably because it focuses less on symptomatic improvement), but is associated with more lasting, and perhaps broader, changes. In the next section, we discuss evidence suggesting that LTPT may be associated with greater changes in underlying vulnerabilities than BPT.

More generally, recent meta-analyses have found evidence for the efficacy and effectiveness of LTPT for patients with so-called "complex" disorders, often including previously unsuccessfully treated (chronic) depressed patients with considerable personality comorbidity.[25,90] Similarly, there is some evidence for the effectiveness of psychoanalysis in the treatment of this group.[89] (de Maat S, De Jonghe F, de Kraker R, et al. The effectiveness of psychoanalysis: a comparison between psychoanalysis (PA) and long-term psychoanalytic psychotherapy (LTPP). Manuscript submitted for publication, 2010.) Importantly, both LTPT and psychoanalysis have been associated with continuing improvement after treatment termination, suggesting that they are associated with changes in vulnerability to depression.[91]

Summary: BPT and LTPT for depression treatment

Overall, findings suggest that BPT should be included in guidelines as a first-line treatment for patients suffering from depressive disorders.[75] LTPT and perhaps psychoanalysis should be considered for patients suffering from complex conditions characterized by (chronic) mood and personality problems. None of the meta-analyses reviewed found differences in effect sizes between controlled trials and naturalistic studies, suggesting that PT for depression can be translated to routine clinical practice without loss of its effects. Future research should concentrate on the cost effectiveness of both BPT and LTPT. A recent review of 8 studies showed that BPT was consistently associated with a significant decrease compared with control conditions in health care costs as expressed in lower physician and hospital costs, reduced medication usage and disability claims, and increases in the proportion of patients returning to work. (Abbass A, Driessen E, Town J. Cost-effectiveness of intensive short-term dynamic psychotherapy. Manuscript submitted for publication, 2011.) More studies focusing on the cost effectiveness of BPT and LTPT in the treatment of depression are needed.

Psychodynamic Psychotherapy and Pharmacotherapy

The evidence base of research comparing the efficacy and effectiveness of PT, pharmacotherapy, and their combination is still relatively limited. Yet, studies in this area seem to be consistent with meta-analyses suggesting few differences in the effects of bona fide psychotherapeutic treatments and pharmacotherapy in the acute treatment of depression and that psychotherapy and combined treatment are associated with better (long-term) outcome.[6,92]

A mega-analysis of 3 RCTs found that BPT was as effective as pharmacotherapy in terms of symptom reduction based on the Hamilton Rating Scale, but patients and therapists considered the effects of BPT to be superior compared with pharmacotherapy.[74] Because this conclusion is based on studies investigating psychodynamic-supportive psychotherapy, results may not generalize to other brief PT. Salminen and colleagues[93] compared a more expressive variant of BPT and fluoxetine in a trial of 51 patients with major depression and found no differences in terms of symptoms and functional ability. BPT was not manualized in this study, so it is possible that therapists differed considerably in their adherence to the therapeutic model. Moreover, follow-up analyses showed that patients with high levels of immature defense styles benefited more from BPT than fluoxetine, suggesting that BPT may be superior to pharmacotherapy when addressing depression in patients with fewer psychologic resources and more severe character pathology.[94] One study found that pharmacotherapy was associated with a more rapid response compared with BPT, but this difference largely disappeared after 8 weeks.[95]

In a small trial (n = 35), Maina and colleagues[96] found that the combination of BPT with pharmacotherapy was superior to the combination of pharmacotherapy with ST. In another study, Maina and collaborators[97] followed up patients that had remission after a trial with either a combination of BPT and medication or medication alone. Remission rates in both conditions were identical (64.1% vs 61.4%, respectively). All patients subsequently received a 6-month continuation treatment with medication alone. At the 48-month follow-up, patients who received the combined treatment, however, showed significantly lower recurrence rates than patients in the medication-alone condition (27.5% vs 46.9%, respectively).

A mega-analysis of 3 RCTs of brief psychodynamic-supportive treatment found that combined treatment was more efficacious than pharmacotherapy alone.[74] Interestingly, again, rates of change were somewhat slower in BPT compared with pharmacotherapy. Finally, Burnand and colleagues[98] found that combined treatment was associated with fewer treatment failures, better work adjustment, better global functioning, and lower hospitalization rates. The costs of psychotherapy were offset by fewer hospitalizations and lost work days in patients receiving the combined treatment.

Although more research is needed, current evidence suggests that BPT is as effective as pharmacotherapy for mild to moderate depression and that combined treatment is more effective and cost effective. Studies show similar findings in patients with comorbid anxiety and depression.[99,100] Moreover, there are also indications that combined treatment is more acceptable to patients than mono-therapy.[101] More long-term follow-up studies are needed. A recent follow-up study, for instance, found no differences in recurrence of depression at 5-year follow-up between BPT alone and combined treatment.[87]

Psychodynamic Therapy in Children and Adolescents

There has been less research on the effectiveness of psychodynamic therapy for children and adolescents than there has been for adults. A recent review, however, provides evidence for both BPT and LTPT in the treatment of young people suffering from various emotional disorders, including depression.[102] Yet, only 2 naturalistic studies[73,103] and 1 randomized trial[104] have specifically targeted children and adolescents with depression as the primary problem. Although this is in line with the more person-centered rather than disorder-focused approach, and children and adolescents do tend to present with a variety of emotional and behavioral problems, more studies of PT that specifically focus on depression are needed. In a study by Trowell and coworkers,[104] depressed adolescents improved more slowly with BPT but made more sustained changes compared with those receiving family therapy. This finding parallels the research focusing on adults with depression who had been treated with PT; results showed slower rates of change but maintenance of effects and even posttreatment improvement. More research in this area is needed. Several ongoing trials, including a trial comparing BPT and CBT in the treatment of adolescent depression,[3] promise to fill this critical gap in our knowledge.

PROCESS AND OUTCOME OF PSYCHODYNAMIC TREATMENT

Little is known about the mutative factors in the range of evidence-based treatments for depression, including PT. Several studies, however, have begun to elucidate those ingredients that promote change. Hilsenroth and colleagues,[105] for instance, using the Comparative Psychotherapy Rating Scale, found a strong association between psychodynamic–interpersonal technique and change in depressive symptoms ($r=.57$, $P<.01$) in patients treated with BPT. Conversely, studies have found that the extent to which psychodynamic techniques were used in other treatments was correlated with good outcome (for an overview, see Shedler[106]). Yet, much more research is needed in this context, particularly as patient, therapist, and alliance factors (and their interactions) may explain more variance in outcome than specific techniques, particularly in brief treatments.

Self-Critical Perfectionism

Blatt and colleagues,[43] for instance, found that self-critical perfectionism, a personality dimension that, as noted, is related to the onset and course of depression, negatively predicted treatment outcome in CBT, Interpersonal Psychotherapy (IPT), and pharmacotherapy in the National Institute of Mental Health Treatment of Depression Collaborative Research Program (TDCRP). Pretreatment levels of self-critical perfectionism were also associated with lower enhanced adaptive capacities, that is, the capacity to manage life stress, at 18-month follow-up, which may explain in part the negative effect of self-critical perfectionism on long-term outcome in this study. Importantly, further analyses showed that pretreatment self-critical perfectionism significantly interfered with therapeutic outcome in the TDCRP by disrupting the development of the therapeutic alliance as well as patients' general social relationships, which left them more vulnerable to stressful life events. Decreases in self-critical perfectionism were significantly associated with a decline in symptoms of depression, which provides further evidence for the role of patient factors in the treatment of depression. More specifically, in the TDCRP, the strength of the therapeutic alliance was significantly associated with changes in self-critical perfectionism, which, in turn, significantly influenced the reduction of depressive symptoms.[107] These findings suggest that the lack of sustained therapeutic gain in the TDCRP may have been the consequence of the failure to address the personality factors involved in vulnerability for depression in all treatment conditions, which then, in turn, negatively affected the therapeutic alliance and, ultimately, treatment outcome. Yet, compared with medication, the 2 psychotherapies (ie, CBT and IPT) led to significantly greater enhanced adaptive capacities and a significantly greater reduction of stress reactivity,[108] which may provide a partial explanation for the superiority of psychotherapy compared with medication in the prevention of relapse of depression.

The negative impact of self-critical perfectionism on outcome in brief treatments has now been replicated in a number of studies.[13,43] The typically externally imposed time-limited treatment may interfere with the strong need for autonomy and control associated with self-critical perfectionism.[109] Patients with these features may also have more difficulty accepting an interpersonal focus,[110] and they may be unable to form a positive therapeutic alliance in such a short timeframe.[43] More generally, in some patients, brief treatments (including BPT), may be associated with relatively high relapse rates because they do not lead to changes in vulnerability factors for depression but only result in a deactivation of maladaptive representations of self and others that are relatively easily re-activated when confronted with stress and adversity.[91] By contrast, LTPT and PA are typically associated with more profound changes as expressed in[106,111]:

1. Increased capacity for self-analysis
2. Ability to experiment with new behaviors, particularly in interpersonal relationships
3. Finding pleasure in new challenges
4. Greater tolerance for negative affect
5. Greater insight into how the past may determine the present

6. Use of self-calming and self-supportive strategies, among which is the use of the representation of the therapist as a supportive good internal object.

Yet, more research that specifically focuses on depression is needed, and studies are needed that investigate whether such changes are causally related to sustained symptom reduction in both brief and long-term treatments.

ACCEPTABILITY AND SUITABILITY OF PSYCHODYNAMIC TREATMENT

BPT is readily accepted by many depressed patients.[2] Patients often prefer combination treatment over medication alone[101] and BPT over pharmacotherapy.[112] Similarly, a study in Germany suggests that LTPT and PA are well accepted by many (chronic) depressed patients and even preferred by at least a substantial subgroup of depressed patients over cognitive behavioral treatment.[113] Yet, cultural factors are likely to determine patient preference.

As for suitability for PT, clinical decision making is seriously hampered by our lack of understanding of therapeutic mechanisms. Clinical lore emphasizes the importance of psychological mindedness, a wish to target the treatment beyond symptom reduction and an openness to consider the antecedents and particularly the relational contexts of current problems.[114] Yet, whether these features are associated with better treatment outcome remains to be investigated, particularly given the broadening scope of PT to more characterologically disturbed patients. Interestingly, in a study by Van and colleagues,[112] there were no differences in outcome after BPT for depression between randomized and by-preference patients. These findings contrast somewhat with findings by Watzke and colleagues[115] that provides some validation for clinical judgment in relation to suitability for psychodynamic psychotherapy. This study also highlights the potential negative effects of unselected assignment to PT and possible iatrogenic factors, at least of PT as practiced in routine clinical care.[114] Basically, Watzke and colleagues[115] found that patients whom clinicians considered suited for PT had better outcome compared with patients who were randomly assigned to PT. No such effect was found for CBT, with patients whom clinicians originally considered to be suited for PT showing similar improvement when they were randomly assigned to CBT compared with patients that initially were considered more suited for CBT. These findings suggest potential limitations in terms of suitability of patients for PT. Yet, they may also suggest limitations of the particular psychoanalytic treatment model that was investigated in this study. More systematic treatment delivery and the ongoing monitoring of intermediate treatment outcomes may lead to improved outcome also in patients that are often considered to be less suited for PT. Moreover, whether these results generalize to depressed patients and all types of PT is unknown. A recent trial in Germany is currently exploring whether randomization versus preference for PT is related to outcome in the long-term psychodynamic treatment of depression.[113]

SUMMARY

Findings reviewed in this article show that PT should be included in treatment guidelines for depression. BPT in particular has been found to be superior to control conditions, equally effective as other active psychological treatments, with treatment effects that are often maintained in the long run, conferring resistance to relapse. Moreover, BPT is as effective as pharmacotherapy in the acute treatment of mild to moderate depression, and, either as monotherapy or combined with medication, BPT is associated with better long-term outcome compared with pharmacotherapy alone. PT is accepted by many depressed patients as a viable and preferred treatment. Furthermore, LTPT and PA have shown promise in treating patients with complex psychological disorders characterized by mood problems, often with comorbid personality problems. Finally, although studies suggest that effects of PT may be achieved somewhat slower compared with other forms of psychotherapy[116] as well as medication[95] in the acute treatment of depression, LTPT appears to be more clinically effective and perhaps more cost effective in the long run, particularly for chronically depressed patients.

As noted, these conclusions need to be interpreted within the context of important limitations. Compared with other treatments, the evidence base for PT in depression remains relatively small, despite a respectable research tradition supporting psychodynamic assumptions with regard to the causation of depression.[64] Moreover, and perhaps most importantly, although more studies now include longer follow-up assessments, our knowledge about the long-term effects of so-called evidence-based treatments of depression remains sketchy at best. In this context, the growing evidence for the efficacy and effectiveness of LTPT is promising.

Overall, it is clear that the future of the treatment of depression may lie in a combined disorder- and person-centered, tailored-made approach, which takes into account, particularly in chronic depression, the broader interpersonal context and life history of the individual. It is clear that psychodynamic therapies have an important role to play in this respect.

ACKNOWLEDGMENTS

The authors wish to thank David L. Mintz and Allan Abbass for constructive comments on an earlier version of this paper and Rose Palmer for her editorial assistance.

REFERENCES

1. Luyten P, Blatt SJ. Psychodynamic approaches of depression: whither shall we go? Psychiatry 2011;74(1):1–3.
2. Lemma A, Target M, Fonagy P. The development of a brief psychodynamic intervention (dynamic interpersonal therapy) and its application to depression: a pilot study. Psychiatry 2011;74(1):41–8.
3. Goodyer I, Tsancheva S, Byford S, et al. Improving mood with psychoanalytic and cognitive therapies (IMPACT): a pragmatic effectiveness superiority trial to investigate whether specialised psychological treatment reduces the risk for relapse in adolescents with moderate to severe unipolar depression: study protocol for a randomised controlled trial. Trials 2011;12(1):175.
4. Driessen E, Cuijpers P, de Maat SCM, et al. The efficacy of short-term psychodynamic psychotherapy for depression: a meta-analysis. Clin Psychol Rev 2010;30(1): 25–36.
5. Wampold BE, Minami T, Baskin TW, et al. A meta-(re)analysis of the effects of cognitive therapy versus 'other therapies' for depression. J Affect Disord 2002; 68(2–3):159–65.
6. Cuijpers P, Van Straten A, Van Oppen P, et al. Are psychological and pharmacologic interventions equally effective in the treatment of adult depressive disorders? A meta-analysis of comparative studies. J Clin Psychiatry 2008;69(11):1675–85.
7. Lambert MJ, Barley DE. Research summary on the therapeutic relationship and psychotherapy outcome. In: Norcross JC, editor. Psychotherapy relationships that work. Oxford: Oxford University Press; 2002. p. 17–32.
8. Blagys M, Hilsenroth M. Distinctive features of short-term psychodynamic-interpersonal psychotherapy: a review of the comparative psychotherapy process-literature. Clinical Psychology: Science and Practice 2000;7:167–88.

9. Lemma A, Roth AD, Pilling S. The competencies required to deliver effective psychoanalytic/psychodynamic therapy. London: University College London, UK; 2009.

10. Luyten P, Mayes LC, Target M, et al. Developmental research. In: Gabbard GO, Litowitz B, Williams P, editors. The American psychiatric publishing textbook of psychoanalysis. 2nd edition. Washington, DC: American Psychiatric Press; in press.

11. Blatt SJ, Luyten P. A structural-developmental psychodynamic approach to psychopathology: two polarities of experience across the life span. Dev Psychopathol 2009;21(3):793–814.

12. Blatt SJ, Luyten P. Depression as an evolutionary conserved mechanism to terminate separation-distress: only part of the biopsychosocial story? [Commentary on Watt & Panksepp]. Neuropsychoanalysis 2009;11:52–61.

13. Luyten P, Fonagy P, Lemma A, et al. Depression. In: Bateman A, Fonagy P, editors. Handbook of mentalizing in mental health practice Washington, DC: American Psychiatric Association; 2012. p. 385–417.

14. Blatt SJ. Experiences of depression: theoretical, clinical and research perspectives. Washington, DC: American Psychological Association; 2004.

15. Gunnar M, Quevedo K. The Neurobiology of stress and development. Annu Rev Psychol 2007;58(1):145–73.

16. Lupien SJ, McEwen BS, Gunnar MR, et al. Effects of stress throughout the lifespan on the brain, behaviour and cognition. Nat Rev Neurosci 2009;10(6):434–45.

17. Champagne FA, Curley JP. Epigenetic mechanisms mediating the long-term effects of maternal care on development. Neurosci Biobehav Rev 2009;33(4):593–600.

18. Balint M. New beginning and the paranoid and the depressive syndromes. Int J Psychoanal 1952;33:214–24.

19. Luyten P, Blatt SJ. Looking back towards the future: is it time to change the DSM approach to psychiatric disorders? The case of depression. Psychiatry 2007;70(2): 85–99.

20. Luyten P, Blatt SJ, Van Houdenhove B, et al. Depression research and treatment: are we skating to where the puck is going to be? Clin Psychol Rev 2006;26(8): 985–99.

21. Luyten P, Blatt SJ. Integrating theory-driven and empirically-derived models of personality development and psychopathology: a proposal for DSM-V. Clin Psychol Rev 2011;31:52–68.

22. Parker G. Beyond major depression. Psychol Med 2005;35:467–74.

23. Slade T. Taxometric investigation of depression: evidence of consistent latent structure across clinical and community samples. Aust N Z J Psychiatry 2007;41(5):403–10.

24. Doidge N, Simon B, Lancee WJ, et al. Psychoanalytic patients in the U.S., Canada, and Australia: II. A DSM-III-R Validation Study. J Am Psychoanal Assoc 2002;50(2):615–27.

25. Leichsenring F, Rabung S. Long-term psychodynamic psychotherapy in complex mental disorders: update of a meta-analysis. Br J Psychiatry 2011;199(1):15–22.

26. Freud S. The complete letters of Sigmund Freud to Wilhelm Fliess: 1887–1904. Cambridge (MA): Harvard University Press; 1985.

27. Freud S. On narcissism: an introduction. In: Strachey J, editor. The standard edition of the complete psychological works of Sigmund Freud. London: Hogarth Press; 1914. p. 67–104.

28. Freud S. Mourning and melancholia. In: Strachey J, editor. The standard edition of the complete psychological works of Sigmund Freud. London: Hogarth Press; 1915. p. 237–58.

29. Sandler J. From safety to the superego: selected papers of Joseph Sandler. New York: Guilford Press; 1987.

30. Bibring E. The mechanism of depression. In: Greenacre P, editor. Affective disorders. New York: International Universities Press; 1953. p. 13–48.
31. Klein M. A contribution to the psychogenesis of manic-depressive states. The writings of Melanie Klein, vol. I: Love, guilt and reparation. London: Hogarth Press (1975); 1935. p. 236–89.
32. Bowlby J. Attachment and loss: separation. New York: Basic Books; 1973.
33. Luyten P, Van Houdenhove B. Common versus specific factors in the psychotherapeutic treatment of patients suffering from chronic fatigue and pain disorders. Journal of Psychotherapy Integration, in press.
34. Freud S. Group psychology and the analysis of the ego. In: Strachey J, editor. The standard edition of the complete psychological works of Sigmund Freud. London: Hogarth Press; 1921. p. 69–143.
35. Blatt SJ. Levels of object representation in anaclitic and introjective depression. The Psychoanalytic Study of the Child 1974;29:107–57.
36. Blatt SJ, Zuroff DC. Interpersonal relatedness and self-definition: two prototypes for depression. Clin Psychol Rev 1992;12:527–62.
37. Zuroff DC, Mongrain M, Santor DA. Conceptualizing and measuring personality vulnerability to depression: commentary on Coyne and Whiffen (1995). Psychol Bull 2004;130:453–72.
38. Beck AT. Cognitive therapy of depression: new perspectives. In: Clayton PJ, Barrett JE, editors. Treatment of depression: old controversies and new approaches. New York: Raven Press; 1983. p. 265–90.
39. Arieti S, Bemporad J. Psychotherapy of severe and mild depression. Northvale (NJ): Jason Aronson; 1978.
40. Luyten P, Corveleyn J, Blatt SJ. The convergence among psychodynamic and cognitive-behavioral theories of depression: a critical overview of empirical research. In: Corveleyn J, Luyten P, Blatt SJ, editors. The theory and treatment of depression: towards a dynamic interactionism model. Mahwah (NJ): Lawrence Erlbaum Associates; 2005. p. 107–47.
41. Blatt SJ, Homann E. Parent-child interaction in the etiology of dependent and self-critical depression. Clin Psychol Rev 1992;12:47–91.
42. Soenens B, Vansteenkiste M, Luyten P. Towards a domain-specific approach to the study of parental psychological control: distinguishing between dependency-oriented and achievement-oriented psychological control. J Pers 2010;78(1):217–56.
43. Blatt SJ, Zuroff DC, Hawley LL, et al. Predictors of sustained therapeutic change. Psychother Res 2010;20:37–54.
44. Shahar G, Priel B. Active vulnerability, adolescent distress, and the mediating/suppressing role of life events. Pers Indiv Diff 2003;35(1):199–218.
45. Luyten P, Kempke S, Van Wambeke P, et al. Self-critical perfectionism, stress generation and stress sensitivity in patients with chronic fatigue syndrome: relationship with severity of depression. Psychiatry 2011;74(1):21–30.
46. Heim C, Newport DJ, Mletzko T, et al. The link between childhood trauma and depression: Insights from HPA axis studies in humans. Psychoneuroendocrinology 2008;33(6):693–710.
47. Hammen C. Stress and depression. Ann Rev Clin Psychol 2005;1(1):293–319.
48. Panksepp J, Watt D. Why does depression hurt? Ancestral primary-process separation-distress (PANIC/GRIEF) and diminished brain reward (SEEKING) processes in the genesis of depressive affect. Psychiatry 2011;74(1):5–13.
49. Mikulincer M, Shaver PR. Attachment in adulthood: Structure, dynamics and change. New York: The Guilford Press; 2007.

50. Roisman GI, Holland A, Fortuna K, et al. The adult attachment interview and self-reports of attachment style: an empirical rapprochement. J Pers Soc Psychol 2007;92(4):678–97.

51. Bifulco A, Moran PM, Ball C, et al. Adult attachment style. I: Its relationship to clinical depression. Soc Psychiatry Psychiatr Epidemiol 2002;37:50–9.

52. Bifulco A, Moran PM, Ball C, et al. Adult attachment style. II: Its relationship to psychosocial depressive-vulnerability. Soc Psychiatry Psychiatr Epidemiol 2002;37:60–7.

53. Conradi HJ, de Jonge P. Recurrent depression and the role of adult attachment: a prospective and a retrospective study. J Affect Disord 2009;116(1–2):93–9.

54. Grunebaum MF, Galfalvy HC, Mortenson LY, et al. Attachment and social adjustment: relationships to suicide attempt and major depressive episode in a prospective study. J Affect Disord 2010;123(1–3):123–30.

55. Wichers M, Geschwind N, Jacobs N, et al. Transition from stress sensitivity to a depressive state: longitudinal twin study. Br J Psychiatry 2009;195(6):498–503.

56. Neumann ID. Brain oxytocin: a key regulator of emotional and social behaviours in both females and males. J Neuroendocrinol 2008;20(6):858–65.

57. Carter CS, Grippo AJ, Pournajafi-Nazarloo H, et al. Oxytocin, vasopressin and sociality. Prog Brain Res 2008;170:331–6.

58. DeVries AC, Craft TKS, Glasper ER, et al. Social influences on stress responses and health. Psychoneuroendocrinology 2007;32(6):587–603.

59. Heinrichs M, Domes G. Neuropeptides and social behaviour: effects of oxytocin and vasopressin in humans. Prog Brain Res 2008;170:337–50.

60. Gordon I, Zagoory-Sharon O, Schneiderman I, et al. Oxytocin and cortisol in romantically unattached young adults: associations with bonding and psychological distress. Psychophysiology 2008;45 (3):349–52.

61. Levine A, Zagoory-Sharon O, Feldman R, et al. Oxytocin during pregnancy and early postpartum: individual patterns and maternal-fetal attachment. Peptides 2007;28 (6):1162–9.

62. Insel T, Young L. The neurobiology of attachment. Nat Rev Neurosci 2001;2:129–36.

63. Feldman R, Weller A, Zagoory-Sharon O, et al. Evidence for a neuroendocrinological foundation of human affiliation: plasma oxytocin levels across pregnancy and the postpartum period predict mother-infant bonding. Psychol Sci 2007;18(11):965–70.

64. Luyten P, Fonagy P, Lemma A, et al. Mentalizing and depression. In: Bateman A, Fonagy P, editors. Mentalizing in mental health practice. Washington, DC: American Psychiatric Association; in press.

65. Hudson JI, Arnold LM, Keck PE Jr, et al. Family study of fibromyalgia and affective spectrum disorder. Biol Psychiatry 2004;56(11):884–91.

66. Van Houdenhove B, Luyten P. Customizing treatment of chronic fatigue syndrome and fibromyalgia: the role of perpetuating factors. Psychosomatics 2008;49(6):470–7.

67. Eisenberger NI, Lieberman MD, Williams KD. Does rejection hurt? An FMRI study of social exclusion. Science 2003;302(5643):290–2.

68. Davanloo H, editor. Short-term dynamic psychotherapy. New York: Jason Aronson; 1980.

69. Malan DH. A study of brief psychotherapy. New York: Plenum Press; 1963.

70. Mann J. Time-limited psychotherapy. Cambridge, MA: Harvard University Press; 1973.

71. Sifneos PE. Short-term dynamic psychotherapy: evaluation and technique. New York: Plenum Press; 1979.

72. Strupp HH, Binder JL. Psychotherapy in a new key: a guide to time-limited dynamic psychotherapy. New York: Basic Books; 1984.
73. Target M, Fonagy P. The efficacy of psychoanalysis for children: prediction of outcome in a developmental context. J Am Acad Child Adolesc Psychiatry 1994;33: 1134–44.
74. de Maat S, Dekker J, Schoevers R, et al. Short psychodynamic supportive psychotherapy, antidepressants, and their combination in the treatment of major depression: a mega-analysis based on three randomized clinical trials. Depression and Anxiety 2008;25(7):565–74.
75. Abbass A, Driessen E. The efficacy of short-term psychodynamic psychotherapy for depression: a summary of recent findings. Acta Psychiatr Scand 2010;121(5):398.
76. Lewis AJ, Dennerstein M, Gibbs PM. Short-term psychodynamic psychotherapy: review of recent process and outcome studies. Aust N Z J Psychiatry 2008;42: 445–55.
77. Gloaguen V, Cottraux J, Cucherat M, et al. A meta-analysis of the effects of cognitive therapy in depressed patients. J Affect Disord 1998;49(1):59–72.
78. Leichsenring F, Kruse J, Rabung S. Efficacy of psychodynamic psychotherapy in specific mental disorders: a 2010 update. In: Luyten P, Mayes LC, Fonagy P, et al, editors. Contemporary psychodynamic approaches to psychopathology. New York: The Guilford Press; in press.
79. Abbass A, Town J, Driessen E. The efficacy of short-term psychodynamic psychotherapy for depressive disorders with comorbid personality disorder. Psychiatry: Interpersonal and Biological Processes 2011;74(1):58–71.
80. Mulder RT. Personality pathology and treatment outcome in major depression: a review. Am J Psychiatry 2002;159(3):359–71.
81. Maina G, Forner F, Bogetto F. Randomized controlled trial comparing brief dynamic and supportive therapy with waiting list condition in minor depressive disorders. Psychother Psychosom 2005;74(1):43–50.
82. McCallum M, Piper WE. A controlled study of the effectiveness and patient suitability for short-term group psychotherapy. Int J Group Psychother 1990;40:431–52.
83. Piper WE, McCallum M, Joyce AS, et al. Patient personality and time-limited group psychotherapy for complicated grief. Int J Group Psychother 2001;51:525–52.
84. Koelen J, Luyten P, Eurelings-Bontekoe EH, et al. The impact of personality organization on treatment response: a systematic review. Psychiatry, in press.
85. Cuijpers P, van Straten A, Bohlmeijer E, et al. The effects of psychotherapy for adult depression are overestimated: a meta-analysis of study quality and effect size. Psychol Med 2010;40(2):211–23.
86. Westen D, Novotny CM, Thompson-Brenner H. The empirical status of empirically supported psychotherapies: assumptions, findings, and reporting in controlled clinical trials. Psychol Bull 2004;130(4):631–63.
87. Koppers D, Peen J, Niekerken S, et al. Prevalence and risk factors for recurrence of depression five years after short term psychodynamic therapy. J Affect Disord 2011;134:468–72.
88. Knekt P, Lindfors O, Härkänen T, et al. Randomized trial on the effectiveness of long-and short-term psychodynamic psychotherapy and solution-focused therapy on psychiatric symptoms during a 3-year follow-up. Psychol Med 2008;38(05):689–703.
89. Knekt P, Lindfors O, Laaksonen MA, et al. Quasi-experimental study on the effectiveness of psychoanalysis, long-term and short-term psychotherapy on psychiatric symptoms, work ability and functional capacity during a 5-year follow-up. J Affect Disord 2011;132(1):37–47.

90. Leichsenring F, Rabung S. Effectiveness of long-term psychodynamic psychotherapy: a meta-analysis. JAMA 2008;300(13):1551–65.

91. Luyten P, Blatt SJ, Mayes LC. Process and outcome in psychoanalytic psychotherapy research: the need for a (relatively) new paradigm. In: Levy RA, Ablon JS, Kächele H, editors. Handbook of evidence-based psychodynamic psychotherapy bridging the gap between science and practice. 2nd edition. New York: Humana Press/Springer; in press.

92. Cuijpers P, Dekker J, Hollon SD, et al. Adding psychotherapy to pharmacotherapy in the treatment of depressive disorders in adults: a meta-analysis. J Clin Psychiatry 2009;70(9):1219–29.

93. Salminen J, Karlsson H, Hietala J, et al. Short-term psychodynamic psychotherapy and fluoxetine in major depressive disorder: a randomized comparative study. Psychother Psychosom 2008;77(6):351–7.

94. Kronström K, Salminen JK, Hietala J, et al. Does defense style or psychological mindedness predict treatment response in major depression? Depression and Anxiety 2009;26(7):689–95.

95. Dekker JJM, Koelen JA, Van HL, et al. Speed of action: the relative efficacy of short psychodynamic supportive psychotherapy and pharmacotherapy in the first 8 weeks of a treatment algorithm for depression. J Affect Disord 2008;109:183–8.

96. Maina G, Rosso G, Crespi C, et al. Combined brief dynamic therapy and pharmacotherapy in the treatment of major depressive disorder: a pilot study. Psychother Psychosom 2007;76(5):298–305.

97. Maina G, Rosso G, Bogetto F. Brief dynamic therapy combined with pharmacotherapy in the treatment of major depressive disorder: long-term results. J Affect Disord 2009;114(1):200–7.

98. Burnand Y, Andreoli A, Kolatte E, et al. Psychodynamic psychotherapy and clomipramine in the treatment of major depression. Psychiatr Serv 2002;53(5):585–90.

99. Bressi C, Porcellana M, Marinaccio PM, et al. Short-term psychodynamic psychotherapy versus treatment as usual for depressive and anxiety disorders: a randomized clinical trial of efficacy. J Nerv Ment Dis 2010;198(9):647–52.

100. Martini B, Rosso G, Chiodelli DF, et al. Brief dynamic therapy combined with pharmacotherapy in the treatment of panic disorder with concurrent depressive symptoms. Clin Neuropsychiatry 2011;8(3):204–11.

101. de Jonghe F, Kool S, van Aalst G, et al. Combining psychotherapy and antidepressants in the treatment of depression. J Affect Disord 2001;64(2–3):217–29.

102. Midgley N, Kennedy E. Psychodynamic psychotherapy for children and adolescents: a critical review of the evidence base. J Child Psychother 2011;37(3):1–29.

103. Horn H, Geiser-Elze A, Reck C, et al. Efficacy of psychodynamic short-term psychotherapy for children and adolescents with depression. Prax Kinderpsychol Kinderpsychiatr 2005;54(7):578–97.

104. Trowell J, Joffe I, Campbell J, et al. Childhood depression: a place for psychotherapy. An outcome study comparing individual psychodynamic psychotherapy and family therapy. Eur Child Adolesc Psychiatry 2007;16(3):157–67.

105. Hilsenroth M, Ackerman SJ, Blagys MD, et al. Short-term psychodynamic psychotherapy for depression: an examination of statistical, clinically significant, and technique-specific change. J Nerv Ment Dis 2003;191(6):349–57.

106. Shedler J. The efficacy of psychodynamic psychotherapy. Am Psychol 2010;65(2): 98–109.

107. Hawley LL, Ho M-HR, Zuroff DC, et al. The relationship of perfectionism, depression, and therapeutic alliance during treatment for depression: latent difference score analysis. J Consult Clin Psychol 2006;74(5):930–42.

108. Hawley LL, Ho M-HR, Zuroff DC, et al. Stress reactivity following brief treatment for depression: differential effects of psychotherapy and medication. J Consult Clin Psychol 2007;75(2):244–56.

109. Reis S, Grenyer BFS. Fearful attachment, working alliance and treatment response for individuals with major depression. Clinical Psychol Psychother 2004;11:414–24.

110. McBride C, Atkinson L, Quilty LC, et al. Attachment as moderator of treatment outcome in major depression: a randomized control trial of interpersonal psychotherapy versus cognitive behavior therapy. J Consult Clin Psychol 2006; 74(6):1041–54.

111. Falkenstrom F, Grant J, Broberg J, et al. Self-analysis and post-termination improvement after psychoanalysis and long-term psychotherapy. J Am Psychoanal Assoc 2007;55(2):629–74.

112. Van HL, Dekker J, Koelen J, et al. Patient preference compared with random allocation in short-term psychodynamic supportive psychotherapy with indicated addition of pharmacotherapy for depression. Psychother Res 2009;19:205–12.

113. Leuzinger-Bohleber M. Zum Stand der LAC Depressionsstudie. Mitgliederversammlung der DGPT. Halle, Germany; 2011.

114. Fonagy P. Psychotherapy research: do we know what works for whom? Br J Psychiatry 2010;197(2):83–5.

115. Watzke B, Rüddel H, Jürgensen R, et al. Effectiveness of systematic treatment selection for psychodynamic and cognitive-behavioural therapy: randomised controlled trial in routine mental health care. Br J Psychiatry 2010;197(2):96–105.

116. Knekt P, Lindfors O, editors. A randomized trial of the effects of four forms of psychotherapy on depressive and anxiety disorders: design methods and results on the effectiveness of short term spychodynamic psychotherapy and solution focused therapy during a 1-year follow-up. Helsinki: Social Insurance Institution; 2004.

Evidence-Based Somatic Treatment of Depression in Adults

Daniel Carlat, MD*

KEYWORDS

- Antidepressants • Selective serotonin reuptake inhibitors
- Serotonin–norepinephrine reuptake inhibitors
- Efficacy studies • STAR-D trial

This article reviews recent studies and controversies about the effectiveness of antidepressant medications for depression. These medications are used for treatment of a wide variety of nondepressive conditions. Most notably, selective serotonin reuptake inhibitors (SSRIs) and serotonin–norepinephrine reuptake inhibitors (SNRIs) are often prescribed for most anxiety disorders, and they are clearly effective in this sphere, with robust differences between active drugs and placebos in controlled clinical trials. As one studies the contentious literature on antidepressants for depression, it is important to not lose sight of the fact that the very term "antidepressant" has become anachronistic. These drugs are actually broad-spectrum emotional and physical pain-relieving agents with efficacy in depression, anxiety, insomnia, as well several nonpsychiatric pain syndromes such as migraines, irritable bowel syndrome, neuropathies, and fibromyalgia.

This review is divided into three broad topics: (1) the heated controversy regarding how one should interpret "efficacy studies" of antidepressants, that is, the standard placebo-controlled double-blind studies used by drug companies to gain Food and Drug Administration (FDA) approval; (2) "effectiveness studies," open-label studies enrolling types of patients who are excluded from efficacy studies, focusing on one enormous study in particular—the STAR-D trial; and (3) the evidence base that can guide clinicians in the choice of antidepressants for particular patients.

Disclosure: Dr Carlat has nothing to disclose regarding the topic of this article.
Department of Psychiatry, Tufts University School of Medicine, 800 Washington Street, Boston, MA 02111, USA
* Carlat Publishing, PO Box 626, Newburyport, MA 01950.
E-mail address: drcarlat@comcast.net

Psychiatr Clin N Am 35 (2012) 131–142
doi:10.1016/j.psc.2011.11.002
0193-953X/12/$ – see front matter © 2012 Elsevier Inc. All rights reserved.

EFFICACY STUDIES OF ANTIDEPRESSANTS: ARE ANTIDEPRESSANTS SIMPLY PLACEBOS WITH SIDE EFFECTS?

Psychologist Irving Kirsch has published papers and a recent book (*The Emperor's New Drugs: Exploding the Antidepressant Myth*)[1] arguing that antidepressants work no better than placebos. Kirsch is neither an "antipsychiatrist" nor a scientologist. Instead, he is a well-respected professor of psychology with a keen understanding of research methodology, which is why his articles have led to serious debate among both professionals and patients who have a stake in depression treatment.

In a series of papers over a long career, Kirsch has taken a magnifying glass to the gold standard research trials in antidepressant research—the placebo-controlled double-blind studies. In a nutshell, he has argued that, when averaged together, such studies actually show only a very small benefit of active treatment, and even this small benefit can likely be explained as an artifact of the side effects of antidepressants.

Many practicing psychiatrists are tempted to discount this claim automatically. After all, patients regularly appear to improve dramatically on antidepressants. But the history of medicine is filled with examples of treatments that were widely assumed to be effective based on individual clinical experience, which turned out to have little effect whatsoever. Benjamin Rush, for example, who is commonly considered the "Father of American Psychiatry," believed strongly in the effectiveness of bloodletting and purging with ipecac to "cure" a range of psychiatric illnesses.[2] Such dramatic treatments likely did lead to improvements, but subsequent experience and study revealed that these treatments were nonspecific—and that any effectiveness was due to placebo factors such as expectancy and hopefulness.

It was not until the mid-1930s that medical researchers began to compare treatments with placebo controls—inactive treatments that were packaged to look identical to active treatments. Such trials were able to subtract out the placebo effect and therefore empirically prove that a supposedly effective treatment was, indeed, effective. The first fully randomized placebo-controlled trials in medicine were first performed by psychiatrists in the 1950s in studies of thorazine and lithium.[2] Eventually, the FDA formalized the importance of these methods, when in 1980 it adopted a requirement that any drug submitted for approval must include at least two "pivotal" trials, generally meaning placebo-controlled trials.

The Kirsch Findings

More than a dozen antidepressants have been FDA approved within these strict guidelines, leading most people, both patients and physicians, to assume that these agents are genuinely effective. But in 1998, Kirsch and his colleagues published the first of many papers questioning these studies. His work culminated in a recent meta-analysis on all clinical trials submitted to the FDA in support of four antidepressants: fluoxetine, venlafaxine, nefazodone, and paroxetine.[3] In summarizing the results of all these trials, they found that the average improvement on the Hamilton Depression Scale (HamD) was 9.6 points for patients randomly assigned to medications versus a mean improvement of 7.8 points for patients assigned to placebo, yielding a mean drug–placebo difference of 1.8. This corresponded to an average effect size of 0.31, considered small.

Although acknowledging that there is a statistically significant benefit of antidepressants over placebos, Kirsch argued that this separation was not clinically significant. To put this in perspective, consider that the Hamilton Depression Scale used in most studies is a 17-item scale with a maximum score of 51 points. The higher the score is, the worse the depression. Mild depression is generally defined as a score of 8 to 13, moderate depression, 14 to 18; severe depression, 19 to 23; and very severe depression greater than 23. The 2-point difference reported by Kirsch (rounded up from 1.8) may not seem like much. As Kirsch notes in his book, a 2-point difference on the Hamilton scale "can be obtained by no longer waking during the night, or by no longer waking early in the morning, or by being less fidgety during the interview, or by eating better." These appear, indeed, to be clinically rather trivial improvements. Kirsch also cites guidelines from the United Kingdom's National Institute for Health and Clinical Excellence (NICE), which considers a minimum of a 3-point difference on the HamD between drug and placebo as being clinically significant.

Nor is Kirsch the only researcher to report these small differences. Erick Turner (a psychiatrist and former FDA analyst) and colleagues conducted a larger analysis, looking at data on all 12 antidepressants approved by the FDA between 1987 and 2004 (this included 8 SSRIs, 2 SNRIs, Wellbutrin, and Serzone). Although Turner and colleagues did not calculate the mean differences in HamD scores (because these data were not available for all of the studies they analyzed), they did calculate the average effect size. They reported an effect size of 0.32, nearly identical with Kirsch's 0.31.[4] This number, too, falls well short of NICE guidelines, which set an effect size of 0.5 as being the minimum to be considered clinically significant.

Are Antidepressants Placebos with Side Effects?

In his book *The Emperor's New Drugs* Kirsch goes even further in his skepticism of antidepressant efficacy. He believes that even the small, clinically questionable benefit of antidepressants that he calculated may be a meaningless artifact of the side effects of antidepressants. Placebo-controlled studies are based on how successfully patients and physicians are fooled into believing a placebo might be the active drug. But active drugs such as antidepressants often cause side effects that can clue patients to their treatment assignments. This risks "unblinding" the study, and might give the active treatment an unfair advantage, in the sense that patients might be more hopeful of improvement if they believe they are receiving a real drug. This would neutralize the scientific integrity of a placebo-controlled trial.

Indeed, there is some evidence that in clinical trials, patients respond better to antidepressants when they notice more side effects,[5] implying that studies may become unblinded and therefore less valid. Is it possible that antidepressants are seemingly more effective than placebos purely because they cause side effects? Are patients responding to side effects, and not to the antidepressant?

Another study analyzed the effect of so-called "active placebos," which are sometimes used in antidepressant trials. In such studies, patients assigned to placebo are given a drug such as atropine, which has no inherent antidepressant effect but causes anticholinergic effects such as dry mouth and constipation. If antidepressants work via their side effect alone, one would expect no difference between antidepressants with side effects and placebos with side effects. However, a review of nine such clinical trials did not find this. In this meta-analysis, the average antidepressant versus active placebo effect size was 0.39, larger than the antidepressant versus regular placebo effect size of 0.31 reported by Kirsch.[6]

Defining "Clinical Significance"

It seems likely, therefore, that antidepressants do, in fact, exert a specific antidepressant effect—but what of the charge that their effects are so small as to be clinically negligible? In an editorial, Turner and Rosenthal reviewed Kirsch's data and discussed the appropriateness of his dependence on the United Kingdom's NICE's criteria as a benchmark for clinical significant. They argued that NICE's cutoff of an effect size of 0.5 is arbitrary because "effect size" is a continuous measure. Even the father of effect sizes, Cohen (the effect size is sometimes called "Cohen's *d*"), acknowledged when he proposed effect size benchmarks that "the values chosen had no more reliable a basis than my own intuition."[7]

For the average clinician, the concepts of Hamilton depression scores and effect sizes are somewhat abstract. The outcomes that seem more clinically relevant are the response rate (the percentage of patients who show a 50% or more decrease in HamD score) and the remission rate (percentage of patients with final scores below 7).

In a recent comprehensive review of the literature, Levkovitz and colleagues analyzed all published studies from 1980 to 2009 of antidepressants for either major depressive disorder or dysthymia.[8] These studies included 28,807 patients randomized to medication versus 16,887 patients randomized to placebo. For major depressive disorder, the pooled response rate (RR) for antidepressants was 54.3% versus 37.9% for placebo, resulting in a number needed to treat (NNT) of 6.1. The NNT is a practical measure of the effectiveness of a treatment, and refers to the number of patients one would have to treat with a medication to yield one response beyond what would be produced by placebo. For dysthymia (for which there was far fewer data), the pooled RR for antidepressants was 52.4% versus 29.9% for placebo, for an NNT of 4.4.

These significant differences in response rates appear more impressive than the very small differences in HamD scores. One caveat of this study, however, is that the researchers reviewed only data that had been published. Drug companies must submit at least two positive studies to receive FDA approval, but they typically conduct many more to account for the possibility of negative studies—that is, studies showing no significant difference between drug and placebo. They are not required to publish negative studies, and the aforementioned research by Turner and colleagues[4] found that studies with positive outcomes were 12 times more likely to be published than studies with negative outcomes. Further, they found that 94% of published antidepressant trials were positive (drug superior to placebo), but when both published and unpublished trials were pooled, only 51% of all antidepressant trials were positive. Overall, they computed that selective publication inflated the apparent effect size of antidepressants by 32%. Nonetheless, even including the negative data, they reported that all 12 antidepressants were statistically superior to placebo.

Generalizability of Clinical Trials

A serious critique of any meta-analysis that focuses on placebo-controlled trials is that such trials are not representative of the kinds of patients practitioners see in clinical settings. Controlled trials exclude a wide range of patients, including those with comorbid anxiety, substance abuse, bipolar disorder, psychosis, personality disorders, and suicidality. In addition, patients whose depression is too mild or too severe, or who have active medical problems, will also often be excluded. One study found that only 14% of patients presenting to a clinic for depression treatment would be enrolled in a typical randomized controlled trial.[9]

What is the implication of this lack of generalizability? Many of the patients barred from these studies are the patients clinicians see in their offices every day. These are patients with "messy" symptom pictures, some with multiple disorders and others with atypical symptoms that may not qualify for an official *Diagnostic and Statistical Manual* (DSM) category. There are few studies of antidepressant efficacy in such patients, but even in the absence of clear evidence, one must treat patients who seek help. Rightly or wrongly, many clinicians tend to use the results of randomized controlled trials (RCTs) as rough indicators of a "signal" of antidepressant efficacy, and then assume that if drugs work in these rarified populations, they will presumably also work for their patients.

Researchers have called for companies to conduct studies more representative of actual patient populations, but it is unclear that companies will heed the call. The more heterogeneous the patient mix, the harder it is to demonstrate a clear difference between drug and placebo—and therefore the harder it is to recoup the millions of dollars spent on clinical trials.

Effect of Depression Severity

A number of studies, including one conducted by Kirsch and colleagues, have indicated that antidepressants work most robustly for patients with the most severe depression. Kirsch found that the higher the baseline HamD score, the more antidepressants separated from placebo. However, he also reported the interesting finding that this greater benefit for more severely depressed patients was due more to a lower placebo response than a greater response to medication.[3]

A more recent study reported similar results, in which patients with a baseline HamD score of 25 or more benefited more from antidepressants than less severely depressed patients.[10]

EFFECTIVENESS STUDIES OF ANTIDEPRESSANTS: THE STAR*D TRIALS

Thus far, this article has reviewed only studies that meet the "gold standard" of clinical trials—that is, randomized, double-blind, placebo-controlled. In 2006, the first results of the STAR-D (Sequenced Treatment Alternatives to Relieve Depression) trial were published. This was the largest clinical trial for depression ever conducted, as well as one of the few large trials performed without industry funding and thus with less potential for strategic biases in research design that might favor one drug over another.[11] STAR-D was designed as an "effectiveness" trial as opposed to an "efficacy" trial. The researchers recently provided an excellent explanation of the unique features of this type of trial:

> "STAR*D has key features that define it as an effectiveness trial. Design elements such as broadly inclusive selection criteria and enrollment of patients from primary and specialty settings and with multiple concurrent medical and psychiatric illnesses give STAR*D results high external validity. Comparison of STAR*D participants with the U.S. population highlights the generalizability. The racial-ethnic composition of the enrolled participants approximates that of the U.S. population on the basis of data from the 2000 Census, and the distribution of depressive severity seen in STAR*D participants is consistent with the spectrum reported by Kessler and colleagues in a nationally representative sample (10% mild, 38% moderate, 39% severe, and 13% very severe). Both facts suggest that the sample was representative of depressed patients in the United States."[12]

There were other elements of the STAR-D methodology that make the results unusually generalizable to real-world practice. For example, there was no placebo condition. As is true in real practice settings, both physicians and patients knew which drugs were being taken. Although patients were randomly assigned to different drugs in STAR-D, they were allowed some input into the kind of treatment they received.

On the other hand, these methodologic decisions may well have backfired on the study designers, as there is much debate regarding whether the STAR-D results have provided any information of true value to clinicians, as noted later.

Table 1		
Results of augmentation		
Celexa plus . . .	**Remission (HRSD-17, %)**	**Response (QIDS-SR-16, %)**
BuSpar	30.1	26.9
Wellbutrin SR	29.7	31.8

STAR-D Level 1: Monotherapy with Celexa

In Level 1 of the trial, 4041 patients were enrolled and started to receive Celexa up to 60 mg/d for up to 12 weeks. After an average length of treatment of 10 weeks, and on an average dose of 41.7 mg/d, patients receiving Celexa had a response rate of 47% (as measured by a nonstandard outcome measure, the 16-item Quick Inventory of Depressive Symptomatology-Self-Report [QIDS-SR]) and a remission rate of 27% (as measured by the standard HAM-D). How does this compare to other antidepressant trials? As noted in the previous section, the average response rates in placebo-controlled trials is 54.3%, so in this population Celexa appeared to be somewhat less effective than might be expected. On the other hand, this was a more treatment-resistant population than patients enrolled in typical trials, so it is difficult to compare these numbers with other studies.

STAR-D Level 2: Augmentation Versus Switching

While 30% of STAR*D patients remitted on Celexa alone, 70% did not. Of these remaining patients, many discontinued participation in the study for various reasons, but 1474 remained and were assigned to one of three different groups, based on patient preference: 565 to augmentation treatment, 727 to a switch strategy, and 182 to cognitive therapy (either alone or added to Celexa).

Augmentation track

Patients who chose augmentation were assigned to treatment with either Wellbutrin SR (279 patients, mean dose 267.5 mg/d) or BuSpar (286 patients, mean dose 40.9 mg/d), and remained on their Celexa. Remission took an average of 6.3 weeks for the Wellbutrin SR patients and 5.4 weeks for those assigned to BuSpar (not a statistically significant difference). The remission and response numbers are in **Table 1**.

Although both BuSpar and Wellbutrin SR augmentation produced about 30% remission, various aspects of effectiveness and tolerability, reproduced in **Table 2**, place Wellbutrin SR slightly ahead of BuSpar.

Switch track

Patients who chose the switching track were assigned to switch from Celexa to one of three agents: Effexor XR, Wellbutrin SR, or Zoloft. **Table 3** provides the results of the switching arm; there were no statistically significant differences between the treatments.

Table 2			
Wellbutrin SR Versus BuSpar for augmentation			
	Reduction in QIDS-SR Depression Score (%)	**Time Adhered to Treatment**	**Rate of Discontinuation due to Side Effects**
Wellbutrin SR	25.3	10.2 weeks	12.5%
BuSpar	17.1	9.2 weeks	20.6%

All differences are statistically significant.

Table 3		
Results of switching antidepressants in level 2 of STAR-D		
Switch from Celexa to . . .	**Remission (HRSD-17, %)**	**Response (QIDS-SR-16, %)**
Effexor XR	24.8	28.2
Wellbutrin SR	21.3	26.1
Zoloft	17.6	26.7

Finally, a relatively small number of patients (182) chose the cognitive behavior therapy arm of the study, with a remission rate of 31%.

STAR-D Levels 3 and 4: More Augmentation and Switching

At Level 3, patients were offered the opportunity of continuing in the study through two more levels of treatment, though relatively few did so. There were no significant differences between switching patients to Remeron (mirtazapine) or nortriptyline, though patients augmented with triiodothyronine (T3) had marginally better results than those augmented with lithium and experienced fewer side effects. Finally, at heroic Level 4, a very small number of patients were randomized to either "California Rocket Fuel" (Effexor XR plus Remeron) or the monoamine oxidase inhibitor Parnate (tranylcypromine), with no significant outcome differences between these two agents.

A 67% Cumulative Remission?

In a press release by the American Psychiatric Association announcing the first results of the STAR*D trial, the lead was "In STAR*D, the nation's largest depression treatment study, results indicate that 67 percent of patients who complete from one to four treatment steps can reach remission." But recent papers have closely analyzed these results and found that they were significantly inflated as a result of post hoc changes in the statistical plan. The two main changes were: (1) a decision to drop the original primary outcome variable, the HAMD remission rate, and to replace it with the QIDS, a patient-rated scale that yielded higher remissions; and (2) another post hoc decision to include the most mildly depressed patients in the final analysis (those with initial HamD scores of less than 14). Thus the actual cumulative remission rate is unclear, but is likely less than 40% according to the original analytic plan. Further, looking at the 12-month continuation care results, only 108 of the original 4041 (2.6%) survived the trial without dropping out or relapsing.[13]

Lessons of STAR-D

The goal of STAR-D was to provide us with evidence-based guidelines for how to proceed with treatment when a patient does not respond to an initial SSRI trial at a robust dose continued for 2 to 3 months. What is the next step in treating such patients?

Before STAR-D, most experts on treatment resistant depression would answer this question with, "If the patient has responded at least partially to the first medication, add a second. But if your patient's symptoms have not budged at all, switch to a different treatment." This reasonable approach was based on cobbling together various small studies, mostly without control groups. The great hope was that NIMH-funded study would finally provide the answer.

But as the authors of STAR-D recently acknowledged:

"The data collected did not allow direct comparison of the benefits of switching versus augmenting. Patient preferences were a part of the equipoise randomization strategy, and most patients preferred either augmentation or switching at level 2. Consequently, patient groups were not equivalent at the point of randomization at the beginning of level 2; the augmentation group at level 2 was somewhat less depressed than the group that switched."[12]

In other words, STAR-D's design was excellent for recruiting many real-world patients, but was poor for creating clinical guidelines. It does not indicate which patients should be switched to a different antidepressant or which patients augmented. But assuming that a decision is made to switch or to augment—does STAR-D help us to choose the best medication? In a one sense, it does because it provides the valuable information that *it does not really matter which medication one chooses*—they are all equally effective. One can reasonably switch patients to an SNRI, Wellbutrin, or another SSRI; and one can reasonably augment with either Wellbutrin or BuSpar (though Wellbutrin might be a better choice in terms of side effects).

For more treatment-resistant patients, we learn from STAR-D that switching to Remeron or nortriptyline is identical, and that augmenting with lithium or T3 are similar (though one might lean toward thyroid in terms of tolerability). Finally, "California Rocket Fuel" (Effexor XR plus Remeron) or Parnate will provide similar benefits for the most treatment resistant. In a sense, STAR-D enhances our confidence in a clinical truism that has lasted for decades—that all antidepressants are created equal.

Choosing an Antidepressant

Thus far, we have found that gold standard placebo-controlled studies show a small advantage of antidepressants over placebo for patients with mild to moderate depression, and the advantage is larger and more convincing as the severity of depression deepens. In real patient populations with comorbidities and with depressive symptoms that may not qualify for a specific diagnosis, we have no clear guidance for how well antidepressants will work, though most clinicians assume that the "signal" of efficacy from RCTs implies that they will be efficacious for other patients.

In addition, the largest trial of antidepressants in history provided relatively little clinical guidance, but did indicate a lack of difference between different antidepressant choices, whether for augmentation or switching.

The following paragraphs consider the information obtained from head-to-head studies of antidepressants.

SNRIs Versus SSRIs

For a time, the SNRI Effexor (venlafaxine) was thought to be somewhat more effective than SSRIs, based on a famous 2001 meta-analysis.[14] In this study, based primarily on studies comparing Effexor with Prozac (fluoxetine), Effexor registered a 45% remission rate versus a 35% rate for SSRIs, an NNT of 10. However, over time, more Effexor has been compared with more agents, and the magnitude of its advantage has narrowed. In 2008, a company-sponsored meta-analysis found that the NNT of venlafaxine over SSRIs is 17, meaning that a clinician would have to treat 17 patients with venlafaxine to find one additional patient who would not have responded to an SSRI.[15] Generally, any NNT above 10 is considered to be clinically insignificant, although, as for the NICE criteria for clinical significance, this is a judgment call.

The most recent meta-analysis was not funded by a manufacturer (it was funded as a health technology assessment by the German government), and was likely the most comprehensive review yet compiled, including both published and unpublished data of comparisons among duloxetine, venlafaxine, SSRIs, and tricyclic antidepressants (TCAs).[16] The analysis included 10 randomized controlled trials comparing Cymbalta to SSRIs, 31 trials comparing Effexor to SSRIs, and 11 trials comparing Effexor to TCAs.

The researchers found that response rates were statistically significantly higher for Effexor than for SSRIs—but by only a small margin (66.5% vs 61.3%). There was no advantage in terms of remission rates. Effexor did not differ from either Cymbalta or TCAs on response or remission, nor did Cymbalta differ from SSRIs or TCAs. Both Effexor (11.8% vs 9.2%) and Cymbalta (8.4% vs 5.8%) had higher rates of discontinuation due to adverse events than did SSRIs. Effexor's adverse event–related discontinuation rates were not different from rates on TCAs.

The authors of this German study reported that data from several additional unpublished studies had been included in a different meta-analysis sponsored by the manufacturer of Effexor.[15] When they asked for these data, Wyeth declined to release them, casting doubt on the validity of the earlier findings that Effexor had a higher remission rate than SSRIs.

Overall, the most recent findings imply that there is little to no efficacy advantage of SNRIs over SSRIs, at least for the selected patients enrolled in randomized clinical trials. Because of the worse tolerability of SNRIs, they should continue to be considered second-line agents.

Choosing Among the SSRIs

Given that SSRIs continue to be our first-line antidepressants, are there any reasons to choose one over the other? Many head-to-head studies of antidepressants have been conducted over the years, and recently two groups of researchers have assembled these trials and have performed meta-analyses.

The two studies used different methods of choosing studies and doing their analyses, and they therefore came up with somewhat different conclusions. The first study was arguably the more careful of the two. It was commissioned by the Agency for Healthcare Research and Quality, and surveyed a wide range of studies using different potential methods for comparing drugs. In addition to analyzing 105 head-to-head studies, they also analyzed 66 placebo-controlled studies. They found that no single antidepressant was more efficacious than the others. If this was the extent of the findings, the study would have been of limited use.

But this is only where the interesting results began. Among the clinically useful results were the following:

- Mirtazapine has a significantly faster onset of action than citalopram, fluoxetine, paroxetine, or sertraline.
- Meta-analysis of 15 fair-quality studies indicates that venlafaxine is associated with a higher rate of nausea and vomiting than SSRIs as a class (33% vs 22%).
- Evidence from 15 fair-quality studies indicates that sertraline is associated with a higher incidence of diarrhea than bupropion, citalopram, fluoxetine, fluvoxamine, mirtazapine, nefazodone, paroxetine, or venlafaxine (11% vs 8%).

- Seven fair-quality trials indicate that mirtazapine leads to higher weight gain than citalopram, fluoxetine, paroxetine, or sertraline (0.8–3.0 kg after 6–8 weeks).
- A good-quality systematic review provides evidence that paroxetine and venlafaxine have the highest rates of the discontinuation syndrome; fluoxetine has the lowest (data not reported).
- Evidence from five fair-quality trials provide shows that bupropion causes significantly less sexual dysfunction than fluoxetine, paroxetine, or sertraline. Among SSRIs, paroxetine has the highest rates of sexual dysfunction. Overall, more than 50% report sexual dysfunction.[17]

Cipriani and coworkers took a different approach to their meta-analysis, limiting the articles reviewed to 117 head-to-head comparisons (and omitting trials comparing single drugs vs placebo, observational trials, and pooled trials, all of which were included in the paper by Gartlehner and colleagues). Although less comprehensive, this analysis allowed the researchers to produce rankings of different antidepressants

Table 4
Second-generation antidepressants

Medication	Indications (Includes Long-Acting Forms)	Evidence-Based Features
Bupropion (Wellbutrin, Zyban, Generic)	MDD, seasonal affective disorder, smoking cessation	Less sexual dysfunction, no weight gain
Citalopram (Celexa, Generic)	MDD	
Desvenlafaxine (Pristiq)	MDD	
Duloxetine (Cymbalta)	MDD, diabetic peripheral neuropathy, fibromyalgia, GAD	Unique efficacy for pain in dispute
Escitalopram (Lexapro)	MDD, GAD	Particularly high efficacy/tolerability
Fluoxetine (Prozac, Sarafem, Generic)	MDD, OCD, bulimia nervosa, PMDD, panic disorder	Lower risk of discontinuation syndrome
Fluvoxamine (Luvox, Generic)	OCD	
Mirtazapine (Remeron, Generic)	MDD	High weight gain, somnolence; fast onset of action
Paroxetine (Paxil, Generic,)	MDD, OCD, panic, social phobia, GAD, PTSD	High sexual dysfunction, weight gain, discontinuation symptoms
Sertraline (Zoloft, Generic)	MDD, OCD, panic, PTSD, PMDD	Particularly high efficacy/tolerability/low cost; high diarrhea
Venlafaxine (Effexor, Generic)	MDD, GAD	Efficacy advantage over SSRIs now disputed; high nausea/vomiting, discontinuation symptoms
Vilazodone (Viibryd)	MDD	

Abbreviations: GAD, generalized anxiety disorder; MDD, major depressive disorder; OCD, obsessive–compulsive disorder; PMDD, premenstrual dysphoric disorder; PTSD, posttraumatic stress disorder.

in terms of efficacy, tolerability, and economics. They concluded that venlafaxine, mirtazapine, sertraline, and escitalopram were slightly more effective than the eight other new-generation antidepressant medications examined. Among these, escitalopram and sertraline had the best tolerability, while sertraline was the most economical; sertraline therefore took the "grand prize" by scoring high in efficacy, tolerability, and price.[18] However, the methodology of this article has been critiqued because all of the trials were phase 4 trials sponsored by manufacturers, and it is possible that some drug companies were more skillful than others in designing trials to best their competitors. Nonetheless, the results seem intuitively consonant with the experiences of many clinicians.

SUMMARY

The efficacy of antidepressants has become a contentious topic over the last decade, and yet a review of the literature shows that they are consistently more effective than placebo. Although the average magnitude of this effect is unclear, many individual patients respond well to a course of antidepressants, and relapse when the medication is discontinued.

Choosing the right antidepressant for a given patient remains more art than science, but the studies reviewed here provide some helpful guidance. **Table 4** lists the second-generation antidepressants along with potential reasons for choosing one over the other (based on side effects, costs, or possible therapeutic advantages.)

Based on these data, the following conclusions can be drawn:

- For an all-around first-line antidepressant, sertraline is hard to beat, given its combination of efficacy, tolerability, and low expense. Once escitalopram becomes generic, it will join sertraline in this category.
- Bupropion is often a first-line alternative to sertraline, because of its lack of sexual side effects; although it has less efficacy for anxiety disorders, it is helpful for other comorbidities, such as tobacco dependence and attention-deficit/hyperactivity disorder.
- Both paroxetine and mirtazepine are often maligned because of side effects of sedation and weight gain; however, these side effects may be advantageous for those whose depressive symptoms include insomnia and excessive weight loss.
- Although not specifically reviewed in this article, certain antidepressants are liable to cause more drug–drug interactions than others; the most prominent of these are fluoxetine, paroxetine, and fluvoxamine.

REFERENCES

1. Kirsch I. The emperor's new drugs: exploding the antidepressant myth. Philadelphia: Basic Books; 2010.
2. Healy D. The antidepressant era. Cambridge (MA): Harvard University Press; 2000. p. 91.
3. Kirsch I, Deacon BJ, Huedo-Medina TB, et al. Initial severity and antidepressant benefits: a meta-analysis of data submitted to the Food and Drug Administration. PLoS Med 2008;5:e45.
4. Turner EH, Matthews AM, Linardatos E, et al. Selective publication of antidepressant trials and its influence on apparent efficacy. N Engl J Med 2008;358:252–60.
5. Greenberg RP, Bornstein RF, Zborowski MJ, et al. A meta-analysis of fluoxetine outcome in the treatment of depression. J Nerv Ment Dis 1994;82:547–51.
6. Moncrieff J, Wessely S, Hardy R. Active placebos versus antidepressants for depression. Cochrane Database Syst Rev 2004;1:CD003012.

7. Turner E, Rosenthal R. Efficacy of antidepressants. BMJ 2008;336:516–7.
8. Levkovitz Y, Tedeschini E, Papakostas G. Efficacy of antidepressants for dysthymia: a meta-analysis of placebo-controlled randomized trials. J Clin Psychiatry 2011;72(4): 509–14.
9. Zimmerman M, Mattia JI, Posternak MA. Are subjects in pharmacological treatment trials of depression representative of patients in routine clinical practice? Am J Psychiatry 2002;159:469–73.
10. Fournier JC, DeRubeis RJ, Hollon SD et al. Antidepressant drug effects and depression severity: a patient-level meta-analysis. JAMA 2010;303(1):47–53.
11. Trivedi MH, Rush AJ, Wisniewski SR, et al. Evaluation of outcomes with citalopram for depression using measurement-based care in STAR*D: implications for clinical practice. Am J Psychiatry 2006;163:28–40.
12. Gaynes BN, Warden D, Trivedi MH, et al. What did STAR*D teach us? Results from a large-scale, practical, clinical trial for patients with depression. Psychiatr Serv 2009; 60:1439–45.
13. Pigott HE, Leventhal AM, Alter GS, et al. Efficacy and effectiveness of antidepressants: current status of research. Psychother Psychosom 2010;79:267–79.
14. Thase ME, Entsuah AR, Rudolph RL. Remission rates during treatment with venlafaxine or selective serotonin reuptake inhibitors. Br J Psychiatry 2001;178:234–41.
15. Nemeroff CB, Entsuah R, Benattia I, et al. Comprehensive Analysis of Remission (COMPARE) with Venlafaxine versus SSRIs. Biol Psychiatry 2008;63(4):424–34.
16. Schueler YB, Koesters M, Wieseler B, et al. A systematic review of duloxetine and venlafaxine in major depression, including unpublished data. Acta Psychiatrica Scand 2011; 23:247–65.
17. Gartlehner G, Gaynes BN, Hansen RA. Comparative benefits and harms of second-generation antidepressants: background paper for the American College of Physicians. Ann Intern Med 2008;149:734–50.
18. Cipriani A, Furukawa TA, Salanti G, et al. Comparative efficacy and acceptability of 12 new-generation antidepressants: a multiple-treatments meta-analysis. Lancet 2009; 373:746–58.

How (Not What) to Prescribe: Nonpharmacologic Aspects of Psychopharmacology

David L. Mintz, MD*, David F. Flynn, MD

KEYWORDS

- Depression • Psychopharmacology • Treatment resistance
- Doctor-patient relationship • Alliance • Treatment outcome

Over the past 2 decades psychiatry has benefited from an increasingly evidence-based perspective and a proliferation of safer and more tolerable antidepressant treatments. Despite these advances, however, there is no evidence that treatment outcomes are better than they were a quarter of a century ago. New psychiatric medications come on the market every year, often with great enthusiasm, only to be tempered by the realities of clinical practice. More recently, it seems that novel antidepressants have not even been able to generate much fanfare. This phenomenon is not particularly surprising considering that the widely publicized STAR*D trial[1,2] reported relatively underwhelming performances of various psychopharmacologic agents when applied in real-world settings. One possible explanation for the failed promise of psychopharmacology rests in the fact that the field has been so enthusiastic about biological treatments that psychosocial aspects of psychopharmacology have been almost entirely neglected in recent years.

There is a growing body of evidence that suggests that nonpharmacologic or nonspecific factors in psychopharmacology are at least as potent as the putative active ingredients in the medication. Metaanalyses reviewing US Food and Drug Administration databases (which include a relatively unbiased sample of both published and unpublished data from antidepressant clinical trials) suggest that 75% to 81% of drug response can be attributed to nonpharmacologic effects, such as placebo.[3–5] Other research from well-designed placebo-controlled trials show that a strong pharmacotherapeutic alliance is an even more powerful antidepressant than the actual drugs that are prescribed.[6]

McKay and colleagues,[7] in their groundbreaking analysis of outcome data from the Treatment of Depression Collaborative Research Program, an extensive, National Institute of Mental Health–funded multicenter placebo-controlled trial of the treatment

The authors have nothing to disclose.
The Austen Riggs Center, 25 Main Street, PO Box 962, Stockbridge, MA 01262, USA
* Corresponding author.
E-mail address: david.mintz@austenriggs.net

Psychiatr Clin N Am 35 (2012) 143–163
doi:10.1016/j.psc.2011.11.009
0193-953X/12/$ – see front matter © 2012 Elsevier Inc. All rights reserved.

of depression found a provocative prescriber effect. They were able to stratify outcomes by prescriber, despite the fact that experimental conditions tightly controlled most aspects of the doctor-patient engagement. One-third of the psychiatrists in the study could be described as highly effective, achieving superior results with active drug. Another one-third of prescribers exhibited average performance, and another one-third were relatively ineffective. More striking perhaps is the fact that the most effective one-third of prescribers achieved better outcomes with placebos than the least effective one-third of prescribers got with active antidepressants. This result suggests that *how* the doctor prescribes is even more important that *what* the doctor prescribes.

Whereas there is overwhelming evidence identifying the contributions from nonpharmacologic factors in drug response, forces inside and outside of organized psychiatry have tended to promote a model of treatment that tends toward biological reductionism.[8–10] These forces include optimism about neuroscientific advances as well as the domination of managed care and its promotion of a model that incentivizes simplified and split treatments promising short-term cost savings. It is perhaps telling that, of 26 English language studies in the past 2 decades exploring interventions to promote antidepressant adherence, 25 of those studies came from primary care departments and only one came from organized psychiatry.[11]

This article is an effort to provide some balance and offer some guidance to psychiatric prescribers about how to prescribe in order to promote better treatment outcomes. Where possible, the authors cite evidence pertaining directly to the literature on the treatment of depression. In some cases, recommendations are extrapolated from findings with other psychiatric conditions. It is likely, given the seeming universality of nonspecific factors in healing, that the recommendations made here pertain to the range of psychiatric conditions and not just depression.

THE PROBLEM OF TREATMENT RESISTANCE

As our awareness of the limitations of medications grows, so too does awareness of the problem of treatment resistance. Over the past 3 decades, references to treatment resistance in the psychiatric literature have outpaced the total number of references by a factor of 16.[8] STAR*D and other studies[12–14] suggest that a minority of patients with depression will fully recover with pharmacologic treatment. The mainstream media have begun to reflect the growing disenchantment with psychopharmacology with skeptical articles about antidepressants appearing in a wide variety of major news outlets in the last several years. Without a transformative shift in our approach to depression, the field may unwittingly move from the era of psychopharmacology and into an era of treatment resistance.

THE MEANING OF MEDICATION

Nonpharmacologic factors contributing to patient response in medication trials are well-established, although these findings are often sequestered in the psychology literature. In their comprehensive review of the placebo response, Fisher and Greenberg[15] lay out a compelling body of evidence examining the nonpharmacologic aspects of drug response. Factors ranging from the color[15–17] or expense[18] of the pill to the route of administration,[19] the setting in which the pill is administered,[15] and the attitude of the prescriber[15,20] all seem to influence outcome (**Table 1**). Similarly, mounting evidence suggests that the prescribing process equals or exceeds the clinical import of the putative active ingredient of the antidepressant. However, our field is only beginning to understand what the most effective prescribers do. As

Table 1	
Medication characteristics affecting treatment outcome	
Medication Characteristics	**Evidence**
Color	de Craen et al,[17] 1996
	Fisher & Greenberg,[15] 1997
Expense	Waber et al,[18] 2008
Setting of Administration	Fisher & Greenberg,[15] 1997
Route of Administration	de Craen et al,[19] 2000

interpersonal processes cannot be patented, psychopharmacology process research has unfortunately received only a miniscule fraction of the investment that has been made into researching the effectiveness of specific drugs. Such process research, central to the study of the psychotherapies, is much needed if the field of psychiatry is truly committed to improving treatment outcomes in pharmacotherapy.

The impact of the physical characteristics of the medication, the symbolic aspect of taking (or refusing) a medicine, and the interpersonal relationship tied to a medication (eg, pill as substitute contact with the doctor) can be integrated into a phenomenon called meaning effects. Despite the considerable evidence suggesting these meaning effects are central to medication response, there is no widely accepted method for incorporating them into clinical practice. Psychodynamic psychopharmacology[21,22] is one attempt to integrate these factors to help anticipate therapeutic roadblocks and pitfalls. It emphasizes how to prescribe rather than what to prescribe. It complements the traditional objective-descriptive approach of prescribing that considers how patients are similar (diagnostic criteria) and explicitly acknowledges, incorporates, and addresses the central role of meaning and interpersonal factors in psychopharmacology. Psychodynamic psychopharmacology is organized around six technical principles. Whereas these six principles are informed by a psychodynamic attitude, they are applicable in any treatment setting. These principles are the organizing framework for this article, although many or most of the recommendations here could not be considered the sole province of psychodynamics.

1. Avoid mind-body split.
2. Know who the patient is.
3. Attend to ambivalence about loss of symptoms.
4. Cultivate the therapeutic alliance.
5. Attend to countertherapeutic uses of medications.
6. Identify, contain, and use countertransference.

AVOID A MIND-BODY SPLIT
Think Integratively, Not Reductionistically

It seems likely that a first step, before making any behavioral interventions that might facilitate treatment, involves developing an attitude toward pharmacotherapy that integrates biological and psychosocial perspectives. Most fundamentally, a prescriber must grasp that depression and recovery represent interplays of biological and psychosocial factors that are so complex that a full understanding is likely to elude doctor and patient. For example, when a patient benefits following the introduction of a new antidepressant, it is impossible to know the relative contributions of the active medication, the placebo effect, the alliance, the patient's expectations and desire for change, and a multitude of other factors. However, an ability to respond flexibly to meaning factors in psychopharmacology and to use them to enhance outcomes is conditioned on an ability to hold an integrated perspective.

This response and use may be easier said than done, because there are many pressures toward reductionism in the practice of psychopharmacology. Culturally, mind-body dualism is embedded in Western metaphors since Descartes at least and constrains our possibilities of thought. On a personal level, doctors may be pulled toward a reductionistic understanding to escape anxiety and ambiguity or because a simplified field allows the doctor to address the patient with greater certainty and authority. Professional pressures to fall onto one side of the mind-body split include allegiances to a particular model of treatment (eg, biological vs psychotherapeutic) underlying metaphors in medicine[23] as well as pressures intrinsic to the current model of health care delivery (ie, managed care), which often pushes biologically focused or split treatments. How often, for example, in a managed care review, does the treater face pressure to add another medication when a more helpful intervention would be to assist the patient in addressing a family member about some intolerable aspect of his or her living situation? Reductionistic pressures may also derive from patients, particularly when they are defensively invested in the experience of not being responsible for illness behaviors[21] and, thus, present their symptoms in the form of an argument for a biological explanation.

Recognize the Patient as Both Subject and Object

Within the psychoanalytic paradigm, patients were seen as responsible for the production and alleviation of symptoms. This position, when held dogmatically, had the potential to leave the patient feeling blamed for the illness. Under the sway of a more biological model, patients are more likely now to be seen as victims of an inexorable biology and treated as if they have no internal resources that they can recruit in the service of recovery. The treatments that follow (the prescription of an antidepressant) invest all of the healing power in the doctor and his tools. Instructions regarding the proper use of medications are too infrequently buttressed with adequate instruction regarding healthy behaviors on the part of the patient.[24]

Much is lost when the patient is not seen as a potential agent and ally in the process of recovery. Ironically, it is often not in psychiatry but in primary care medicine and related fields that "bio" gets linked with "psychosocial" in the recognition that the way the patient lives and approaches the illness can make all the difference between a treatment success and a treatment failure. As with diabetes or hypertension, the treatment contract for patients with depression should emphasize that patients have a central role in managing the disease, maximizing patients' authority in relation to their illness.

There are a variety of lifestyle factors that can impact the outcome of depression. These are often neglected in favor of purely pharmacologic approaches. In addition to psychotherapy, lifestyle variables such as exercise,[25] adequate social supports,[26] and religion[26] have all been shown to enhance outcomes with depression. By recognizing the patient's agency, the prescriber and patient can multiply the tools in the treatment armamentarium and enhance the chances of a good outcome.

The prescriber might also recognize that the patient is not simply an ally in the treatment. Because of ambivalence about illness, secondary gains, or negative feelings about the doctor, treatment, or medication, the patient may also be an adversary.[21] Recognition of these aspects of the patient's subjectivity may allow mental health professionals to address and ameliorate those resistances to treatment.

Consider Nonpharmacologic Factors in Treatment Response

When a patient improves on medications, or fails to improve or worsens, it may be useful (and it is certainly the most honest) to recognize that the reasons are always somewhat obscure. The patient's improvement on an antidepressant may be related to the medication's direct effects on serotonin and other neurotransmitters. However, it is just as easily attributable to the placebo response,[3–5] the treatment alliance,[6,27–29] the patient's expectations and wishes, and a myriad of other nonpharmacologic factors. Similarly, if a patient worsens on medications, it may be the result of side effects but could just as easily represent a nocebo response (see following), a defensive reaction, or a manifestation of disempowerment based on meanings attributed to treatment. Keeping these possibilities in mind helps treaters resist the pull to biological reductionism and to remain flexible in their thinking and approach to patients.

Incorporate Psychosocial Factors in the Treatment Agreement

Providing informed consent and educating the patient about his or her illness can involve educating the patient about potency of psychosocial factors in psychopharmacology. Depending on the patient's needs, this education may include discussions of the power of the placebo effect, treatment alliance, the patient's expectancies, and desire for change. The ultimate task here is to balance the instillation of hope with an honest and realistic humility regarding the actual limitations of our medications. Patients are thus encouraged to mobilize their own agency and become partners in the pursuit of health.

Construct an Integrated Treatment Frame

With fewer psychiatrists providing psychotherapy, split treatments have become the norm. If the prescriber and therapist differ widely in their beliefs about medications and goals of treatment, it is not likely that their shared patient will recover, especially if this disagreement is communicated in any way to the patient. However, just because a treatment is split does not mean that it is unintegrated, fragmented, or conflictual. Collaborative working relationships involving shared goals, a supportive position toward other health care providers' work, and necessary communication are possible and important, particularly when working with patients with treatment-refractory depression or significant character pathology. A broad evidence base suggests that models of collaborative care, which might include teamwork between therapists and prescribers[21,22] or comprehensive treatment teams involving physician extenders,[30] which provide more opportunities for clinical contact, have been shown to significantly improve outcomes in depressed patients. It is also worth noting that combined treatments, with one provider administering both medications and psychotherapy, are not necessarily integrated. A single provider can easily wear these two hats in such a way that pharmacologic and psychotherapeutic approaches are almost completely divorced.

KNOW WHO THE PATIENT IS

Within a biologically reductionistic model, the prescriber is concerned primarily with what the patient is (ie, the clinical diagnosis). Knowledge of the clinical characteristics of the depression (duration, severity, recurrence, clinical features, and somatic sensitivities) can certainly help the prescriber know what to prescribe for the average patient but may not adequately guide the doctor in prescribing for this unique patient with his or her particular history, character, and concerns. There are a variety of

Table 2	
Patient characteristics affecting treatment outcome	
Patient Characteristics	**Evidence**
Neuroticism	Joyce & Paykel,[31] 1989
	Scott et al,[32] 1995
	Bagby et al,[26] 2002
	Steunenberg et al,[33] 2010
Defensive Style	Kronström et al,[34] 2009
Locus of Control	Reynaert et al,[35] 1995
Autonomy	Peselow et al,[36] 1992
Sociotropy	Peselow et al,[36] 1992
Social Disadvantage	Hahn,[37] 1997
Acquiescence	McNair et al,[38] 1968
	McNair et al,[39] 1970
	Fast & Fisher,[40] 1971
Attachment Style	Ciechanowski et al,[41] 2001
	Ciechanowski et al,[42] 2006
	Comninos & Grenyer,[43] 2007
Expectations of Treatment	Meyer et al,[44] 2002
	Krell et al,[45] 2004
	Aikens et al,[46] 2005
	Gaudiano & Miller,[47] 2006
	Sneed et al,[48] 2008
Treatment Preferences	Lin et al,[49] 2005
	Iacoviello et al,[50] 2007
	Kocsis et al,[51] 2009
	Raue et al,[52] 2009
	Kwan et al,[53] 2010
Ambivalence About Medications	Sirey et al,[54] 2001
	Aikens et al,[55] 2008
	Warden et al,[56] 2009
Secondary Gains Associated With Illness	van Egmond & Kummeling,[57] 2002
Autonomous Motivation for Treatment	Zuroff et al,[58] 2007
Readiness to Change	Beitman et al,[59] 1994
	Lewis et al,[60] 2009

nonclinical patient characteristics (**Table 2**) that affect pharmacologic treatment outcome. Understanding the patient more fully can help the prescriber to know not only what to prescribe, but how to prescribe it.

Personality and Temperament Factors Affecting Pharmacologic Outcomes

A wide variety of psychological and psychosocial factors have been shown to impact outcome in the pharmacologic treatment of depression (see **Table 2**). Neuroticism, a characterologic tendency toward worry and dysphoria coupled with relatively immature defenses was among the first personality characteristics found to impact pharmacologic treatment outcome. The vast majority of studies examining the relationship between neuroticism and pharmacologic treatment outcome have found negative correlations in both short-term and long-term response to antidepressant treatment,[31,32] as well as risk of recurrence.[33] This result is consistent with other findings that immaturity of defenses is a poor prognostic sign for psychopharmacologic treatment.[34] Curiously, a few studies conducted since 2000 have not found a correlation between neuroticism and pharmacologic nonresponse.[61,62] It is not clear why these later studies show different results, although they may reflect the particular measurement instrument used in these contemporary studies.

Autonomy (a sense of self-efficacy) and sociotropy (an orientation toward others for assistance and focus on pleasing others so as to secure interpersonal attachments) are personality characteristics that have also been found to impact pharmacologic treatment outcome, the former directly and the later inversely.[36] Patients exhibiting high autonomy and low sociotropy showed a response rate of 74.1% to antidepressant, whereas high-sociotropic/low-autonomous patients responded at half that rate (38.5%). It is intriguing to consider that sociotropic patients may paradoxically impair themselves in the context of pharmacologic treatment, handing too much responsibility for cure over to the doctor and emptying themselves of personal efficacy. Similarly, patients with an internal locus of control also fare significantly better with antidepressants than patients with an external locus of control.[35]

Attachment styles,[63] defined as fundamental modes of relating to others that are shaped in part by early caregiving relationships, also significantly affect the ways that medications are used. People with secure attachments are able comfortably to connect to and separate from important others and have a basic sense of trust. Anxious-fearful attachment patterns, similar to sociotropy, are characterized by an anxious attachment and worries about evoking a negative response from important others. People with dismissive or avoidant attachments, on the other hand, readily disconnect from others at the first disappointment. These are the "one strike and you're out" patients who often show particular difficulty with treatment adherence.[41] Patients with disorganized attachments are comfortable neither in proximity nor at a distance and tend to experience chaotic shifts in relationships as a result. Patients with secure attachments show an earlier response to antidepressants[43] compared with patients with fearful attachments.

An understanding of the patient's attachment style may guide treatment decisions. Difficulties with adherence that are associated with dismissive attachments can be reversed by particularly good communication on the part of the doctor.[41] These patients may also respond better to a team-based collaborative care approach[42] that offers extended support.

Patient Expectations of Treatment

Patients who expect more from pharmacologic treatment are likely to reap more benefits from it. This expectation is the reason that placebo controls are necessary in pharmacologic research. Patients who are enrolled in studies in which they know they will receive an antidepressant show antidepressant response rates of approximately 60%. The antidepressant response rate drops to 46% when patients are aware that they might receive placebo.[48]

The unique expectations that a patient brings to treatment also exert a significant effect on outcomes. For example, Krell and colleagues[45] found that patients with high expectations of pharmacologic treatment showed an impressive 90% antidepressant response rate, whereas patients who had only moderate expectations of treatment responded only 33% of the time. This effect was not moderated by adherence. Aikens and colleagues[46] found that initial skepticism about the appropriateness of pharmacologic treatment resulted in significant increases in antidepressant discontinuation (although, curiously, these skeptical, nonadherent patients did not have worse outcomes). The vast majority of other studies examining the role of expectations, however, have found a correlation between high expectations and outcome, although this effect may be moderated through effects on the therapeutic alliance in the treatment of major depression[44] or bipolar disorder.[47]

There are several technical implications of these findings. One is that it can be helpful to discuss a patient's expectations of treatment, which can inform patient and doctor about prognosis and provide opportunities to address irrational expectations that interfere with treatment response. The doctor can also use psychoeducational and supportive strategies to increase expectations. Such an intervention is incorporated into the model of interpersonal psychotherapy,[64] in which treaters are directed to encourage patients regarding their prognosis. When skepticism about medications is deeper and more irrational, psychotherapeutic interventions may be needed to enhance expectancies (eg, helping a patient differentiate himself or herself from a chronically mentally ill parent who failed to benefit from medications).

Nocebo Responders

Just as patients who expect to be helped benefit especially from medications (the placebo response), patients who harbor explicit or unconscious expectations of harm are more likely to develop side effects from medications (the nocebo response). Whereas it is not a simple matter to differentiate chemical sensitivity and abnormalities in drug metabolism from nocebo responsiveness, there are a number of psychosocial factors that are known to predispose patients to side effects. Most directly, there are conscious expectations of harm. Such expectations could be elicited in discussions of patient expectations of treatment. More neurotic patients may be prone to increased side effect reporting.[65] An experience of powerlessness seems also to be particularly fertile ground for nocebo responses. Individuals from socially disadvantaged groups (minorities, women, low socioeconomic status) are more nocebo-prone,[37] as are acquiescent patients.[38–40] Acquiescence is a personality trait of easily surrendering to the will of others. It is as if these patients, unable to say no with their voices, do so instead with their bodies. Discussing the conditions of nocebogenesis before side effects emerge may give the patient and doctor some room to think about options (besides discontinuation) if side effects emerge.[8,21]

CULTIVATE THE PHARMACOTHERAPEUTIC ALLIANCE

Although every medical student learns that the doctor-patient relationship (**Table 3**) is of central importance in the practice of medicine, it typically receives far less attention than the more specific treatments that the doctor offers. However, given that the therapeutic alliance seems to contribute more potently to pharmacologic treatment outcomes than does the actual drug used,[6] it is essential to focus on and cultivate a strong therapeutic alliance. This effort toward alliance means not only gaining the patient's respect through a combination of competence, presence, tact, and empathy, but also respecting the patient's capacities as a participant in the therapeutic endeavor and actively engaging conditioned distortions (transferences) that the patient brings into pharmacotherapy regarding prescribers and/or caregiving figures in general.

Support the Patient's Agency

One potential danger of pharmacologic treatment of depression is that the patient, feeling stricken by a biological disease beyond his or her control, may surrender

Table 3
Characteristic of the doctor-patient relationship promoting improved outcomes

Outcome-Enhancing Characteristics of the Doctor-Patient Relationship in Pharmacotherapy	Evidence
Overall Effectiveness of the Doctor	McKay et al,[7] 2006
The Doctor's Positive Attitude About the Medication	Downing et al,[20] 1973
Therapeutic Alliance	Krupnick et al,[6] 1996
	Weiss et al,[27] 1997
	Klein et al,[28] 2003
	Blatt & Zuroff,[29] 2005
Good Communication	Lin et al,[66] 1995
	Bultman & Svarstad,[24] 2000
	Bull et al,[67] 2002
Involvement of the Patient in Decision-Making	Clever et al,[68] 2006
	Loh et al,[69] 2007
	Woolley et al,[70] 2010
Agreement About Diagnosis	Woolley et al,[70] 2010
Autonomy-Promoting	Zuroff et al,[58] 2007

personal agency, passively awaiting cure by the doctor's medications. Such a passive orientation does not bode well for the patient. Patients who are sociotropic[36] or who manifest an external locus of control[35] are less likely to benefit from antidepressant treatment. Conversely, patients who view their depression as nonbiological seem to benefit more from antidepressant treatment, at least for milder forms of depression.[71]

Biologically reductionistic explanations of the patient's illness, although relieving more masochistic patients of self-blame, may in the long run promote treatment resistance. The negotiation of a treatment agreement is a complicated process, instilling hope while maintaining a realistic humility about the limits of medications, and emphasizing the role that patients can play in their own recovery while sensitively trying to help them not to feel blamed for illness.

The attitude and behavior of the prescriber can have wide-ranging effects on patients' relationship toward their illness and treatment. Patients who perceive their doctors as supporting their autonomy feel more inwardly (as opposed to externally) motivated for treatment. This in turn is a strong predictor of treatment outcome; perhaps even stronger than therapeutic alliance itself.[58]

Alliance, Not Compliance

In pharmacotherapy, it is not uncommon for alliance to be confused with compliance[72] and for patients to be seen as in alliance with the doctor when they take their medication. Conversely, patients may also believe they have a good alliance with their doctor when the doctor gives them the medications they want, regardless of the physician's misgivings. Alliance, however, is a two-way street, a negotiation in which neither participant submits to the will of the other and both find a way to feel invested in the treatment plan. The model of doctor as ultimate authority on the patient's health is frequently more harmful than helpful. Similarly, is it not useful to conceptualize the doctor as servant, because the customer is not always right. A model of shared inquiry and partnership is ideal and seems to promote long-term adherence.[73]

Focus on Communication

Communication style and skills are important ingredients of a therapeutic alliance. Effective doctor-patient communication is not only clear but also collaborative, involving active listening and a nonauthoritarian orientation to problem-solving and conflict resolution.[24] Clear and collaborative communication enhances medication adherence.[24,66] Skilled communication may be especially important with specific populations, such as patients with a dismissive attachment style.[41] Discussions regarding medication should have clear explanations regarding time course of response and recommended duration of treatment.[66] Discussion of anticipated side effects also promotes adherence.[67] Many of these recommendations border on the obvious but can easily be neglected by the harried provider. Less obvious, perhaps, is the finding that adherence is increased when communication with the depressed patient involves encouragement to engage in pleasurable activities.[24,66]

Elicit Patient Preferences for Type of Treatment

Within the bounds of reason and conscience, it is useful to give the patient the treatment that he or she wants, particularly if the patient holds strong preferences for one form of treatment over another.[52] When patients prefer medications to psychotherapy, they should be offered medications. The converse is even more true: patients who prefer psychotherapy should be offered psychotherapy, because they are unlikely to benefit from medications. Kocsis and colleagues[51] found that patients receiving their preferred treatments remitted approximately 45% to 50% of the time. However, when receiving nonpreferred treatments, patients getting psychotherapy showed a 22.2% remission rate, whereas patients receiving medications remitted only 7.7% of the time. Patients receiving preferred treatments seem also to benefit more rapidly than patients receiving nonpreferred treatments.[49]

It may be that treatment preferences exert their effects on outcome indirectly through effects on other variables such as adherence and alliance. Patients assigned to nonpreferred treatments are more likely not even to start treatment and are more likely to drop out after starting,[52] particularly when treatment preferences are strong. Additionally, patients receiving nonpreferred treatments attend fewer scheduled appointments with treaters, accounting for as much as 16% of outcome variance,[53] whereas those receiving medications who prefer psychotherapy show significant decreases in alliance over the course of treatment.[50]

Involve the Patient in Decision-Making

Beyond the type of treatment (medications vs therapy), there are other ways to involve the patient in decision-making, including selection of treatment goals, medication, and dosing schedule. Involving the patient in this way enhances the alliance and increases patient satisfaction with treatment.[69]

More important, involving the patient in treatment decisions enhances utilization of treatment. In one study,[70] depressed inpatients and outpatients who were involved in treatment decisions were 2.3 times more likely to continue taking their medications. These patients were also twice as likely to discontinue treatment when they did not agree with the doctor's diagnosis. When patients disagreed with the diagnosis and felt uninvolved in decision-making, they were 7.3 times more likely to discontinue treatment against recommendations. Patients involved in decision-making have substantially better 18-month treatment outcomes,[68] with the degree of involvement directly correlated with the degree of improvement. Involving patients in decision-making also benefits treatments in more subtle ways, promoting treatment regimens that are ulti-mately more guideline-concordant.[68]

Even involvement in relatively minor treatment decisions such as the dosing schedule for the medication can exert significant effects. For example, patients given a choice between once daily and 3 times daily dosing of an antidepressant medication were significantly more likely to adhere to prescribed regimens. It is perhaps worth noting that such a negotiation is a place where the doctor might make rational concessions to the patient's irrational wishes for the sake of promoting an alliance and a positive outcome. The art of forging an alliance often involves thoughtfully choosing one's battles.

The busy prescriber might protest that there is insufficient time to elicit patients' preferences and involve them in clinical decision-making. However, the available evidence suggests that this negotiation does not actually increase the time required for a consultation.[69]

Increase the Dose . . . of the Doctor

When patients fail to respond to medications, common treatment algorithms might suggest an increase in medication dose to a therapeutic maximum, if not beyond. However, it might be just as helpful to make alliance-enhancing interventions such as increasing the dose, not of the medication, but of the doctor.[74] More frequent contact with treaters is likely an ingredient of a strong alliance and a factor in improved antidepressant adherence.[67] This benefit may be especially true when frequent contact is paired with a supportive environment and involvement with family mem-bers.[73] Indeed, it may be that nonpharmacologic factors, such as regular contact, are of sufficient importance that a treatment cannot truly be called evidence-based unless it follows the meeting schedule of the original study that forms the evidence base,[74] a schedule that typically involves weekly or biweekly meetings with the doctor or the doctor's representatives.

Address Problems in the Alliance/Negative Transferences

Either as a result of previous experiences with medications and caregivers or unconstructive interactions with the current prescriber, patients may harbor negative feelings toward the doctor. These feelings are often not articulated and may not even be conscious. These negative feelings may be expressed as poor adherence, treatment nonresponse, or nocebo effects. The maintenance of an alliance requires the prescriber to develop comfort with hearing the patient's criticism and negative feelings and the ability to address those feelings nondefensively. It may be helpful to remember that in any enduring relationship, injuries, however small, will always occur.

ATTEND TO THE PATIENT'S AMBIVALENCE

Patients may be ambivalent about their doctors. This ambivalence may emerge from transference-based expectations of caregivers or may be the result of problems in the real relationship between doctor and patient, or both, and may lead patients to resist treatment. It is more common that patients are ambivalent about their medications. This ambivalence may be particularly ubiquitous regarding psychiatric medications, which carry the standard side effect risk common to all medications but are also infused with threats to identity and stigmatizing social meanings.[75] Not surprising, perceived stigma is known to predict antidepressant nonadherence.[54]

In a content analysis of patients' representations of antidepressant medications, ambivalence was the most common of 15 themes to emerge.[76] In the average patient, perception of dangerousness and addictiveness easily balanced therapeutic effects. Whereas 44% saw antidepressants as soothing and 39% saw them as improving mood, 47% saw them as causing dependence, and 56% saw them as having adverse effects. Often the deck is stacked against medication adherence before the patient even begins treatment. Patients who express early ambivalence are twice as likely to discontinue medications prematurely and three times more likely to stop medications prematurely in the context of side effects.[56]

Inquire Specifically About Ambivalence

Given potential risks of medications (both somatic and psychosocial), the prescriber knows that patients have reason to be ambivalent. However, to understand the varying degrees of ambivalence and patterns of ambivalence, it is important to ask. The types of questions are important, because they yield very different types of information. When patients are asked broad, general questions about ambivalence toward medications, only 2% to 4% will identify ambivalence about taking medications as a significant issue. However, when asked more specific questions (eg, if you develop side effects, how likely are you to stop medications, or if you perceive no benefits in 1 month, how likely are you to stop), 23% to 36% of patients will signal their ambivalence.[56]

Inoculate the Ambivalent Patient

Like the patient with a dismissive attachment style,[65] these ambivalent patients may require particular attention and very clear communication. Patients who worry about side effects may benefit from knowing that the prescriber is sensitive to and concerned about side effects, and adherence may be increased with thorough psychoeducation about the time course of side effects (especially when tolerance is likely to develop to side effects) and strategies to manage side effects. Similarly, the ambivalent patient especially needs to understand that lack of immediate benefit does not signal a negative outcome and that these medications typically take 3 to 6 weeks to show a beneficial effect.[56] Some prescribers may seek to avoid discussions of potential side effects in an effort not to generate further ambivalence. It seems, however, that it is better to address these issues head-on. When adverse reactions are discussed with the prescriber, patients are actually less likely to discontinue antidepressants.[67]

Shape Prescribing Strategies to the Patient's Ambivalence

In a thoughtful and well-controlled study of ambivalence, Aikens and colleagues[55] explored medication adherence as a function of the patients' reasoned assessment of the balance of risks and benefits. The investigators identified four categories of patients. Depressed, medication-accepting patients saw antidepressants as necessary and were not particularly concerned about negative effects. At the opposite pole, skeptical patients had low expectations of antidepressants and high degrees of concern. Ambivalent patients saw medications as necessary for treatment of depression but also were quite concerned about the potential for negative consequences. The fourth group, indifferent patients, were not especially worried about medications, but neither did they expect much. The investigators suggest that each of these types of patients would benefit from a different treatment strategy. Accepting patients are likely to adhere to medications, whatever the approach. Indifferent patients will need to see results to be convinced of the importance of adherence. Because they are not especially concerned about side effects, an aggressive built-for-speed approach designed to bring about a rapid and complete response may be preferable. On the other hand, ambivalent patients, whose adherence is affected by concern about side effects, may benefit more from a start low, go slow approach that is designed-for-comfort. Skeptical patients may best be treated with nonpharmacologic interventions unless their illness unfolds in such a way as to increase their perceived need for medications or psychotherapeutic interventions ameliorate negative transferences or dysfunctional attitudes about medications.

Ambivalence About Illness

Perhaps more insidious and difficult to treat are those cases in which the patient is ambivalent not so much about medications as about getting better. A traditional conceptualization of medical illness takes for granted that the patient wants to get better. Whereas it is true that patients vote with their feet when they seek treatment, it is worth challenging this basic assumption.

Studies of illness benefits (or secondary gain) suggest that approximately half of patients can identify secondary benefits that derive from the sick role and/or treatment-seeking.[77,78] A study involving depressed students and psychiatric outpatients found that 44% of students and 64% of community participants identified benefits to their illness.[77] The health implications of this result are significant, because patients who expect some gain from their illness are much less likely to experience remission of symptoms.[57] When patients are treatment-refractory, ambivalence about illness should be considered as a possible source of treatment resistance.

Maintain Neutrality and Empathy

Whereas sometimes there is an overt and cynical interest in remaining (or acting) ill (eg, in order to secure remuneration for illness), secondary gains from the sick role are often subtle and may not even be conscious. Patients who become truly depressed typically do not do so in order to derive secondary gains; however, once ill, they may discover that the sick role confers certain benefits. The dynamic model of symptoms as partial solutions becomes useful in this regard. Symptoms and illness behaviors may come to represent the patient's best effort at managing overwhelming affect, communicating something that cannot be put into words or allowing for the assumption of a role in a family that would otherwise be intolerable.[21]

These patients often evoke frustration, if not condemnation, from treaters, and the capacity of treaters to remain empathic is often strained. It is perhaps useful to remember that patients who cleave to the sick role generally do so at tremendous personal cost to themselves. To understand the reasons that patients would give up so much for the seemingly meager benefits of the sick role is to restore empathy and establish a therapeutic frame in which a true exploration of ambivalence can occur.

The patient's ambivalence about recovery is not presented readily. Although 42% of patients seeking psychiatric help expect some secondary gain from treatment, only 9% reveal this expectation to their treaters.[78] It can be useful to inquire, during the initial assessment phase of pharmacotherapy, about what a patient stands to lose if treatment works. It is less useful to ask the same question later in treatment, because it is then more likely to come from a place of frustration, sparking the patient's defensiveness and shutting down awareness of ambivalence.

Even with the treater's sensitive curiosity, patients may not be willing to say (or know) they are ambivalent. Patients often feel ashamed or humiliated by a conscious wish to remain sick. More often, however, these aspects remain largely out of the patient's awareness. Generally, psychotherapeutic interventions are called for if patients are to get to a place where they might best be able to make use of medications in the service of recovery. An appreciation by the treater for the patient's ambivalence about the loss of symptoms may also influence the timing of interventions (pharmacologic or psychotherapeutic), because there is some evidence that a patient's readiness to change may be a powerful variable in treatment response.[59,60]

It is through attentive, nonjudgmental, and open investigation that the patient may begin to connect with underlying ambivalence. These investigations, aimed at a fuller appreciation for the patient's current situation and underlying motivations, are an essential aspect of working collaboratively with a patient. In the course of these explorations, patients may be helped to see more clearly their attachment to the sick role and the losses they have experienced as a result of that attachment. In addition to social costs, there may be psychological costs (such as guilt over unearned benefits of the sick role) that enter into the patient's changing understanding of the economy of gain.[79] These explorations can enhance alliance, which can improve pharmacologic outcome on its own.[6] The adoption of a neutral, curious, and empathic stance can be difficult to achieve and may be nearly impossible when patients or social systems put the treater in the position of gatekeeper for access to concrete rewards for illness (eg, disability benefits).

ADDRESS COUNTERTHERAPEUTIC USES OF MEDICATIONS

Clinicians are often attentive to signs that their patient is misusing a prescribed medication that has effects on the brain's reward systems (opiates and benzodiazepines in particular). Physicians are less likely to consider medication misuse when those medications are not seen as rewarding or intoxicating, such as occurs when patients use antipsychotics recreationally.[80] It may be harder still to identify signs that a prescribed medication has been turned to serve more subtle countertherapeutic ends, particularly when the patient experiences the medication as helpful and there is evidence of attenuation of some symptoms.

Treatment Resistance from Medications

One sign of a countertherapeutic use of medications might be when a patient who feels better with certain medications does not seem to get better. Overall functioning does not improve, or worsens, or perhaps the prescriber merely senses, with a feeling of apprehension or guilt, that the patient is in the process of becoming chronic. In these cases it is useful to consider whether medications are being used in ways that interfere with the developmental task of treatment.

There are a number of ways that prescribed medications may unintentionally contribute to treatment resistance. In some cases the medication (or the diagnosis that comes with the medication) may serve as an inexact interpretation[81,82] that patients seize on to bolster unhealthy defenses, interfering with the patient's adaptability or self-awareness.

One common example of this inexact interpretation is when primitively organized and character-disordered patients who rely on splitting and projective dynamics receive a prescription of mood stabilizers for bipolar disorder. Such patients tend to see things strictly in black and white and often defend against feeling intolerably and completely bad by displacing all of the "badness" onto the "other" in a relationship. Such a patient, prone to splitting as a defense, will often experience an immediate reduction in dysphoria at receiving a bipolar diagnosis. A psychopharmacologist who is inclined to think both psychodynamically and biologically will recognize that the reduction in dysphoria may be occurring not because of the medication but because it allows the patient to create a stable split within which he or she can remain good, while all badness is located in "my bipolar." Although patients may feel better, they actually do worse. No longer feeling personally responsible for symptomatic behavior, they give their worst instincts free rein, exacerbating personal and interpersonal chaos. Substances can be used defensively to disavow responsibility for feelings and actions.[83]

Medications can be used defensively in myriad other ways. Patients who experience people as dangerous and unreliable may attempt to replace people with pills, turning to medications instead of people to deal with ordinary frustrations and injuries. Although pills may help them to manage, their medicalized universe becomes increasingly depopulated. This patient is not likely to emerge from depression. Still other patients may believe that any negative feeling is pathologic and should be extinguished. In a sense, these patients no longer have feelings that they should learn from. Instead they have symptoms that become the purview of the doctor. If accepted at face value, this situation can lead a well-meaning psychiatrist toward an ever more complex and burdensome medication regimen that actually contravenes healthy developmental aims.

When pills are used to manage developmentally appropriate feelings like loneliness, disappointment, sadness, frustration, or anger, patients lose important opportunities that might lead to improved internal controls and increased affective or interpersonal competence. Patients who turn too much to their doctors to solve their problems of living may not only be treatment-resistant *to* their medications but also may become treatment resistant *from* their medications.[35,36,71]

Think Like a Mental Health Professional

One's ability to recognize countertherapeutic uses of medications may be conditioned on one's conceptualization of the therapeutic task. With a singular focus on symptoms and symptom reduction, a great many providers have inadvertently become mental *illness* professionals, pursuing symptoms while losing sight of larger developmental aims. In contrast, a mental *health* professional is concerned not just with the absence of illness, but even more with the promotion of health. By prescribing in a way that fosters the patient's agency and overall adaptive capacity, a mental health professional does not miss the forest for the trees and is more likely to be attuned to defensive and disempowering uses of medications.

IDENTIFY AND CONTAIN COUNTERTRANSFERENCE PRESCRIBING

A hallmark of countertransference prescribing is its focus on managing the experience of the prescriber rather than the experience of the patient. Although the image of a rational and methodical prescriber may be appealing, the emotional response of the prescriber is sometimes the primary impetus for a prescription.[84] Especially in those cases in which the patient's dysphoria is infectious, provoking intense feelings of anger, hopelessness, helplessness, or even despair in the doctor, prescriptions may unconsciously be aimed at decreasing those feelings. In the same way that resistance from medications interferes with the developmental task of treatment, unexamined countertransference prescribing runs the risk of becoming a chronic form of nontreatment. Understood, however, instances of countertransference prescribing can become valuable sources of data about the patient's experience and relationships outside the treatment.

Colleagues are Crucial

Managing the impulse to prescribe out of countertransference or recognizing that one is already prescribing out of countertransference often requires an outside perspective. The role of consultation with other colleagues cannot be underestimated when working with patients who evoke strong countertransference reactions. Systems, however, are in no way immune to prescribing enactments in the face of strong feelings.[85] Colleagues with some distance from the intensity of the case can best offer a connection to a standard of practice that a prescriber can lose touch with amid an enactment.

Develop a Dynamic Formulation

A dynamic formulation can also exert a containing and conservative effect, orienting the prescriber and others under the pressure of strong disorganizing affect. A self-aware prescriber with a formulation of repetitive patterns in the patient's life will be more likely to anticipate prescribing enactments (eg, when the prescriber recreates the dynamic of the parents who cannot tolerate the strong affects of their child). A dynamic formulation may also help providers to maintain empathy toward the patient. Both psychodynamic and cognitive-behavioral formulations of symptoms have empathogenic effects. However, benefits accruing from a psychodynamic formulation seem to persist, whereas the benefits of cognitive-behavioral understandings decline to nonsignificance over time.[86]

A dynamic formulation need not be a thousand-word document. A brief focused formulation of the patient's relationship to medications and/or treaters is generally sufficient for the prescriber. Such a formulation might, for example, predict that a patient with deep-seated issues around control would attempt to wrest control of the medications from the doctor or anticipate that a patient who could neither bear nor articulate a desperate feeling of helplessness would powerfully evoke that same feeling in the treater. When in the thrall of strong countertransference feelings the prescriber can then call on the formulation, which may allow the prescriber to identify and contain potential irrational processes in the pharmacotherapeutic relationship.

Similarly, a dynamic formulation that contains a systems perspective, if shared, can help the prescriber to contain irrational processes in the larger treatment system. If this sharing works well, the prescriber will benefit from only having to deal with uncontained irrationality on one front: the patient. A brief dynamic formulation, included in the patient's chart, is also a way to pass on accumulated wisdom about a patient and to inoculate future treaters from predictable enactments.

SUMMARY

Despite advances in psychopharmacology over the past several decades, treatment outcomes for depression have not substantially improved. Depression is not being eradicated. If anything, the evidence suggests that the problem of depression and treatment-resistant depression is growing, not shrinking.[87] As biologically reductionistic approaches dominate psychiatric practice, patient care has steered away from considering the potent effects of meaning and relationships in the psychopharmacologic treatment of our patients. By construing patients as passive recipients of concrete, specific, and straightforward medical interventions, the field has succumbed to a delusion of precision,[88] and unwittingly moved into an era of treatment resistance in which some of our most potent tools are wasted. In such a model we have settled for treating a disorder rather than a whole person. This article is intended as a step toward remedy. Meaning effects, therapeutic alliance, ambivalence, and patient autonomy, among others, have a powerful and measurable impact on the use of medication that should be considered if we are to treat the whole person. Bringing these elements together into a coherent model of treatment, however, is only a starting point. More research is needed if we are to understand the effects these elements have when used together in an integrated model that is simultaneously personalized and evidence-based.

REFERENCES

1. Trivedi MH, Rush AJ, Wisniewski SR, et al. Evaluation of outcomes with citalopram for depression using measurement-based care in STAR*D: implications for clinical practice. Am J Psychiatry 2006;163:28–40.
2. Rush AJ, Trivedi MH, Wisniewski SR, et al. STAR*D Study Team. Bupropion-SR, sertraline, or venlafaxine-XR after failure of SSRIs for depression. N Engl J Med 2006;354:1231–42.
3. Kirsch I, Sapirstein G. Listening to Prozac but hearing placebo: a meta–analysis of antidepressant medication. Prevention and Treatment 1998;1(2):Article 2a.
4. Khan A, Warner HA, Brown WA. Symptom reduction and suicide risk in patients treated with placebo in antidepressant clinical trials: an analysis of the Food and Drug Administration database. Arch Gen Psychiatry 2000;57:311–7.
5. Kirsch I, Moore TJ, Scoboria A, et al. The emperor's new drugs: an analysis of antidepressant medication data submitted to the U.S. Food and Drug Administration. Prevention and Treatment. 2002;5:Article 23.
6. Krupnick JL, Sotsky SM, Simmens S, et al. The role of therapeutic alliance in psychotherapy and pharmacotherapy outcome: findings in the National Institute of Mental Health Treatment of Depression Collaborative Research Program. J Consult Clin Psychol 1996;64:532–9.
7. McKay KM, Imel ZE, Wampold BE. Psychiatrist effects in the psychopharmacological treatment of depression. J Affect Disord 2006; 92:287–90.
8. Mintz D. Meaning and medication in the care of treatment-resistant patients. Am J Psychother 2002;56:322–37.
9. Plakun EM. A view from Riggs: Treatment resistance and patient authority: I. A psychodynamic perspective. J Am Acad Psychoanal Dyn Psychiatry 2006;34: 349–66.
10. Mojtabai R, Olfson M. National trends in psychotherapy by office-based psychiatrists. Arch Gen Psychiatry 2008;65,962–97.
11. Chong WW, Aslani P, Chen TF. Effectiveness of interventions to improve antidepressant medication adherence: a systematic review. Int J Clin Pract 2011;65:954–75.
12. Rush AJ, Trivedi MH. Treating depression to remission. Psychiatr Ann 1995;25: 704–9.
13. Berlim MT, Turecki G. What is the meaning of treatment resistant/refractory major depression (TRD)? A systematic review of current randomized trials. Eur Neuropsychopharmacol 2007;17:696–707.
14. Thase ME, Friedman ES, Biggs MM, et al, Cognitive therapy versus medication in augmentation and switch strategies as second step treatments: a STAR*D report. Am J Psychiatry 2007;164:739–52.
15. Fisher S, Greenberg RP. The curse of the placebo: fanciful pursuit of a pure biological therapy. In: Greenberg RP, Fisher S, editors. From placebo to panacea. New York: Wiley; 1997. p. 3–56.
16. Schapira K, McClelland HA, Griffiths NR, et al. Study on the effects of tablet colour in the treatment of anxiety states. BMJ 1970;1:446–9.
17. de Craen AJ, Roos PJ, Leonard de Vries A, et al. Effect of colour of drugs: systematic review of perceived effect of drugs and of their effectiveness. BMJ 1996;313:1624–6.
18. Waber RL, Shiv B, Carmon Z. Commercial features of placebo and therapeutic efficacy. JAMA 2008;299:1016–7.
19. de Craen AJ, Tijssen JG, de Gans J, et al. Placebo effect in the acute treatment of migraine: subcutaneous placebos are better than oral placebos. J Neurol 2000;247: 183–8.

20. Downing RW, Rickels K, Dreesmann H. Orthogonal factors vs. interdependent variables as predictors of drug treatment response in anxious outpatients. Psychopharmacologia 1973;32:93–111.

21. Mintz DL, Belnap BA. A view from Riggs: treatment resistance and patient authority - III. What is psychodynamic psychopharmacology? An approach to pharmacologic treatment resistance. J Am Acad Psychoanal Dyn Psychiatry. 2006;34:581–601.

22. Mintz DL, Belnap BA. What is psychodynamic psychopharmacology? An approach to pharmacological treatment resistance. In: Plakun EM, editor. Treatment resistance and patient authority: an Austen Riggs reader. New York: Norton; 2011. p. 42–65.

23. Mintz, D. The distancing function of language in medicine. J Med Humanit 1991;13: 223–33.

24. Bultman DC, Svarstad BL. Effects of physician communication style on client medication beliefs and adherence with antidepressant treatment. Patient Educ Couns 2000;40:173–85.

25. Ströhle A. Physical activity, exercise, depression and anxiety disorders. J Neural Transm 2009;116:777–84.

26. Bagby RM, Ryder AG, Cristi C. Psychosocial and clinical predictors of response to pharmacotherapy for depression. J Psychiatry Neurosci 2002;27:250–25.

27. Weiss M, Gaston L, Propst A, et al. The role of the alliance in the pharmacologic treatment of depression. J Clin Psychiatry 1997;58:196–204.

28. Klein DN, Schwartz JE, Santiago NJ, et al. Therapeutic alliance in depression treatment: controlling for prior change and patient characteristics. J Consult Clin Psychol 2003;71:997–1006.

29. Blatt SJ, Zuroff DC. Empirical evaluation of the assumptions in identifying evidence based treatments in mental health. Clin Psychol Rev 2005;25:459–86.

30. Vergouwen AC, Bakker A, Katon WJ, et al. Improving adherence to antidepressants: a systematic review of interventions. J Clin Psychiatry 2003;64:1415–20.

31. Joyce PR, Paykel ES. Predictors of drug response in depression. Arch Gen Psychiatry 1989;46:89–99.

32. Scott J, Williams JM, Brittlebank A, et al. The relationship between premorbid neuroticism, cognitive dysfunction and persistence of depression: a 1-year follow-up. J Affect Disord 1995;33:167–72.

33. Steunenberg B, Beekman AT, Deeg DJ, et al. Personality predicts recurrence of late-life depression. J Affect Disord 2010;123:164–72.

34. Kronström K, Salminen JK, Hietala J, et al. Does defense style or psychological mindedness predict treatment response in major depression? Depress Anxiety 2009; 26:689–95.

35. Reynaert C, Janne P, Vause M, et al. Clinical trials of antidepressants: the hidden face: where locus of control appears to play a key role in depression outcome. Psychopharmacology 1995;119:449–54.

36. Peselow ED, Robins CJ, Sanfilipo MP, et al. Sociotropy and autonomy: relationship to antidepressant drug treatment response and endogenous-nonendogenous dichotomy. J Abnorm Psychol 1992;101:479–86.

37. Hahn RA. The nocebo phenomenon: concept, evidence, and implications for public health. Prev Med 1997;26:607–11.

38. McNair DM, Kahn RJ, Droppelman RF, et al. Compatibility, acquiescence, and drug effects. In: Brill H, editor. Neuro-psycho-pharmacology: proceedings of the Fifth International Congress of the Collegioum Internationale Neuro-psycho pharmacologicum. New York: Excerpta Medica Foundation; 1968. p. 536–42.

39. McNair DM, Fisher S, Kahn RJ, et al. Drug-personality interaction in intensive outpatient treatment. Arch Gen Psychiatry 1970;22:128–35.

40. Fast GJ, Fisher S. The role of body attitudes and acquiescence in epinephrine and placebo effects. Psychosom Med 1971;33:63–84.
41. Ciechanowski PS, Katon WJ, Russo JE, et al. The patient-provider relationship: attachment theory and adherence to treatment in diabetes. Am J Psychiatry 2001; 158:29–35.
42. Ciechanowski PS, Russo JE, Katon WJ, et al. The association of patient relationship style and outcomes in collaborative care treatment for depression in patients with diabetes. Med Care 2006;44:283–29.
43. Comninos A, Grenyer BF. The influence of interpersonal factors on the speed of recovery from major depression. Psychother Res 2007;17:230–9.
44. Meyer B, Pilkonis PA Krupnick JL, et al. Treatment expectancies, patient alliance, and outcome: further analyses from the National Institute of Mental Health Treatment of Depression Collaborative Research Program. J Consult Clin Psychol 2002;70: 1051–5.
45. Krell HV, Leuchter AF, Morgan M, et al. Subject expectations of treatment effectiveness and outcome of treatment with an experimental antidepressant. J Clin Psychiatry 2004;65:1174–9.
46. Aikens JE, Kroenke K, Swindle RW, et al. Nine-month predictors and outcomes of SSRI antidepressant continuation in primary care. Gen Hosp Psychiatry 2005;27: 229–36.
47. Gaudiano BA, Miller IW. Patients' expectancies, the alliance in pharmacotherapy, and treatment outcomes in bipolar disorder. J Consult Clin Psychol 2006;74:671–6.
48. Sneed JR, Rutherford BR, Rindskopf D, et al. Design makes a difference: a meta-analysis of antidepressant response rates in placebo-controlled versus comparator trials in late-life depression. Am J Geriatr 2008;16:65–73.
49. Lin P, Campbell DG, Chaney EF, et al. The influence of patient preference on depression treatment in primary care. Ann Behav Med 2005;30:164–73.
50. Iacoviello BM, McCarthy KS, Barrett MS, et al. Treatment preferences affect the therapeutic alliance: implications for randomized controlled trials. J Consult Clin Psychol 2007;75:194–8.
51. Kocsis JH, Leon AC, Markowitz JC, et al. Patient preference as a moderator of outcome for chronic forms of major depressive disorder treated with nefazodone, cognitive behavioral analysis system of psychotherapy, or their combination. J Clin Psychiatry 2009;70:354–61.
52. Raue PJ, Schulberg HC, Heo M, et al. Patients' depression treatment preferences and initiation, adherence, and outcome: a randomized primary care study. Psychiatr Serv 2009;60:337–43.
53. Kwan BM, Dimidjian S, Rizvi SL. Treatment preference, engagement, and clinical improvement in pharmacotherapy versus psychotherapy for depression. Behav Res Ther 2010;48(8):799–80.
54. Sirey JA, Bruce ML, Alexopoulos GS, et al. Stigma as a barrier to recovery: perceived stigma and patient-rated severity of illness as predictors of antidepressant drug adherence. Psychiatr Serv 2001;52:1615–20.
55. Aikens JE, Nease DE, Klinkman MS, Explaining patients' beliefs about the necessity and harmfulness of antidepressants. Ann Fam Med 2008;6:23–9.
56. Warden D, Trivedi MH, Wisniewski SR, et al. Identifying risk for attrition during treatment for depression. Psychother Psychosom 2009;78:372–9.
57. van Egmond J, Kummeling I. A blind spot for secondary gain affecting therapy outcomes. Eur Psychiat 2002;17:46–54.

58. Zuroff DC, Koestner R, Moskowitz DS, et al. Autonomous motivation for therapy: a new common factor in brief treatments for depression. Psychother Res 2007;17(2): 137–47.
59. Beitman BD, Beck NC, Deuser WE, et al. Patient stage of change predicts outcome in a panic disorder medication trial. Anxiety 1994;1:64–9.
60. Lewis CC, Simons AD, Silva SG, et al. The role of readiness to change in response to treatment of adolescent depression. J Consult Clin Psychol 2009;77:422–42.
61. Petersen T, Papakostas GI, Bottonari K, et al. NEO-FFI factor scores as predictors of clinical response to fluoxetine in depressed outpatients. Psychiatry Res 2002; 109:9–16.
62. Bos EH, Bouhuys AL, Geerts E, et al. Cognitive, physiological, and personality correlates of recurrence of depression. J Affect Disord 2005;87:221–2.
63. Bartholomew K, Horowitz LM. Attachment styles among young adults: A test of a four-category model. J Personal Soc Psychol 1991;61:226–44.
64. Klerman GL, Weissman MM, Rounsaville BJ, et al. Interpersonal psychotherapy of depression. New York: Basic Books; 1984.
65. Davis C, Ralevski E, Kennedy S, et al. The role of personality factors in the reporting of side effect complaints to moclobemide and placebo: a study of healthy male and female volunteers. J Clin Psychopharmacol 1995;15:5:347–52.
66. Lin EH, Von Korff M, Katon, W, et al. The role of the primary care physician in patients' adherence to antidepressant therapy. Med Care 1995;33:67–74.
67. Bull SA, Hu XH, Hunkeler EM, et al. Discontinuation of use and switching of antidepressants: influence of patient-physician communication. JAMA 2002;288:1403–9.
68. Clever SL, Ford DE, Rubenstein LV, et al. Primary care patients' involvement in decision-making is associated with improvement in depression. Med Care 2006;44: 398–40.
69. Loh A, Simon D, Wills CE, et al. The effects of a shared decision-making intervention in primary care of depression: a cluster-randomized controlled trial. Patient Educ Couns 2007;67:324–32.
70. Woolley SB, Fredman L, Goethe JW, et al. Hospital patients' perceptions during treatment and early discontinuation of serotonin selective reuptake inhibitor antidepressants. J Clin Psychopharmacol 2010;30:716–9.
71. Sullivan MD, Katon WJ, Russo JE, et al. Patient beliefs predict response to paroxetine among primary care patients with dysthymia and minor depression. J Am Board Fam Pract 2003;16:22–3.
72. Gutheil TG, Havens LL. The therapeutic alliance: contemporary meanings and confusions. Int J Psychoanal 1979;6(4):467–81.
73. Frank E, Kupfer DJ, Siegel LR. Alliance not compliance: a philosophy of outpatient care. J Clin Psychiatry 1995;56(Suppl 1):11–6 [discussion: 16–7].
74. Ankarberg P, Falkenström F. Treatment of depression with antidepressants is primarily a psychological treatment. Psychother Theor Res Pract Train 2008;45:329–39.
75. Pound P, Britten N, Morgan M, et al. Resisting medicines: a synthesis of qualitative studies of medicine taking. Soc Sci Med 2005;61:133–55.
76. Piguet V, Cedraschi C, Dumont P, et al. Patients' representations of antidepressants: a clue to nonadherence? Clin J Pain 2007;23:669–75.
77. Dulgar-Tulloch L. An assessment of the positive aspects of depression [PhD dissertation]. Albany (NY): State University of New York at Albany; 2009.
78. Van Egmond J, Kummeling I, Balkom TA. Secondary gain as hidden motive for getting psychiatric treatment. Eur Psychiat 2005;20:416–42.
79. Kwan O, Friel J. Clinical relevance of the sick role and secondary gain in the treatment of disability syndromes. Med Hypotheses 2002;59:129–34.

80. Bogart GT, Ott CA. Abuse of second-generation antipsychotics: what prescribers need to know. Curr Psychiatr 2011;10(5):77–9.
81. Glover E. The therapeutic effect of inexact interpretation: a contribution to the theory of suggestion. Int J Psychoanal 1931;12:397–411.
82. Nevins DB. Psychoanalytic perspectives on the use of medications for mental illness. B Menninger Clin 1990;54:323–39.
83. Gibbons FX, Wright RA. Motivational biases in causal attributions of arousal. J Pers Soc Psychol 1981;40:588–600.
84. Waldinger RJ, Frank AF. Clinicians' experiences in combining medication and psychotherapy in the treatment of borderline patients. Hosp Community Psych 1989; 40:712–8.
85. Swenson CR, Wood MJ. Issues involved in combining drugs with psychotherapy for the borderline inpatient. Psychiatr Clin N Am 1990;13:297–306.
86. Treloar AJ. Effectiveness of education programs in changing clinicians' attitudes toward treating borderline personality disorder. Psychiatr Serv 2009;60:1128–31.
87. Kessler RC, Berglund P, Demler O, et al. The epidemiology of major depressive disorder: results from the National Comorbidity Survey Replication (NCS-R). JAMA 2003;289:3095–105.
88. Gutheil TG. The psychology of psychopharmacology. Bull Menninger Clin 1982;46: 321–33.

Combined Treatment of Depression

Fredric N. Busch, MD[a,b,]*, Larry S. Sandberg, MD[a,b]

KEYWORDS

- Combined treatment • Medication • Psychotherapy
- Depression • Research

Multiple medications and some forms of psychotherapy have demonstrated efficacy in the treatment of depression.[1] However, despite these interventions, many patients continue to respond only partially to available treatments[2] and nonadherence to medication is common,[3,4] adding to the tendency of depression to recur.[5] Many clinicians believe that a combination of medication and psychotherapy provides the greatest potential for long-term relief of depression,[6] and a number of studies have focused on the relative value of combined compared to single treatments.

Given our current state of knowledge, for which patients should a combination of medication and psychotherapy be recommended and employed? The American Psychiatric Association Practice guideline for the treatment of patients with major depressive disorder[1] identifies a broad range of conditions for which combined treatment should be considered (**Box 1**): "Combining a depression-focused psychotherapy and pharmacotherapy may be a useful initial treatment choice for patients with moderate to severe major depressive disorder. Other indications for combined treatment include chronic forms of depression, psychosocial issues, intrapsychic conflict, interpersonal problems, or a co-occurring Axis II disorder. In addition, patients who have had a history of only partial response to adequate trials of single treatment modalities may benefit from combined treatment. Poor adherence with pharmacotherapy may also warrant combined treatment with medications and psychotherapy focused on treatment adherence."[1(p28)]

There are several reasons to believe that medication and psychotherapy should be utilized together for treatment of depression.[7] These approaches probably affect different areas of the brain, potentially creating a synergistic neurophysiologic effect.[8] Given that different patients demonstrate different responses to various treatments, combining two treatments increases the likelihood patients will respond to at least

---

The authors have nothing to disclose.
a Weill Cornell Medical College, 1300 York Avenue, New York, NY 10065, USA
b Columbia University Center for Psychoanalytic Training and Research, 180 Fort, Washington Avenue, New York, NY 10032, USA
* Corresponding author. 10 East 78th Street, #5A, New York, NY 10075.
E-mail address: fnb80@aol.com

Psychiatr Clin N Am 35 (2012) 165–179
doi:10.1016/j.psc.2011.10.002
0193-953X/12/$ – see front matter © 2012 Elsevier Inc. All rights reserved.

Box 1
Recommendations for combined treatment: practice guidelines

- Patients with moderate to severe major depressive disorder
- Chronic forms of depression
- Psychosocial issues, intrapsychic conflict, interpersonal problems
- A co-occurring Axis II disorder
- Partial response to adequate trials of single treatment modalities
- Poor adherence with pharmacotherapy

---

one of them. In addition, the persistent and recurrent nature of depressive syndromes[5,9] and the adverse impact of residual symptoms[10,11] indicate the importance of reducing vulnerability to depression, and psychotherapy and medication may be additive in their impact on this vulnerability. Each modality can potentially enhance the other: medication allowing for more effective use of psychotherapy (eg, through increasing concentration and motivation) and psychotherapy aiding with adherence to medication.[3,12] Combining psychotherapy with medication may allow for reduced doses and a diminished side effect burden of medications, and medication can reduce the need for persistent or more intensive psychotherapy through reduction of symptoms.

However, there are also arguments against combination treatments. Not all patients require medication and psychotherapy to achieve remission of symptoms or prevent recurrence. Therefore combination treatments may expose patients to more treatment and side effects than is necessary. Questions of cost effectiveness arise in the greater expense of psychotherapy plus medication, although potential benefits over the long term need to be considered.[13] Problems in delivery of combined treatments ("split treatment" vs a psychiatrist providing both psychotherapy and medication) may reduce overall effectiveness of one or the other approaches.[14]

Thus, many questions remain regarding the need for and relative efficacy of combined treatment. What types of patients may require a combination approach and which may need only a single treatment? What may be the value of sequencing treatments? Do some forms of depression benefit more from combined treatment than others? What factors may moderate response to combined treatment? What types of psychotherapy are most effective for depression in a combination treatment? How does delivery of combined treatment by a single practitioner compare to a "split treatment" involving a psychotherapist and psychopharmacologist? What do research studies show about combined treatment and how might they aid in clinical decision making? What are limitations and problems with these research studies?

Given these varied viewpoints and remaining questions, clinical decisions are often based on the skill set and belief system of the particular clinician who is treating the patient. In many cases a single treatment is initiated that is changed to a combination treatment if there is a limited response. Through such strategies patients frequently show adequate response to treatment, although many will not achieve remission or will experience a recurrence of depression. In this article we review the literature on combined treatment to develop a rationale for addressing these questions based on theory, clinical experience, and research studies.

THE BIOPSYCHOSOCIAL MODEL IN CONSIDERING COMBINED TREATMENTS

A biopsychosocial model is of particular utility in conceptualizing the value of combining medication and psychotherapy, identifying how biological and psychological interventions can work together in depression treatment.[15] Kendler[16] attempted to further delineate these processes, suggesting a model of bidirectional causality: mental phenomena have an impact on brain function and brain function impacts the mind. Thus medication affects mental phenomena, and psychotherapy becomes a biological treatment affecting brain function. In accord with this model, increasingly studies have identified neurophysiological changes that accompany improvement in depression and anxiety disorders through psychotherapy.[8] This model helps to explain how medication and psychotherapy can operate synergistically.

At the same time, this model can be employed to argue for providing a single treatment. If medication and psychotherapy both affect mind and brain, then why are two treatments necessary? Kendler[16] employs the term "patchy reductionism" in describing how unitary causal models are not sufficient for most mental disorders. The relative value of psychotherapy and medication varies on the basis of the particular form of depressive disorder; the life history, psychology, and environment of the patient; the presence of other disorders; and the particular susceptibility of a given patient to different approaches. Clinical and research efforts are necessary to further identify how to best approach individual patients.

RESEARCH ON COMBINED TREATMENTS

Research studies have attempted to answer the following questions (**Box 2**): Is combined treatment more effective? Does combined treatment provide advantages in the short term, long term, or both? Is there a benefit to sequencing treatments? Do different types of depression respond differentially to combined treatments? What factors moderate treatment outcomes? What types of psychotherapy may be most effective in a combined treatment? This article reviews the status of the research on combined treatments to best provide answers for these questions. The summaries in the text that follows are not meant to be an exhaustive review of the research literature, but are intended to be representative, with a focus on recent studies that are of higher quality. In addition, questions have been raised about the value of evidence-based medicine, including randomized controlled trials (RCTs) and meta-analyses.[17] These issues are not a focus of this article, but call attention to the need for being circumspect in interpreting the research literature.

Box 2
Areas of research

- Comparing combined to single treatments
- Follow-up studies
- Sequencing of treatments
- Types of depression
- Moderators of outcome
- Split versus single treatments

	Type of Study	Effect Size	Other Findings
Table 1 **Recent comprehensive meta-analyses**			
Cuijpers et al[20]	Psychological treatment was compared to the same psychological treatment combined with medication.	0.35 in favor of combined treatment	The difference between CBT and the combined treatment was significantly smaller. At follow-up of 3–6 and 12 months, no significant differences were found.
Cuijpers et al[21]	Medication was compared to a combination of medication and psychotherapy.	0.31 in favor of combined treatment	In patients with dysthymia, the value of adding psychotherapy was significantly less. The dropout rate was significantly lower in combined treatment.
Cuijpers et al[22]	Medication and psychotherapy were compared to psychotherapy and placebo.	0.25 in favor of the combined active treatment	The result indicates that the impact of medication in combined treatment is not just a placebo effect.

Combining Psychotherapy and Medication

Most reviews and meta-analyses[12,18–24] have determined that combined treatment is somewhat more efficacious than a single treatment, although negative studies have raised questions about whether different treatments or patient subgroups affect these results.[20–24] Three recent comprehensive meta-analyses[20–22] demonstrated small but significant advantages of combined treatments and attempted to identify factors that may be relevant to efficacy and treatment choice (**Table 1**). Cuijpers and colleagues[20] reviewed 18 randomized studies in which a psychological treatment was compared to the same psychological treatment combined with medication. This meta-analysis demonstrated a mean effect size of 0.35 in favor of combined treatment, a small but significant advantage. In studies in which cognitive–behavioral therapy (CBT) was examined, the difference between CBT and the combined treatment was significantly smaller, suggesting that CBT may be a more efficacious treatment. In addition, at follow-up of 3 to 6 and 12 months, no significant differences were found.

Cuijpers and colleagues[21] identified 25 randomized trials in which medication was compared to a combination of medication and psychotherapy. A mean effect size in favor of the combined treatment of 0.31 was found, indicating a small but significant advantage for combined treatment compared to medication alone. In patients with dysthymia, the value of adding psychotherapy was significantly less. The dropout rate was significantly lower in combined treatment, indicating that combined treatment may allow for improved adherence. Most recently, Cuijpers and coworkers[22] compared RCTs in which medication and psychotherapy were compared to psychotherapy and placebo to evaluate better the advantage of active medication treatment. In examining 16 studies the authors found an effect size of 0.25 in favor of active medication, again demonstrating a small but significant advantage in the combined active treatment. No subgroup differences were found in this study.

The authors point out that the small to moderate effect sizes found in these meta-analyses, despite their statistical significance, raise a question about the actual degree of clinical advantage of combined treatment. Possible explanations of the relatively small advantage found in these studies[20–22] are the relative effectiveness of combined treatments for certain subgroups, the significant treatment impact of single treatments for many patients, or problems with the quality of studies done thus far. Overall, the data to date show that the average patient will have a better outcome with combined treatment than with unimodal approaches. However, given the relatively small effect sizes, and the potential costs of treatment (in money, time, and side effects), patient preference, clinical features of depression, and various complicating factors should be considered in the clinician's decision to recommend combined treatment.

Assessing Follow-Up

In addition to assessing whether the combination of psychotherapy and medication is superior to single treatments, a critical factor is the impact of these treatments over the long term. Given the persistent and recurrent nature of depression,[5,9] it is important to evaluate whether a combined treatment can reduce vulnerability to these disorders. The capacity to affect persistent symptoms is also relevant to the cost effectiveness of combined treatments. Although Cuijpers and colleagues[20] found that differences between combined treatment and psychotherapy in the short term were lost in follow-up, several recent studies that examined longer term follow-up suggest that these gains may be maintained (**Table 2**).

Schramm and coworkers[25] studied patients hospitalized with major depressive disorder (MDD) in an RCT, comparing 5 weeks of interpersonal psychotherapy (IPT) modified for depressed inpatients plus medication to intensive clinical management plus medication. Patients receiving IPT plus medication showed higher response and remission rates after treatment and higher response rates and Global Assessment of Funtioning (GAF) at 3- and 12-month follow-up. Zobel and coworkers[26] looked at follow-up over 5 years for the patients in the study by Schramm and colleagues.[25] The rate of reduction of symptoms and the percentage of patients who sustained remission over the 5-year period was higher for those receiving IPT (28%) compared to the clinical management group (11%). Combination treatment was more effective for patients with a history of trauma, a finding concordant with that of Nemeroff and colleagues,[27] which is discussed further in the text that follows. Maina and colleagues[28] studied patients with MDD who met criteria for remission after a 6-month treatment with either medication or medication plus brief dynamic therapy (BDT). After the initial treatment there was a 6-month continuation phase with medications alone, followed by an assessment at 48 months. Patients who received combined treatment in the initial phase had significantly lower rates of relapse at 48-month follow-up. Other follow-up studies, involving sequential treatment, are discussed later.[29,30] The emerging data on the value of combined treatment over the long term suggests that it should be more strongly considered, despite the costs of these treatments. Clinicians should remain alert to further follow-up studies in the literature in guiding their decisions.

Sequencing of Treatments

Sequencing of treatments can be employed as an augmenting strategy in the acute phase or as a shift in approaches to treat different phases of the illness. The concept inherent in the latter is that the mechanisms involved in depression onset differ from those contributing to its recurrence, and thus each phase benefits from different interventions.[31] In his review of studies on combined treatment, Petersen found that ". . .sequential use of psychotherapy after induction of remission with acute antidepressant drug therapy may confer a better long-term prognosis in terms of preventing

Table 2
Recent long-term follow-up studies

	Treatments Compared	Length of Follow-Up	Results
Schramm et al[25]	IPT modified for depressed inpatients plus medication to intensive clinical management plus medication	3 and 12 months	IPT plus medication showed higher response rates and GAF.
Zobel et al[26] further follow-up from Shramm et al[25]	IPT modified for depressed inpatients plus medication to intensive clinical management plus medication	5 years	Rate of reduction of symptoms and percentage of patients who sustained remission over the 5-year period was higher for those receiving IPT (28%) compared to the clinical management group (11%).
Maina et al[28]	BDT plus medication compared to medication alone	48 months	Combined treatment had significantly lower rates of relapse at 48-month follow-up.
Bockting et al[29]	Brief CBT added to usual care to usual care alone	5.5 years	CBT plus usual care provided a significant protective effect against relapse/recurrence.

relapse or recurrence and, for some patients, may be a viable alternative to maintenance medication therapy."[7(p19)]

Several studies suggest that a switch to or addition of psychotherapy either does not adversely affect or decreases the risk of depression recurrence (**Table 3**). Segal and colleagues[32] studied patients whose symptoms remitted with antidepressants and then randomized them to eight weekly group sessions of mindfulness based cognitive therapy (MBCT), continuing on medication, or switching to placebo. Among unstable remitters, patients treated with either medication or MBCT showed significantly reduced risk of relapse compared to placebo, suggesting comparable outcomes for the sequencing of treatments. Among stable remitters, there was no difference between the groups. Bockting and colleagues[29] found that brief CBT, when added to usual care and initiated after episode remission in patients with recurrent depression, provided a significant protective effect during a 5.5-year period compared with usual care alone. Kennard and coworkers[33] examined adolescents with MDD who responded to medication treatment and randomized them to either continued medication or medication plus CBT focused on relapse prevention. They found an eightfold reduction in relapse in patients receiving the combined treatment. Fava and colleagues[30,34] studied patients with recurrent depression who had remitted in response to antidepressant medications. Medications were discontinued and patients were randomized to receive either CBT or clinical management. At 6-year follow-up patients receiving CBT had a significantly lower relapse rate (40%) than those receiving clinical management (90%).

Frank and coworkers[35] applied an alternate approach in studying two successive cohorts of women with recurrent major depression. One group was treated with IPT plus medication and the other group was treated first with IPT with the addition of medication if they did not remit. The second group showed a significantly higher remission rate (79%) than those who received combined treatment from the outset (66%). Although the reason for the higher remission rate was unclear and this was not a randomized trial, the study suggests that many patients can benefit from psychotherapy alone, requiring medication only if they are nonresponsive. Overall, studies suggest that sequencing treatment can allow the clinician to identify patients that may need only a single treatment, and that psychotherapy after medication can help to reduce the risk of relapse.

Types of Depression

Subcategories of depression that have been considered to potentially respond differentially to a combination treatment include dysthymia and chronic depression. Interpretation of studies of dysthymia are complicated by the inclusion of many patients who have "double depression" (MDD plus dysthymia), as opposed to "pure" dysthymia.[36] As noted in the preceding text, Cuijpers and colleagues[21] found that the combination of psychotherapy and medication adds little to medication alone in the treatment of dysthymia. Imel and coworkers[36] found medication to have greater efficacy in a meta-analysis of studies comparing psychotherapy and medication in the treatment of dysthymia. Markowitz and colleagues[37] studied 94 subjects with "pure" dysthymia (no episodes of MDD in 6 months before presentation) randomized to 16 weeks of IPT, brief supportive psychotherapy (BSP), sertraline, or sertraline plus IPT. Although subjects were responsive to all of the treatments, responses were higher and at a similar rate with sertraline (58%) and combined treatment (57%) compared to IPT (35%) and BSP (31%).

Patients with chronic depression have been found to be less responsive to treatment.[24] In a landmark study, Keller and colleagues[38] found a significantly higher

Table 3
Studies on sequencing of treatments

	Subjects Studied	Treatments Sequenced/Compared	Results
Segal et al[32]	Patients whose symptoms remitted with antidepressants	Eight weekly group sessions of MBCT, continuing on medication, or switching to placebo	Among unstable remitters, patients treated with either medication or MBCT showed significantly reduced risk of relapse compared to placebo. Among stable remitters, there was no difference between the groups.
Bockting et al[29]	Remitted patients with recurrent depression	Brief CBT added to usual care to usual care alone	CBT plus usual care provided a significant protective effect against relapse/recurrence.
Kennard et al[33]	Adolescents with MDD who responded to medication treatment	Continued medication or medication plus CBT focused on relapse prevention	There was an eightfold reduction in relapse in patients receiving the combined treatment.
Fava et al[30,34]	Patients with recurrent depression who had remitted with antidepressant medications	Medications discontinued and patients randomized to either CBT or clinical management	At 6-year follow-up, patients receiving CBT had a significantly lower relapse rate (40%) than those receiving clinical management (90%).
Frank et al[35]	Women with recurrent major depression	One group IPT plus medication; one group treated first with IPT with medication added if they did not remit	IPT with medication added if they did not remit showed a significantly higher remission rate (79%) than those who received combined treatment from the outset (66%).

rate of response in chronically depressed patients receiving a combination of CBASP (cognitive–behavioral analysis system of psychotherapy) and nefazodone compared to either treatment alone. Subjects were considered to have chronic depression if "(1) criteria for MDE were met continuously for at least 2 years, with no antecedent dysthymia; (2) the MDE was superimposed on antecedent dysthymia; or (3) the MDE was recurrent, with incomplete interepisode recovery, and lasted at least 2 years."[39(p460)] A subsequent reanalysis of the data[39] found that patients receiving the combination treatment showed more rapid remission. Hollon and coworkers,[18] in their review of the literature, suggested that combination treatment may be particularly valuable for patients with chronic depression. In a negative study, Kocsis and colleagues[24] studied chronically depressed patients who did not achieve remission (60% reduction in Hamilton Scale for Depression [HAM-D] score, a 24-item HAM-D total score <8, and no longer meeting DSM-IV criteria for MDD for 2 consecutive visits) and randomized them to either medication alone, medication plus CBASP, or medication plus brief supportive psychotherapy. In their study, 37.5% of patients remitted or showed partial response in phase II, but no differences were found in response to the various treatments. The authors acknowledge that the number of sessions of CBASP received was lower (12.5 vs 16) than in those of Keller and coworkers.[38] Overall, these studies indicate that combined treatment should be strongly considered in cases of chronic depression.

Moderators of Outcome

Two major potential moderators explored in the literature on combined treatment are personality disorders and trauma, addressing the question of whether psychotherapy, in addition to medication, may be necessary to adequately address these factors. Many studies indicate that depression accompanied by personality disorders is less responsive to treatment. For example, Grilo and colleagues[40] studied patients with MDD, assessing for the presence of personality disorders. They found that patients with personality disorders at baseline took a longer time to achieve remission and relapsed much more rapidly after remission compared to patients without personality disorders after achieving remission. Kool and colleagues[41] studied patients with major depression randomized to receive combined medication and short-term psychodynamic psychotherapy or medication alone. In secondary analyses they found that combined treatment was more effective in treating patients who also had personality disorders but not more effective in patients who did not have personality disorders. Maddux and colleagues[42] examined chronically depressed patients treated with CBASP, nefazodone, or their combination. In this study the presence of personality disorders did not have an impact on outcome. However, the study excluded borderline, schizotypal, and antisocial personality disorders.

In the examination by Nemeroff and colleagues[27] of the data of Keller and colleagues,[38] 681 patients with chronic forms of major depression were treated with an antidepressant (nefazodone), CBASP, or the combination. Among those with a history of early childhood trauma (loss of parents at an early age, physical or sexual abuse, or neglect), psychotherapy alone was superior to antidepressant mono-therapy. Moreover, the combination of psychotherapy and pharmacotherapy was only marginally superior to psychotherapy alone among the childhood abuse cohort. In the study by Zobel and coworkers[26] described in the preceding text, combination treatment was found to be more effective for patients with a history of trauma. The results of these studies suggest that psychotherapy may be an essential element in the treatment of depressed patients with a history of childhood trauma and a comorbid personality disorder.

Types of Psychotherapy

Significantly more evidence has been garnered for CBT and IPT compared to psychodynamic psychotherapy with regard to combined treatment of depression.[1] Hollon and colleagues,[18] in their review, surmised that "interpersonal psychotherapy (IPT) appears to have a delayed effect on the quality of interpersonal relationships not found for medications, and cognitive-behavioral therapy (CBT) appears to have an enduring effect that reduces risk for subsequent symptom return even after treatment is over."[18(p456)] As noted in the preceding text, several studies have found that CBT added to medication can reduce the risk of relapse.[29,33] Although research on psychodynamic psychotherapy is more limited, several studies[28,41,43] and recent meta-analyses[19,44] indicate that this treatment can also be effective in achieving remission and reducing relapse. It is unclear at this time what type of psychotherapy in combination with medication may best address co-occurring personality disorders.[45,46]

Single Provider Versus Split Treatment

No studies were located comparing the relative efficacy of a single clinician providing combined treatment and a split treatment. Two studies[47,48] suggest that it is relatively more cost effective to have a psychiatrist providing both treatments. Dewan[47] found that combined treatment by a psychiatrist cost about the same or less than split treatment with either a social worker or psychologist/psychotherapist based on fee schedules of a variety of managed care organizations and Medicare. Goldman and colleagues,[48] reviewing retrospective data of claims from a managed care organization over an 18-month period, found that patients seeing a psychiatrist in combined treatment had lower costs and fewer total visits than patients in a split treatment. These findings are counterintuitive, raising questions about the presumption that split treatment is less expensive.

As noted in the preceding text, the issues of combined treatment delivery is of great significance but relatively ignored in the literature. There are a variety of clinical discussions on managing these situations[14] but minimal research comparing these treatments. A psychiatrist providing psychotherapy and medication has the advantage of avoiding conflicts between two treating clinicians. In addition, the greater frequency of visits to the psychiatrist allows more frequent opportunities to monitor for persistent or recurrent depressive symptoms. There are potential problems with this approach, however, including that a psychiatrist providing psychotherapy can lose sight of the more systematic assessment of symptoms and medication that are done automatically in pharmacologic visits.[14] In addition, psychiatrists often do not have competency in the depression-focused psychotherapies that have been found to be effective for treatment of depression. This could certainly be addressed through additional training.

Several papers have been written that describe the potential areas of conflict in split treatments between the two providers and in patients' experience and perception of these providers.[49,50] Competitive and professional tensions, as well as different theoretical and clinical models, can generate problems in treatment management. Patients may idealize and devalue one or the other of the clinicians, or act out in ways that may be difficult to address. A triadic therapeutic alliance and communication about problems have been recommended as ways of identifying and addressing potential problems.

DISCUSSION

Research studies overall substantiate an advantage of combined treatment over a single treatment for depression and the vulnerability to persistence or recurrence (a

> **Box 3**
> **Recommendations on combined treatments based on clinical experience and research studies**
>
> - Despite an edge in efficacy, the clinician should consider costs of treatment, patient preference, clinical features of depression, and complicating factors (eg, poor treatment adherence, psychosocial problems, co-occurring personality disorders) in recommending combined treatments.
> - Sequencing treatment can allow the clinician to identify patients who may need only a single treatment, and psychotherapy following medication can help to reduce the risk of relapse.
> - Psychotherapy may be a necessary component of treatment in depressed patients with comborbid personality disorders or a history of trauma.
> - Chronic depression appears to respond best to combined treatment, whereas "pure" dysthymia thus far has been found to respond better to medication.
> - Although CBT and IPT have more definitively demonstrated efficacy in the treatment of depression, studies suggest that psychodynamic psychotherapy may be of significant value alone or in combined treatments.
> - Studies have yet to clarify the relative cost effectiveness or efficacy of single practitioner versus split treatment, although each benefits from clinicians being alert to potential clinical problems of each approach.

summary of recommendations is provided in **Box 3**). Further studies are required, however, to better determine the types of patients and treatments for which combined treatments are most appropriate or necessary. From the clinical and research standpoint, the broad range of conditions suggested for combined treatment in the Practice Guideline[1] seems appropriate. Studies thus far suggest an advantage for combined treatment in patients with chronic depression (other than "pure" dysthymia), co-occurring personality disorders, and a history of trauma. Although the Practice Guideline suggests an advantage for combined treatment for dysthymia,[1] research thus far suggests limited value for psychotherapeutic or combined treatment of this disorder. The development of therapies targeted for chronic disorders and the more careful distinction between dysthymia and double depression may affect this recommendation.

From the clinician's standpoint, combination treatment represents a powerful intervention that can be synergistic across the biopsychosocial spectrum. Medication provides rapid relief of symptoms, but includes the problems of persistent side effects and potential for recurrence when medication is discontinued. Psychotherapy may be slower in its impact on symptoms and more labor intensive, but can aid in reduction of persistent symptoms and relapse recurrence. Psychotherapy provides an opportunity to address co-occurring personality disorders, trauma sequelae, and intrapsychic conflicts that can add to persistent depression vulnerability, psychosocial disruption, and suffering. Studies of cost effectiveness are limited,[13] but given the high cost of depression, any form of treatment that diminishes vulnerability over the long term should be given serious consideration. Combined treatment may aid in adherence to both medication and psychotherapy.[3,12,21]

With regard to types of psychotherapy, thus far CBT and IPT have much broader evidence bases for treatment of depression and depression vulnerability, including as part of combined treatment. Given the limited studies, much more research needs to be done before an accurate picture can be obtained comparing psychodynamic psychotherapy to these psychotherapies. Focused psychodynamic psychotherapies for depression are increasingly being developed and more systematic assessment of testable psychodynamic treatments is underway. Difficult as they are, direct comparisons of CBT, IPT, and psychodynamic therapy over the short and long term will be essential to fully clarify the relative value of these treatments. There is reason to believe that psychodynamic psychotherapy, with its broad range of focus on symptom meanings, intrapsychic conflicts, personality dysfunction, and interpersonal relationships and their internal representations may have a broader impact on depression vulnerability than other treatments. A recent meta-analysis[51] suggests that long-term psychodynamic psychotherapy may be valuable for complex mental disorders (personality disorders, chronic illness of at least 1 year's duration, and multiple comorbid disorders).

Further studies are essential to compare the relative efficacy of a single provider versus split treatment. From the clinical standpoint, clinicians should adopt strategies that minimize potential problems with either approach: a single clinician providing both treatments developing a means of regular medication assessment, and communication between providers to address problem areas in a split treatment.

Additional studies are clearly required to delineate further the value of combined versus single treatments in depression. There are no "cookbook" means of approaching depressed patients, although the information discussed can aid clinicians in choosing treatment options. In addition, the evidence base and recommendations continue to shift; for example, an increase in targeted psychotherapy studies led to these treatments being more highly recommended in the most recent Practice Guideline.[1] It is important for clinicians to be knowledgeable about the various interventions available for depression, to be willing to employ more than a single intervention, and to stay informed of ongoing developments regarding these treatments.

REFERENCES

1. American Psychiatric Association. Practice guideline for the treatment of patients with major depressive disorder. 3rd edition. Am J Psychiatry 2010;167(10 Suppl):1–118.
2. Rush AJ, Trivedi MH, Wisniewski SR, et al. Acute and longer-term outcomes in depressed outpatients requiring one or several treatment steps: a STAR*D report. Am J Psychiatry 2006;163(11):1905–17.
3. Bockting CL, ten Doesschate MC, Spijker J, et al. Continuation and maintenance use of antidepressants in recurrent depression. Psychother Psychosom 2008; 77(1):17–26.
4. Simon GE, Von Korff M, Rutter CM, et al. Treatment process and outcomes for managed care patients receiving new antidepressant prescriptions from psychiatrists and primary care physicians. Arch Gen Psychiatry 2001;58:395–401.
5. Judd LL, Akiskal HS, Zeller PJ, et al. Psychosocial disability during the long-term course of unipolar major depressive disorder. Arch Gen Psychiatry 2000;57:375–80.
6. Kornbluh R, Papakostas GI, Petersen T, et al. A survey of prescribing preferences in the treatment of refractory depression: recent trends. Psychopharmacol Bull 2001; 35:150–6.
7. Petersen TJ. Enhancing the efficacy of antidepressants with psychotherapy. J Psychopharm 2006;20:19–28.
8. Goldapple K, Segal Z, Garson C, et al. Modulation of cortical-limbic pathways in major depression: treatment-specific effects of cognitive behavior therapy. Arch Gen Psychiatry 2004;61:34–41.
9. Eaton WW, Shao H, Nestadt G, et al. Population-based study of first onset and chronicity in major depressive disorder. Arch Gen Psychiatry 2008;65:513–20.

10. Judd LL, Akiskal HS, Paulus MP. The role and clinical significance of subsyndromal depressive symptoms(SSD) in unipolar major depressive disorder. J Affect Disord 1997;45(1–2):5–18.
11. Paykel ES, Ramana R, Cooper Z, et al. Residual symptoms after partial remission: an important outcome in depression. Psychol Med 1995;25(6):1171–80.
12. Pampallona S, Bollini P, Tibaldi G, et al. Combined pharmacotherapy and psychological treatment for depression: a systematic review. Arch Gen Psychiatry 2004;61: 714–9.
13. Lynch FL, Dickerson JF, Clarke G, et al. Incremental cost-effectiveness of combined therapy vs medication only for youth with selective serotonin reuptake inhibitor-resistant depression: treatment of SSRI-resistant depression in adolescents trial findings. Arch Gen Psychiatry 2011;68:253–62.
14. Busch FN, Sandberg LS. Psychotherapy and medication: the challenge of integration. Hillsdale (NJ): The Analytic Press; 2007.
15. Engle GL. The need for a new model: a challenge for biomedicine. Science 1977;196: 129–36.
16. Kendler KS. Toward a philosophical structure for psychiatry. Am J Psychiatry 2005; 162:433–40.
17. Gupta M. Does evidence-based medicine apply to psychiatry? Theor Med Bioeth 2007;28:103–20.
18. Hollon SD, Jarrett RB, Nierenberg AA, et al. Psychotherapy and medication in the treatment of adult and geriatric depression: which monotherapy or combined treatment? J Clin Psychiatry 2005;66:455–68.
19. de Maat S, Dekker J, Schoevers R, et al: Short psychodynamic supportive psychotherapy, antidepressants, and their combination in the treatment of major depression: a mega-analysis based on three randomized clinical trials. Depress Anxiety 2008;25: 565–74.
20. Cuijpers P, van Straten A, Warmerdam L, et al. Psychotherapy versus the combination of psychotherapy and pharmacotherapy in the treatment of depression: a meta-analysis. Depress Anxiety 2009;26(3):279–88.
21. Cuijpers P, Dekker J, Hollon SD, et al. Adding psychotherapy to pharmacotherapy in the treatment of depressive disorders in adults: a meta-analysis. J Clin Psychiatry 2009;70(9):1219–29.
22. Cuijpers P, van Straten A, Hollon SD, et al. The contribution of active medication to combined treatments of psychotherapy and pharmacotherapy for adult depression: a meta-analysis. Acta Psychiatr Scand 2010;121:415–23.
23. Vitello B. Combined cognitive-behavioural therapy and pharmacotherapy for adolescent depression: does it improve outcomes compared with monotherapy? CNS Drugs 2009;23(4):271–80.
24. Kocsis JH, Gelenberg AJ, Rothbaum BO, et al. Cognitive behavioral analysis system of psychotherapy and brief supportive psychotherapy for augmentation of antidepressant nonresponse in chronic depression The REVAMP trial. Arch Gen Psychiatry 2009;66:1178–88.
25. Schramm E, van Calker D, Dykierek P, et al. An intensive treatment program of interpersonal psychotherapy plus pharmacotherapy for depressed inpatients: acute and long-term results. Am J Psychiatry 2007;164:768–77.
26. Zobel I, Kech S, van Calker D, et al. Long-term effect of combined interpersonal psychotherapy and pharmacotherapy in a randomized trial of depressed patients. Acta Psychiatr Scand 2011;123:276–82.

27. Nemeroff CB, Heim CM, Thase ME, et al. Differential responses to psychotherapy versus pharmacotherapy in patients with chronic forms of major depression and childhood trauma. Proc Natl Acad Sci USA 2003;100:14293–6.

28. Maina G, Rosso G, Bogetto F. Brief dynamic therapy combined with pharmacotherapy in the treatment of major depressive disorder: long-term results. J Affect Disord 2009;114:200–7.

29. Bockting CL, Spinhoven P, Wouters LF, et al. DELTA Study Group. Long-term effects of preventive cognitive therapy in recurrent depression: a 5.5–year follow-up study. J Clin Psychiatry 2009;70(12):1621–8.

30. Fava GA, Ruini C, Rafanelli C, et al. Six-year outcome of cognitive behavior therapy for prevention of recurrent depression. Am J Psychiatry 2004;161:1872–6.

31. Post RM. Transduction of psychosocial stress into the neurobiology of recurrent affective disorder. Am J Psychiatry 1992;149:999–1010.

32. Segal ZV, Bieling P, Young T, et al. Antidepressant monotherapy vs sequential pharmacotherapy and mindfulness-based cognitive therapy, or placebo, for relapse prophylaxis in recurrent depression. Arch Gen Psychiatry 2010;67:1256–64.

33. Kennard BD, Emslie GJ, Mayes TL. Cognitive-behavioral therapy to prevent relapse in pediatric responders to pharmacotherapy for major depressive disorder J Am Acad Child Adolesc Psychiatry 2008;47(12):1395–404.

34. Fava GA, Rafanelli C, Grandi S, et al. Prevention of recurrent depression with cognitive behavioral therapy: preliminary findings. Arch Gen Psychiatry 1998;55:816–20.

35. Frank E, Grochocinski VJ, Spanier CA, et al. Interpersonal psychotherapy and antidepressant medication: evaluation of a sequential treatment strategy in women with recurrent major depression. J Clin Psychiatry 2000;61(1):51–7.

36. Imel ZE, Malterer MB, Mckay KM, et al. A metaanalysis of psychotherapy and medication in unipolar depression and dysthymia. J Affect Disord 2008;110:197–206.

37. Markowitz JC, Kocsis JH, Bleiberg KL, et al. Research report a comparative trial of psychotherapy and pharmacotherapy for "pure" dysthymic patients. J Affect Disord 2005;89: 167–75.

38. Keller MB, Mccullough JP, Klein DN, et al. A comparison of nefazodone, the cognitive behavioral-analysis system of psychotherapy, and their combination for the treatment of chronic depression. N Engl J Med 2000;342:1462–70.

39. Manber R, Kraemer HC, Arnow BA, et al. Faster remission of chronic depression with combined psychotherapy and medication than with each therapy alone. J Consult Clin Psychol 2008;76:459–67.

40. Grilo CM, Stout RL, Markowitz JC, et al. Personality disorders predict relapse after remission from an episode of major depressive disorder: a 6-year prospective study. J Clin Psychiatry 2010;71:1629–35.

41. Kool S, Dekker J, Duijsens IJ, et al. Changes in personality pathology after pharmacotherapy and combined therapy for depressed patients. J Pers Disord 2003;17:60–72.

42. Maddux RE, Riso LP, Klein DN, et al. Select comorbid personality disorders and the treatment of chronic depression with nefazodone, targeted psychotherapy, or their combination. J Affect Disord 2009;117:174–9.

43. Maina G, Rosso G, Crepi C, et al. Combined brief dynamic therapy and pharmacotherapy in the treatment of major depressive disorder: a pilot study. Psychother Psychosom 2007;76:298–305.

44. Driessen E, Cuijpers P, de Maat SC, et al. The efficacy of short-term psychodynamic psychotherapy for depression: a meta-analysis. Clin Psychol Rev 2010;30(1):25–36.

45. Joyce PR, McKenzie JM, Carter JD, et al. Temperament, character and personality disorders as predictors of response to interpersonal psychotherapy and cognitive-behavior therapy for depression. Br J Psychiatry 2007;190:503–8.

46. Dixon-Gordon K, Turner B, Chapman A. Psychotherapy for personality disorders. Int Rev Psychiatry 2011;23(3):282–302.

47. Dewan M. Are psychiatrists cost-effective? An analysis of integrated versus split treatment. Am J Psychiatry 1999;156(2):324–6.

48. Goldman W, McCulloch J, Cuffel B, et al. Outpatient utilization patterns of integrated and split psychotherapy and pharmacotherapy for depression. Psychiatr Serv 1998; 49:477–82.

49. Busch FN, Gould E. Transference/countertransference in the pharmacotherapy/psychotherapy triangle. Hosp Community Psychiatry 1993;44:772–4.

50. Gould E, Busch FN. Special issues in the psychopharmacology/psychotherapy triangle. Psychoanal Inq 1998;18:730–45.

51. Leichsenring F, Rabung S. Effectiveness of long-term psychodynamic psychotherapy: a meta-analysis. JAMA 2008;300(13):1551–65.

Child and Adolescent Depression: Psychotherapeutic, Ethical, and Related Nonpharmacologic Considerations for General Psychiatrists and Others Who Prescribe

Mary Lynn Dell, MD, DMin[a,b,]*

KEYWORDS

• Children • Adolescents • Depression • Psychotherapy
• Ethics • Multidisciplinary treatment

Depression is among the most common of all illnesses, affecting over 16% of all individuals in the United States at some time in their lives.[1] Because of its recurrent nature, treatment resistance, lack of treatment, or a combination thereof, 85% of those with depression will suffer recurrence within 15 years.[2] Youth experience depression at significant rates as well. Recently published results from the National Comorbidity Study–Adolescent Supplement reveal a lifetime prevalence of major depressive disorder or dysthymia of 11.2% of 13- to 18-year-olds, with a 3.3% lifetime prevalence of a severe depressive disorder in that same age group.[3] The 2008 National Survey on Drug Use and Health, sponsored yearly by the Substance Abuse and Mental Health Services Administration, shows the prevalence of depression among 12- to 17-year-olds to be 8.3%, with girls showing 3 times the prevalence as boys.[4] One-year prevalence rates for major depression are approximately 2% in childhood and 4% to 7% in adolescence.[5] Depression in adolescence is associated with increased risks of substance abuse and dependence and academic, occupational, interpersonal, and other social difficulties.[6–9] Suicide risk is significantly increased in youth with depressive disorders and is the third leading cause of death in adolescents. Data published by the Centers for Disease Control and Prevention report that over a 1-year period of time studied, 13.8% of American adolescents

The author has nothing to disclose.
[a] Case Western Reserve University School of Medicine, 10524 Euclid Avenue, W.O. Walker Building, Suite 1155A, Cleveland, OH 44106, USA
[b] Child and Adolescent Psychiatry Consultation Liaison Service, Rainbow Babies and Children's Hospital/University Hospitals Case Medical Center, Cleveland, OH, USA
* Case Western Reserve University School of Medicine, 10524 Euclid Avenue, W.O. Walker Building, Suite 1155A, Cleveland, OH 44106.
E-mail address: mary.dell@UHhospitals.org

Psychiatr Clin N Am 35 (2012) 181–201
doi:10.1016/j.psc.2011.12.002
0193-953X/12/$ – see front matter © 2012 Published by Elsevier Inc.

psych.theclinics.com

considered killing themselves, 10.9% had made plans, and 6.3% actually reported attempting suicide.[10]

Clearly, a large workforce of well-trained, qualified professionals is needed to provide competent care to the millions of youth affected by psychiatric disorders of all kinds, especially child and adolescent depression. Work force issues have been of prime concern in the American Academy of Child and Adolescent Psychiatry (AACAP). The demand for services by child and adolescent psychiatry was anticipated to increase by 100% between 1995 and 2020, and as of 2009 there were an estimated 7,000 practicing child and adolescent psychiatrists practicing in the United States, far short of the 30,000 predicted to have been needed by 2000, 9 years earlier. Recruitment and funding issues make it unlikely that the numbers of these subspecialty physicians will swell to the estimated 13,000 predicted to be needed to meet demand.

In addition, there are significant distribution concerns within the existing pool of child and adolescent psychiatrists. Rural states and impoverished areas, rural or urban, have poor or limited access to child psychiatric services. It is in these geographical areas that general psychiatrists frequently find seriously ill youth on their patient lists simply because they may be the best qualified physician in the region to care for these children and adolescents.[11] These statistics also portend that pediatricians, family practitioners, nurse practitioners, and general psychiatrists will be called on to assess and treat pediatric depression with increasing frequency in the years to come.

Although this article, for the sole, practical reason of economy of words, predominantly cites general psychiatrists, it also addresses the needs of other clinicians who prescribe for and participate in the care of depressed children and adolescents.

ADULT PSYCHIATRISTS CARING FOR CHILDREN AND ADOLESCENTS: GENERAL CONSIDERATIONS

What preparation do general psychiatry trainees receive in anticipation of rising to the challenge of managing child and adolescent disorders? The Psychiatry Program Requirements determined and published by the Accreditation Council for Graduate Medical Education (ACGME) mandates a minimum of 2 months of full-time equivalent of an organized clinical experience. During this experience, residents are to be "supervised by child and adolescent psychiatrists who are certified by the American Board of Psychiatry and Neurology or judged by the Review Committee to have equivalent qualifications; and provided opportunities to assess development and to evaluate and treat a variety of diagnoses in male and female children and adolescents and their families, using a variety of interventional modalities."[12] Settings vary from inpatient, day treatment, and outpatient, and less commonly, residential settings. Court, school, and other consultative experiences are more challenging to arrange at the general psychiatry level of training. Trainees and supervisors alike are wise to consider child elements of the general training program as exposures to the practice of child and adolescent psychiatry that rarely, if ever, substitute for the breadth and depth of training available in 2-year fellowship programs. Regardless, the completion of a general psychiatry training program does provide a foundational experience that may indeed be that primary preparation for generalists who find themselves treating minors, whether by choice or necessity of their practice setting.

Three distinct, but interrelated, funds of knowledge are essentially important for the general psychiatrist caring for children and adolescents. These include normal development, psychopathology, and treatment, especially the principles and practice of psychopharmacology. Without a developmental perspective, the prescribing psychiatrist can appreciate neither the challenges children and families face as they grow and change

---

Box 1
AACAP practice parameters relevant to the treatment of child and adolescent depression

1. **Current Parameters**

   a. Depressive Disorders (2007)

   b. Assessment of the Family (2007)

   c. Community Systems of Care (2007)

   d. Physically Ill Children (2009)

   e. Prescribing Psychotropic Medication to Children (2009)

2. **Parameters in Development or Updates in Progress**

   a. Assessment of Children and Adolescents (1997–update in progress)

   b. Suicidal Behavior (2001–update in progress)

   c. Psychodynamic Psychotherapy with Children (new parameter under final review)

From the American Academy of Child and Adolescent Psychiatry. Practice Parameters. Available at: http://www.aacap.org/. Accessed December 7, 2011.

---

together, nor psychopathology as it manifests in different age groups and situational contexts. In today's environment of relatively easy access to information, several thorough, clinically helpful reviews of development are available for general clinicians.[13–16] Similarly, several overviews of the psychopathology, assessment, and management of childhood depression are readily available and typically updated every few years.[17–19] Detailed clinical manuals and book chapters on psychopharmacologic treatment of child and adolescent depression are available through several major medical presses and are very helpful resources in clinical work with young patients and their families.[20–29] In addition, the AACAP has helpful documents available in print and online, including approved Practice Parameters for the psychiatric assessment of children and adolescents, the assessment of the family, the assessment and treatment of children and adolescents with depressive disorders, the use of psychotropic medication in children and adolescents, and child and adolescent mental health care in community systems of care (**Box 1**).[30–34]

In many ways, the objective, evidence-based tasks of child and adolescent psychiatry, such as assessment, diagnosis, and medication management are more straightforward and less daunting than in years past. More information is readily available in print and on the internet. Furthermore, telephone consultation can be arranged with experts across the country, and telepsychiatry is becoming increasingly popular with patients and clinicians alike.[35] For the general psychiatrist treating children and adolescents, usually as only a small proportion of his or her practice, the greater challenges are often the "softer," less black or white, matters that have minimal to no evidence base, vary with cultural shifts, and truly are matters of experience and personal and professional judgment. Other challenges arise simply because of the reality that child patients are not of majority age. Consequently, completing assessments, obtaining all necessary information, and communicating with the numerous stakeholders in each case—2 or more parent figures, grandparents, teachers, therapists, probation officers, primary care physicians, and county workers, for instance—takes time and can be messy. Referral sources, treatment collaborators and systems, even the implementation and goals of psychotherapy, are different when treating minors rather than adults. Ethical and cultural considerations may also be more complicated. The rest of this article is devoted to considering work across disciplines with nonmedical professionals who provide mental health services for adolescents, and, exploring cultural, ethical, and regulatory concerns involved in antidepressant treatment of youth.

WHO REFERS DEPRESSED CHILDREN AND ADOLESCENTS TO GENERAL PSYCHIATRISTS AND COLLABORATES IN CONTINUED CARE?

General psychiatrists typically see depressed children and adolescents in consultation for diagnosis, for second opinion or consultation regarding a diagnosis of depression, and for ongoing psychotropic medication management of depression while the young person is in ongoing psychotherapy or behavioral management with a nonphysician mental health clinician. In many ways, this mirrors the roles of child and adolescent psychiatrists who treat children in many practice settings, especially in underserved community, institutional, and forensic settings. Psychiatrists often are only at a given site 1 or more half days a week, have clinics for different types of patients and purposes, and are viewed by systems of care as highly specialized resources whose education and talents are best used tending to tasks few others can do—primarily the prescription of psychotropic medication. Often, however, medication management appointments leave little time to get to know a child or adolescent, his or her relative strengths and weaknesses, issues in the family, and concerns being addressed by therapists and case workers. More so than in general psychiatric work with adults, those who treat children must rely on the skills and conscientiousness of these other clinicians, many of whom are recruited and hired by institutions and systems of care without the input of the psychiatrist. Who are these nonphysician mental health workers who first meet our child patients, identify key issues, interface with the important others in a child's life, and implement the bulk of nonbiological treatments?

Psychologists

Psychologists are a varied group of professionals who study and practice psychological and educational assessments, psychotherapies, behavioral management, parent training, and research. They serve in private practices, community mental health centers, hospitals, schools, residential centers, outpatient settings, residential treatment facilities, and county agencies. They may have master's degrees or doctoral degrees, including PhD's or Doctor of Psychology (PsyD) degrees. Licensure is granted by states and often includes internships and residencies approved by accrediting bodies and required hours of patient contact and supervision. The American Psychological Association is the psychology's primary professional guild. With 154,000 members, it represents psychology in the United States and is the largest association of psychologists worldwide. It is comprised of divisions of specialties within the field, including school psychology, psychotherapy, intellectual and developmental disabilities, the Society of Clinical Child and Adolescent Psychology, and Society of Pediatric Psychology, which focuses on health behaviors. Nationwide, psychologists comprise one of the largest groups of professionals that refer children and adolescents to general psychiatrists for medication assessment and management.[36]

Social Workers

Social workers are another group of professionals heavily involved in the care of youth referred to general psychiatrists. Also licensed by the states, with minimum education, supervision, and continuing education requirements, social workers commonly have master's degrees, though increasingly, leadership and academics will have a PhD or Doctor of Social Work (DSW) degree. Social workers have diverse job descriptions, including individual psychotherapy, abuse work, patient advocacy, and interfacing with services in the community needed by youth and their families. They work in hospitals, community mental health centers, private practices, medical offices, county offices, and agencies. Social workers are represented, among other organizations, by the 145,000-member National Association of Social Workers, headquartered in Washington, DC. The mission of the National Association of Social Workers is to "enhance professional growth of its members, to create and maintain professional standards, and to advance sound social policy."[37]

Marriage and Family Therapists

Another group of mental health professionals who work with psychiatrists, especially in areas with child psychiatrist shortages, are marriage and family therapists. This is a more diverse group of individuals, consisting of psychologists, social workers, nurses, educators, pastoral counselors, and others who identify themselves based on the patient or client population and services they provide instead of their discipline of origin. Certification is state regulated, though with more variability than other fields. Two years of clinical supervision is customarily required, and the American Association for Marriage and Family Therapy also conducts a national examination.[38]

Pastoral Counselors

Finally, pastoral counselors, pastoral psychotherapists, and clergy comprise a large, but diverse, group of mental health care collaborators for the general psychiatrist. Education and formal training varies greatly, ranging from no formal psychological training to second-career clergy who may have been mental health professionals earlier during their working lives. Religious professionals may counsel individuals in their congregation as part of their pastoral responsibilities, or work in churches or synagogues, private practices, or larger pastoral care centers as full-time therapists. Pastoral counselors vary with regard to how much religious and spiritual content they introduce or encourage their clients to discuss in sessions. The most reputable professional association for pastoral counselors is the American Association of Pastoral Counselors. Professional certification by American Association of Pastoral Counselors requires a 3-year professional seminary degree, a master's or doctoral degree in a mental health field, approximately 1400 hours of supervised clinical experience with 250 hours of direct supervision by approved supervisors. Religious professionals and parish clergy may provide much of the nonmedical mental health assessments and care in the very same geographical areas in which general psychiatrists may see higher proportions of adolescent patients because of shortages of child and adolescent psychiatrists.[39,40]

SCHOOLS AND THE GENERAL PSYCHIATRIST

All psychiatrists who care for children and adolescents must have an up-to-date familiarity with public and private primary and secondary schools in their practice locations. General psychiatrists often treat adolescents with mood and psychotic disorders who are still in high schools and may be struggling academically and socially.

The school setting has much to offer regarding adolescent mental health. School convenes daily, and, because everyone is required to go, is often a less stigmatizing location to receive care. Schools and their communities are committed to promoting qualities that enhance academic achievement, such as proper identification and treatment of psychiatric illness. They are also committed to minimizing risky behaviors that often accompany or predispose to behavioral health concerns, such as substance abuse, antisocial behaviors, and unhealthy sexual activity.[41] Mental health care in the school setting can improve access for minorities, help reduce the stigma of requesting and obtaining care, and facilitate service delivery in areas that otherwise have few treatment options.[42–44] Service provision in school may lead to improved attendance and fewer behavioral concerns.[45] In addition, adults serving youth in school settings typically are educated, have devoted their professional lives to education, and are invested in the total well-being of their students. School professionals, therefore, are valuable collaborators, multidisciplinary team members, and even rich patient referral sources for general psychiatrists who offer pharmacotherapy to adolescents. And, even in the current age of geographical mobility, schools know countless families over many years, provide continuity for the adolescent, and are valuable sources of longitudinal information and observation for treating clinicians.

General psychiatrists who care for children and adolescents will be remiss not to be in touch with schools, if only to confirm the history provided to them by child and parents. Regular contact is often a necessity for monitoring the course and treatment of the illness. Depressed youth may be in regular or special education classes. The teachers in both settings are rich sources of historical information for diagnosis and following treatment. Many schools now have school psychologists. Their jobs may include individual and group therapy, psychological or achievement testing, running social skills groups, and developing individualized education plans (IEPs) in collabo-ration with school-based colleagues. In many school settings, guidance counselors see students individually in addition to their instructional advising duties. Some larger schools may have a full-time nurse, whereas smaller or financially struggling districts may assign nurses to multiple sites. In addition, depending on initial diagnosis, some patients may be working with occupational, physical, and speech and language therapists provided through the schools.

Ongoing interactions of the general psychiatrist and schools can take one of several forms or models. The physician may prescribe antidepressant medication only, and only be available to the school as an emergency contact on registration forms. Psychiatrists may prescribe for children receiving their psychotherapy from a school psychologist or guidance counselor. The physician may have a contract or arrangement with the school district whereby the psychiatrist, with parental consent, evaluates and prescribes psychotropic medication at the school. Another possible arrangement is one in which the psychiatrist consults to the school about systems and programmatic issues, instead of providing services for the individual child. This is perhaps more fitting for and commonly done by child and adolescent than general psychiatrists, although not always the case in rural, underserved areas, in which adult psychiatrists provide this service out of necessity. General psychiatrists are also in the ranks of many who offer their time for screening, assessment, and emergency care of students in crisis situations, such as student or teacher deaths, incidents of violence, or natural disasters.

General psychiatrists must be familiar with a few basic terms and statutes fundamental to education if they treat adolescents on a regular basis. The *Americans with Disabilities Act*, passed in 1990 and amended in 2008, states that students with disabilities cannot be denied educational services or be discriminated against after they are enrolled. *Accommodations* are changes in the learning or school environment to assist the student in overcoming the particular disability. Common examples for adolescent patients include providing a classroom aide for an autistic individual or personalized organization of the desk or work space area to remove distractors and enhance attention and concentration for a teen with severe attention deficit hyperactivity disorder. Accommodations often are agreed to formally in a *504 Plan*, from Section 504 of the *Rehabilitation Act of 1973*. The *Education for All Handicapped Children Act,* or *Public Law 94-142,* now revised as the *Individual with Disabilities Education Act (IDEA)* includes children and adolescents with severe psychiatric and physical illnesses and handicaps. The IDEA guarantees these individuals a free public education with special instruction and services required to meet their educational needs up to the age of 22 years. The IDEA guarantees an IEP, which parents can attend and provide their input and consent. Should the parent or guardian disagree with their child's IEP or educational placement, they are afforded due process and appeal.[41,46]

Identical to communication with all outside sources, the general psychiatrist must obtain consent from the patient's parent or guardian before communicating with the school. Many severely ill adolescents and young adults between the ages of 18 and 22 years may be enrolled in special education programs, and the clinician will need to establish whether the parent obtained guardianship after the young person's 18th birthday so that proper consent for communication is obtained. Even if the patient cannot give consent, obtaining their assent or agreement for the psychiatrist to speak and cooperate with the school is very important in maintaining and strengthening the therapeutic relationship between the psychiatrist and the young adult patient. As youth approach their late teens and beyond, the school setting remains just as important as their family life. Strong partnerships with their patients' educational institutions are essential for general psychiatrists who prescribe for children and adolescents, regardless of the psychiatric diagnosis.

CHILD AND ADOLESCENT DEPRESSION AND COMMON PSYCHOTHERAPIES

As noted previously, the role of many general psychiatrists in the treatment of pediatric depression is the assessment for and ongoing management of antidepressant medication. They will be collaborating with a host of other mental health professionals who provide psychotherapy, behavioral, and case management. For optimal treatment of depression, it is imperative that the physician in these collaborative treatment arrangements understand the essentials of psychotherapies commonly used in the field, particularly as they pertain to adolescents. Four individual therapies commonly used by mental health professionals from other disciplines are reviewed: individual psychodynamic, cognitive-behavioral, interpersonal, and psychoeducation.

Individual Psychodynamic Psychotherapy

Practically speaking, individual psychotherapy often is used as an umbrella term to encompass supportive psychotherapy, brief psychotherapy, and insight-oriented, psychodynamic psychotherapy. In addition, clinicians in different disciplines describe their psychotherapeutic orientations and techniques in many ways. Therefore, it is important for the psychiatrist collaborating with a therapist to understand as completely as possible what is occurring under the rubric of individual psychotherapy.

The use of individual psychodynamic psychotherapy in children and adolescents is bolstered by a long and rich case-based literature and a wealth of clinical experience. A major advantage is that the focus, content, and, to a certain extent, the therapeutic techniques can be flexible to address developmental, family, peer, academic, and other concerns. These therapies are compatible with medication management and can also allow for therapeutic attention to more existential, less quantifiable concerns, such as the meaning of life and issues of the adolescent's emerging worldview.

However, evidence-based support, although emerging and promising, is still rather limited.[30,47] Costs, time commitment, and therapist availability may limit access and use by youth and families struggling with the recent socioeconomic downturn and multiple obligations at home and work. However, psychiatrists will recognize the use of psychodynamic psychotherapy principles in even brief interventions by therapists of all backgrounds and across the continuum of outpatient care.

Cognitive–Behavioral Therapy

Cognitive–behavioral therapy (CBT), based on Beck's depression paradigms and psychotherapy techniques, long has been accepted as efficacious in the treatment of depressed adults, adolescents, and children.[48–51] CBT acknowledges the biopsychosocial contributors to depression, including genetics, temperament, and family environment, then addresses cognitive distortions and vulnerabilities and negative and automatic thoughts. Interventions include mood monitoring, goal setting, activity scheduling, problem solving, parent training, attention to social skills, and relapse prevention.

As psychotherapies for depressed youth go, CBT is the most studied, with numerous clinical trials, protocols, and meta-analyses of studies to support its superiority over other nonpharmacologic interventions.[48,50–54] CBT gained large-scale national endorsements, especially after black box warnings regarding increased suicidality were issued for antidepressants.[55] However, the Treatment for Adolescents with Depression Study (TADS) called into question the infallibility of CBT in the treatment of some youths at certain points in the course of their depressive disorders. TADS was a multicenter, randomized, controlled trial of 439 adolescents, ages 12 to 17 years, with major depressive disorder. Study subjects were randomly placed into the following arms: fluoxetine, CBT, combined fluoxetine and CBT, and placebo. For the first 12 weeks of treatment, fluoxetine alone and the combination of fluoxetine and CBT were more effective than placebo, but CBT alone was not. Interestingly, at the 18-week mark of the study, the CBT-only arm showed similar improvements to the fluoxetine-alone or combined fluoxetine and CBT groups. Several publications detail additional important findings from the TADS study group.[56–59] TADS did not show that CBT was ineffective or unhelpful in the treatment of adolescent depression, as has been misunderstood by some when the initial 12-week data were presented. However, it may be that CBT is more effective when administered at various points in treatment, its benefits may be appreciated at different points in the course of the illness and its treatment, and certain adolescents will benefit to different degrees than others from CBT alone.

Interpersonal Psychotherapy

Interpersonal psychotherapy (IPT) was developed as a brief, time-limited therapy for adult outpatients with unipolar, nonpsychotic depression. It is based on the straightforward observation that when one is depressed, interpersonal relationships are affected, and conversely, the quality of one's interpersonal relationships affect one's mood. General goals of IPT are to decrease depressive symptoms and improve the functioning of the depressed individual within important relationships with others. IPT for depressed adolescents (IPT-A) is a manualized, evidence-based psychotherapy that capitalizes on the importance of interpersonal relationships as a developmental cornerstone of typical adolescence. IPT-A is well suited to address common adolescent issues, such as separation/individuation from parents, peer pressure, facing deaths of relatives or friends, and developing dyadic relationships. Gunlicks-Stoessel and colleagues[60] and Mufson and colleagues[61–64] conducted randomized, controlled trials and published extensively on IPT-A. This 12-session program has been used with depressed adolescents in clinical and school settings, with demonstrated maintenance of symptom improvement and social functioning at 1-year follow-up visits. IPT-A is compatible with antidepressant treatment and includes adaptations for use with depressed prepubertal children; pregnant teens; youths with self-injurious, nonsuicidal behaviors; and in group settings.[60-64]

Psychoeducation

Although many clinicians consider psychoeducation to be any information about a psychiatric disorder and its treatment that is conveyed to a patient or family member, the term properly refers to a more formal, standardized curriculum and procedures, typically in manualized form. It stresses education about the disorder, problem solving, and communication skills vital to symptom recognition, management, and appropriate service use. This modality uses principles from CBT, social support, client-centered, and learning theories, among others. It is used most effectively as an adjunctive treatment with pharmacotherapy. Psychoeducation with depressed adolescents and their families has demonstrated changes in dysfunctional understandings about depression and improvement in social functioning and parent–child relationships.[65-68]

PRESCRIBING FOR CHILDREN AND ADOLESCENTS: THE PSYCHODYNAMICS OF PSYCHOPHARMACOLOGY

The act of writing a prescription for a psychotropic medication for a child or adolescent is more than pen meeting a small piece of specially treated paper or printing out a form from the electronic medical record. The child or adolescent patient, parents, siblings, and extended family members, peers, teachers, and significant others may ascribe particular meanings to the circumstances culminating in the act of prescribing an antidepressant. Is the core depressive illness the result of wrongdoing, inadequacy, weakness, or sin on the part of the child or the parent? Is there an understanding of illness as multifactorial, including genetics, medical contribution, and psychosocial factors that contribute to the particular timing, expression, and severity of the patient's presentation? Was the parent neglectful in any way, in the past or the present, perhaps not seeking timely and appropriate assessment for earlier symptom expressions of the mood disorder? Do the youth and his illness remind a mother of another prominent person in her past, such as the child's abusive father? Are the parents resistant to having their teenager on an antidepressant because of embarrassment about not being able to pay for it or the difficulties they anticipate in committing to appropriate follow-up visits? The meanings ascribed to medications have the potential to determine how it is used (or not) and whether the medication helps or hurts, as discussed by Mintz in this issue.

Although most commonly associated with traditional forms of family therapy, the term *identified patient* remains a potentially helpful concept for clinicians prescribing medications for children and adolescents. According to Minuchin, the identified patient is the member of the family or system first put forth as the problem or the focus of the turmoil. Therapeutic intervention is expected to be directed at that individual, with the expectation that the therapist will change him or her and the troubling symptoms or behaviors. The therapist, on the other hand, views the entire family or system as symptomatic, and seeks to reverse or affect change in ineffective transactions and dysfunctional patterns of behaving within the entire family system that produce heightened affect and potential scapegoating. In essence, the identified patient can be understood as the *symptom bearer* for unhealthy individual, dyadic, and multiple-person interactions within the family context.[69,70] Although contemporary family therapies have become more evidence based and use practice standards and integrative treatment strategies with individual, school, and community collaborations and interventions, the identified patient concept remains helpful—even for those clinicians who prescribe medications but do not provide individual or family psychotherapeutic treatments.[71–77]

When deciding on antidepressant medication, the prescribing clinician must be sure she is diagnosing and treating true symptoms of the youth and not those projected on them as the family's symptom bearer. In addition to biological diatheses to affective changes, irritability, anger, and other emotions, family functioning may play a prominent part in the origin of the child's symptoms. This should always be suspected if medication responses are poor or incomplete, in addition to the pharmacologic concerns regarding drug selection, dosing, side effects, possible need for augmentation, and related questions all prescribers must always keep in mind.

Even when assessment, diagnosis, and pharmacologic treatment are performed carefully and competently by physicians, children and adolescents who are the identified patients in tumultuous family settings may still hear messages implicitly or overtly that they must take medicine because they are bad or others cannot deal with them. In some family systems, even expression of what may be a normal range of affect and emotion may be reported to doctors as pronounced symptoms of mood disorders. Youth who have been the symptom bearers for their families of origin may benefit from individual psychotherapy as young adults to process and reframe their experience of what it meant to be the identified patient and the benefits, burdens, and meanings of being prescribed psychotropic medication in that context (David L. Mintz, MD, Stockbridge, MA, personal communication, October 2011). When prescribing physicians suspect unhealthy family dynamics, and the child's family is not already in active treatment, appropriate referrals to qualified therapists should be offered.

Psychiatrists must not overlook the meaning of the physical attributes of the medication itself. Children may attribute meanings to the color, size, shape, letters, and form of medicine, whether a tablet that must be swallowed whole, an under-the-tongue meltaway, liquid, or intramuscular form. A larger pill or a frequent dosing schedule can be misperceived as meaning the child is "sicker" than if only taking a small tablet every morning, or some may be relieved that taking a larger pill several times daily is greater help or a better treatment. The adolescent's relationship with and regard for the prescribing clinician can influence her enthusiasm about adhering to medication instructions. Although children and teens typically do not need to take antidepressants during the school day, extracurricular activities, evening jobs, leisure activities, and stigma from peers can discourage reliable medication adherence in the evening or at bedtime.

Adolescence is a period of burgeoning autonomy and independence. If the teen shares a therapist or a psychiatrist with family members or others they know through school, extracurricular activities, or employment settings, he may express his individuality by refusing to attend the appointment, have the prescription filled, or taking the medication at all. It is always wise to inquire about these potential conflicts before or during the assessment of an adolescent, and certainly before contemplating prescribing an antidepressant. If this appears to be an issue that may interfere with treatment, referring to a different psychiatrist for pharmacotherapy should be considered to hasten symptom remediation. As noted previously, in many rural and inner city areas there is a shortage of child psychiatrists, and available general psychiatrists may choose not to prescribe for individuals less than 18 years of age. In situations in which treatment by another psychiatrist is not possible, perhaps because of clinician shortage or restrictive provider lists of third-party payers, the trust and confidentiality concerns inherent to an adolescent and another family member being cared for by the same psychopharmacologist should be discussed openly with all concerned before writing the first prescription.

In addition to developmental and family considerations, general psychiatrists treating depressed children and adolescents should keep in mind the ever-increasing cultural and religious plurality of the communities in which they practice. Clinicians should inquire in greater detail about these issues whenever the psychodynamics, treatment adherence, or the relationships of prescriber, minor patient, and parent or guardian require further reflection.[77-79]

ETHICAL ASPECTS OF CHILD AND ADOLESCENT PHARMACOTHERAPY
Basic Ethical Principles

Several reviews exist regarding basic ethical principles in child and adolescent psychiatry clinical practice and research.[80-83] In general, the application of the principles of beneficence and nonmaleficence are quite similar in prescribing psychotropic medications for children, adolescents, and adults. All clinicians are obligated to seek out and to provide the best possible care for their patients (beneficence), and in so doing, fulfill the duty or moral obligation to avoid harm. Indeed, the physician's cardinal rule is "primum non nocere," or "do no harm." No psychotropic medications, including antidepressants, have so few risks to be considered beneficial in all situations. Even when using medications with relatively few side effects compared with other agents in the treatment of pediatric depression, prescribers must weigh the potential risks with the potential harms of medication side effects, potential drug interactions, and deleterious effects on growth and development.[84-86]

Justice has taken on much greater significance in recent years as the prescription of psychotropic medications to children and adolescents has come under greater scrutiny. In the discipline of philosophy, justice signifies fairness, or similar regard or treatment of individuals in comparable circumstances. In psychiatry and pediatrics, the term justice often is used to signify the narrower concept of distributive justice, or the fair distribution and access to care and treatment as determined by the norms, policies, and procedures of society and its processes for determining these guidelines.[84,87] Perhaps no other medical specialty faces issues of distributive justice more so than child and adolescent psychiatry. Psychiatrically ill youth are one of the largest marginalized groups in health care, and justice issues and inadequate access to services contribute to the rates of depression, recurrence, and suicide. In addition, fairness and distributive justice, or lack thereof, are key considerations in the economics and business of health care and pharmaceuticals, all of which affect the type, amount, and quality of antidepressants on insurance and third-party payer formularies available to treat depression and other psychiatric illnesses in children.[88-92]

Over the last decade, data about psychotropic medication prescription practices in the United States has provided food for thought regarding justice and mental health care for youth. The overall rate of psychotropic medication use increased from 1.4 per 100 children in 1987 to 3.9 per 100 children in 1996. These figures reflected increases not only for antidepressants but for all medications except benzodiazepines and antipsychotics.[93] Looking specifically at antidepressants, prescription rates for selective serotonin reuptake inhibitors increased until 2000, whereas those for tricyclic antidepressants decreased. In 2002, an estimated 0.3% to 0.9% of adolescents were prescribed a selective serotonin reuptake inhibitor, and prescription rates were higher for whites than Hispanics but comparable in boys and girls.[94,95]

Other researchers have examined sex and racial patterns for psychotropic prescription in children and adolescents. One study of Medicaid databases in 7 states found that 2.3% of preschoolers received 1 or more prescriptions in 2001, double the rate calculated for 1995. Boys were twice as likely to receive prescriptions as girls, whites 2 times more likely than African Americans and 4 times more likely than Hispanics. In this particular Medicaid preschooler study, atypical antipsychotics and antidepressants accounted for the most significant increases in prescriptions.[92] In general, studies in all practice settings consistently report that boys are 2 to 4 times as likely as girls to receive a psychotropic medication.[96,97] Although this difference may be attributed at least in part to the epidemiology of certain entities, with some Axis I disorders, such as attention deficit hyperactivity disorder, known to be more common in boys than girls, epidemiologic arguments do not explain other ethnic disparities. Data also are emerging on psychotropic prescription rates for vulnerable children, such as those in foster care. Zito and coworkers[98] discovered that children in foster care insured by Medicaid received significantly more prescriptions than children matched for age and sex who were also covered by Medicaid but not in foster care. Forty-three percent of the foster care children received prescriptions for 3 or more classes of agents during 2004 alone. Antidepressants were the most commonly prescribed medications, with psychostimulants and antipsychotics prescribed somewhat less often.[98]

Although no single, clear-cut, evidence-based explanation exists for the degree of unevenness of care across socioeconomic and cultural groups, from a philosophical point of view, this issue can be conceptualized at the following levels: (1) the pediatric patient and his or her family, (2) the individual practitioner in any given clinical encounter, (3) organized medicine, medical education, and systems of care as elements of the larger US health care system, and (4) the values and priorities of American society in general. For instance, are there particular ways in which pediatric depression presents or the symptoms are expressed or reported in nonmajority populations that predispose them to receive prescriptions for medications at a higher rate than other children? Are there language and cultural barriers that limit recommendations for and acceptance of nonpharmacologic treatments modalities? Are there significant differences in training, experience, and supervision of physicians prescribing for minority youth? Are there common elements or characteristics of these clinicians that, when compared with clinicians treating majority youth, distinguish their practice and prescribing patterns, potentially contributing to different psychopharmacologic treatments for different groups of patients? The medical community as a whole may be a factor in discrepant rates of prescription in different patient groups.

Efforts to improve access to high-quality care to underserved patient populations, to increase the number of child and adolescent psychiatrists nationally, and to supplement training and expertise of primary care physicians and general psychiatrists in the area of pediatric psychopharmacology are certainly underway. Although data on these initiatives are not yet available, one would like to be optimistic that these efforts will improve access to higher-quality care for all pediatric mental health concerns.

At a societal level, for just and equitable care for depressed children and adolescents to become the rule for all youth, the issue must not only be kept in the forefront of public awareness but also at the top of the "to do" or "must have" lists of voting citizens, school boards, and government at all levels—local, state, and federal. If justice in the area of care for childhood and adolescent depression means reasonable access for all children and families to quality of care supported by evidence-based practices, all must make the need known and insist on its availability—patients, families, clinicians, schools, professional guilds, and societal groups advocating and determining policies for health care access and systems of care.

Certainly, more work needs to be done in epidemiology of psychiatric disorders, standardization of accurate diagnostic methods and tools, and service delivery and economics to increase mental health care and access to appropriately prescribed psychotropics to those youth who need them. More work also needs to be done to decrease unnecessary or inappropriate prescriptions to those who do not need or are unlikely to benefit.

Informed Consent and Assent

According to expert ethicists, informed consent consists of 5 elements: (1) competence, (2) disclosure, (3) understanding, (4) voluntariness, and (5) consent.[99] Building on the work of Appelbaum and coworkers,[100] the American Academy of Pediatrics enumerated the following elements of informed consent:

1. "Provision of information: Patients should have explanations, in understandable language, of the nature of the ailment and condition; the nature of proposed diagnostic steps and/or treatment(s) and the probability of their success; the existence and nature of risks involved; and the existence, potential benefits, and risks of recommended alternative treatments (including the choice of no treatment)."
2. Assessment of the patient's understanding of the above information.
3. Assessment, if only tacit, of the capacity of the patient or surrogate to make the necessary decision(s).
4. "Assurance, insofar as is possible, that the patient has the freedom to choose among the medical alternatives without coercion or manipulation."[101]

In the majority of cases, parents and guardians provide informed consent for depressed minors to be treated for their illness and to receive antidepressant medications. Children who are in foster care, incarcerated, or for other reasons wards of the county or state have their consent for care given by an authorized person(s) of the custodial entity, sometimes with input from a parent or other family member. The consent process may be complicated and lengthy when multiple adults and agencies are involved. Regardless of who gives legal consent—parent, guardian, or other designated authority—several compelling reasons exist for obtaining assent, or agreement, on the part of the identified child patient when psychotropic medication is recommended.[85] The American Academy of Pediatrics has named 4 essential components of assent, all very relevant to antidepressant treatment for youth:

1. "Helping the patient achieve a developmentally appropriate awareness of the nature of his or her condition"
2. Telling the patient what he or she can expect with test(s) and treatment(s)
3. Making a clinical assessment of the patient's understanding of the situation and the factors influencing how he or she is responding (including whether there is inappropriate pressure to accept testing or therapy)
4. "Soliciting an expression of the patient's willingness to accept the proposed care."[101]

If the child or adolescent does not assent to the treatment, or if there is extreme reluctance to give assent, the prescribing psychiatrist should take the time to understand the patient's concerns and work through them patiently with her. Often, an impasse can be worked through given additional time and developmentally appropriate education about the mood disorder, its treatments, and the benefits of treatment.

From time to time, the general psychiatrist will treat an individual younger than 18 years who can legally consent to treatment, including pharmacotherapy. The term *emancipated minor* applies to individuals less than 18 years of age who are in the armed services, married, are parents themselves or who are living outside the home of their family of origin and are in charge of their own finances and affairs. Exact criteria for the status of emancipation vary across jurisdictions, so clinicians should consult local or state officials for guidance when initially treating these young people.[85]

Reviewing written information about childhood and adolescent depression and antidepressant medication with the parent and youth at the time of obtaining informed consent and assent can strengthen therapeutic relationships, provide visual input in addition to the listening element of consent/assent, and permit review and reflection on the same material after they leave the office or hospital setting. Several easily understood references for parents and developmentally appropriate information sheets for children and adolescents are available, authored and furnished by reputable clinicians and professional organizations.[102–104]

BLACK BOX WARNINGS AND OFF-LABEL PRESCRIBING

Black box warnings refer to warnings placed by the US Food and Drug Administration (FDA) regarding important concerns about the safety of medications. The concerns may relate to particular characteristics of the patient population involved, the condition(s) being treated, or serious or life-threatening side effects, either short or long term. Over the last decade, several medications in multiple drug classes commonly prescribed to treat child and adolescent psychiatric disorders have been given black box warning status.

In 2003, a possible association between paroxetine and suicidal ideation was noted in controlled trials in child and adolescent populations.[105] Based on this concern, the FDA asked all manufacturers of antidepressants to resubmit safety data from controlled trials in pediatric populations. In a meta-analysis of the safety data from 24 pediatric antidepressant trials, a 4% risk of suicidality was demonstrated by youth on active medication compared with a 2% risk of the same in patients on placebo. In 2004, based on this meta-analysis, the FDA issued a black box warning for all antidepressant use in children and adolescents, regardless of the disorder for which they were actually prescribed. In addition, guidelines were issued recommending patient monitoring consisting of weekly face-to-face visits with the clinician for 4 weeks, followed by biweekly meetings for the next 4-week period, and then monthly appointments.[106] The effect of the 2004 black box warning was a significant decrease in the prescription of antidepressants to children and adolescents.[107] A subsequent meta-analysis of data from approximately 77,000 subjects in 295 placebo-controlled trials found similar increased risk of suicidality in young adults up to the age of 24 years. As a result, the black box warning for antidepressants was extended to 24-year-olds in December 2006.[108] As might be predicted, both the rates of depression diagnosis and the prescription of antidepressants have declined since the requirement for black box warnings for antidepressant therapy for patients under the age of 25 years.[109–111] As some opponents of the black box warnings feared, the decrease in antidepressant prescriptions has been correlated to an increase in completed suicides in this population in the years immediately after the issuance of these black box warnings.[112]

Off-label prescribing refers to using a drug to treat an illness or condition or a particular patient population for which the drug is not approved by the FDA. Just because a medication has been approved for use in one patient population for a specific disorder does not mean that it is effective or safe to use in the same or comparable condition in a different population.[113] This is often the case in the treatment of childhood depression. Fluoxetine has an FDA approval for the treatment of major depressive disorder in children 8 years and older, and escitalopram has an FDA approval for the treatment of depression in youth 12 years and older. With those 2 exceptions, use of all other pharmacologic agents to treat depressed pediatric patients is indeed off-label. Clinicians must use their medical fund of knowledge, clinical experience, and wisdom to weigh the risks and benefits of treatment and which specific antidepressant to prescribe. Parents and caregivers should be informed if the recommended treatment is FDA approved or off label, as well as the reasons the physician is recommending the particular medication being prescribed.[22] The passage of key federal legislation, including that US Food and Drug Administration Modernization Act of 1997, the Best Pharmaceuticals for Children Act in 2002, and the Pediatric Research Equality Act of 2003, has required and encouraged multicenter trials of psychotropic medications in pediatric patient populations. National Institutes of Health initiatives have also incentivized more scientifically rigorous research in pediatric psychopharmacology. Information and experience gleaned from these multicenter studies should enlighten prescribers on both the benefits and risks of antidepressants, give greater direction about which medications to try, in particular, contexts with certain individual patients, and be helpful to prescribers and parents as we all attempt to act in the child's best interests.[114]

Kratochvil has offered a clinically and ethically reasonable approach to the issue of youth and young adult depression, antidepressant prescription, and the black box warnings. He stated that astute informed clinicians will know how to interpret relevant data about risks and benefits of a treatment, even if information is still coming forward. The clinician will share with patients and families the benefits and risks of potential treatments, of not treating, and what and how monitoring for treatment effects should be accomplished. Treatment with antidepressants may require flexibility on the prescriber's part, perhaps even first trying alternatives to the physician's first recommendation. Regardless, close monitoring of the patient's condition is essential.[77]

SUMMARY

Depression is a common, recurring disorder affecting millions of youth at some point before they reach mature adulthood. Given the shortage of and uneven distribution of psychiatrists who have completed specialized fellowships in child and adolescent psychiatry, a significant number of depressed youth will receive their pharmacotherapy from general psychiatrists and other prescribers with varying degrees of interest, training, and even willingness to treat children and adolescents. For general psychiatrists who will prescribe antidepressants for minors, knowledge of the training and expertise of nonphysician mental health professionals, the psychotherapies they may employ, and familiarity with school services are essential. Physicians who typically work only with adults will also need familiarity with differing ethical, legal, and regulatory issues and standards applicable to pediatric psychopharmacology. General psychiatrists, pediatricians, family physicians, nurse practitioners, and others contribute greatly to the care of depressed children, adolescents, and their families, and many find this work to be a very rewarding part of their professional practices.

ACKNOWLEDGMENTS

The author gratefully acknowledges the assistance of Jennifer Staley, MLIS, librarian at the Pediatrics Learning Center at Rainbow Babies and Children's Hospital.

REFERENCES

1. Kessler RC, Berglund P, Demler O, et al. The epidemiology of major depressive disorder: results from the national Comorbidity Survey Replication (NCS-R). JAMA 2003;289:3095–105.
2. Mueller TI, Leon AC, Keller MB, et al. Recurrence after recovery from major depressive disorder during 15 years of observational follow-up. Am J Psychiatry 1999;156: 1000–6.
3. Merikangas KR, He J, Burstein M, et al. Lifetime prevalence of mental disorders in U.S. adolescents: results from the National Comorbidity Study—Adolescent Supplement(NCS-A). J Am Acad Child Adolesc Psychiatry 2010;49:980–9.
4. The Substance Abuse and Mental Health Services Administration (SAMHSA). National survey on drug use and health (NSDUH). Available at: http://www.nimh.nih.gov/statistics/1MDD_CHILD.shtml. Accessed October 1, 2011.
5. Costello EJ, Pine DS, Hammen C, et al. Development and natural history of mood disorders. Biol Psychiatry 2002;52:529–42.
6. Rao U, Ryan ND, Birmaher B, et al. Unipolar depression in adolescents: clinical outcome in adulthood. J Am Acad Child Adolesc Psychiatry 1995;34:566–78.
7. Weissman MM, Wolk S, Goldstein RB, et al. Depressed adolescents grown up. JAMA 1999;17:7–13.
8. Bardone AM, Moffitt T, Caspi A, et al. Adult mental health and social outcomes of adolescent girls with depression and conduct disorder. Dev Psychopathol 1996;8: 811–29.
9. Lewinsohn PM, Pettit JW, Joiner TE, et al. The symptomatic expression of major depressive disorder in adolescents and young adults. J Abnorm Psychol 2003;112: 244–53.
10. Centers for Disease Control and Prevention, National Center for Injury Prevention and Control. In: Web-based Injury Statistics Query and Reporting System (WISQARS). Atlanta (GA): Centers for Disease Control and Prevention; 2010. Available at: http://www.cdc.gov/ncipc/wisqars. Accessed October 2, 2011.
11. American Academy of Child and Adolescent Psychiatry. AACAP workforce fact sheet. Available at: http://www.aacap.org/cs/root/legislative_action/aacap_workforce_fact_sheet. Accessed October 1, 2011.
12. Accreditation Council for Graduate Medical Education (ACGME). Psychiatry program requirements, 2007. Available at: www.acgme.org/acWebsite/RRC_400/400_prIndex.asp. Accessed October 1, 2011.
13. Dell ML, Dulcan MK. Childhood and adolescent development. In: Stoudemire S, editor. Clinical psychiatry for medical students. 3rd edition. Philadelphia: JB Lippincott; 1998. p. 261–317.
14. Gemelli R. Normal child and adolescent development. Washington, DC: American Psychiatric Press, Inc; 1996.
15. Gemelli R. Normal child and adolescent development. In: Hales RE, Yudofsky SC, Gabbard GO, editors. Textbook of psychiatry. 5th edition. Arlington (VA): American Psychiatric Publishing, Inc; 2008. p. 245–300.
16. Lewis M, Volkmar F. Clinical aspects of child and adolescent development. 3rd edition. Philadelphia: Lea and Febiger; 1990.

17. Birmaher B, Brent D. Assessment and treatment of child and adolescent depressive disorders. In: Martin A, Scahill L, Kratochvil CJ, editors. Pediatric psychopharmacology: principles and practice. 2nd edition. New York: Oxford University Press; 2010. p. 453–65.

18. Birmaher B, Brent DA. Depression and dysthymia. In: Dulcan MK, editor. Dulcan's textbook of child and adolescent psychiatry. Arlington (VA): American Psychiatric Publishing, Inc.; 2010. p. 261–78.

19. Zalsman G, Brent DA, Weersing VR. Depressive disorders in childhood and adolescence: an overview. Child Adolesc Psychiatric Clin N Am 2006;15:827–41.

20. Cohen D, Gerardin P, Mazet P, et al. Pharmacological treatment of adolescent major depression. J Child Adolescent Psychopharmacol 2004;14:19–31.

21. Crawford GC, Cozza SJ, Dulcan MK. Treatment of children and adolescents. In: Hales RE, Yudofsky SC, Gabbard GO, editors. Textbook of psychiatry. 5th edition. Arlington (VA): American Psychiatric Publishing, Inc; 2008. p. 1377–448.

22. Croarkin PE, Emslie GJ, Mayes TL. Antidepressants I: selective serotonin reuptake inhibitors. In: Martin A, Scahill L, Kratochvil CJ, editors. Pediatric psychopharmacology: principles and practice. Second edition. New York: Oxford University Press; 2010. p. 275–85.

23. Dulcan MK, Lake MB. Concise guide to child and adolescent psychiatry. Fourth edition. Arlington (VA): American Psychiatric Publishing, Inc; 2012.

24. Emslie GJ, Croarkin P, Mayes TL. Antidepressants. In: Dulcan MK, editor. Dulcan's textbook of child and adolescent psychiatry. Arlington (VA): American Psychiatric Publishing, Inc; 2010. p. 701–24.

25. Findling RL, editor. Clinical manual of child and adolescent psychopharmacology. Arlington (VA): American Psychiatric Press, Inc; 2008.

26. Gottfried R, Frosch E, Riddle M. Antidepressants II: other agents. In: Martin A, Scahill L, Kratochvil CJ, editors. Pediatric psychopharmacology: principles and practice. Second edition. New York: Oxford University Press; 2010. p. 286–96.

27. Green WH. Child and adolescent clinical psychopharmacology. Philadelphia (PA): Lippincott, Williams, and Wilkins; 2006.

28. McVoy M, Findling R. Child and adolescent psychopharmacology update. Psychiatr Clin N Am 2009;32:111–33.

29. Moreno C, Roche AM, Greenhill LL. Pharmacotherapy of child and adolescent depression. Child Adolesc Psychiatric Clin N Am 2006;15:977–98.

30. American Academy of Child and Adolescent Psychiatry. Practice parameter for assessment and treatment of children and adolescents with depressive disorders. J Am Acad Child Adolesc Psychiatry 2007;46:1503–26.

31. American Academy of Child and Adolescent Psychiatry. Practice parameters for the assessment of the family. J Am Acad Child Adolesc Psychiatry 2007;46:922–37.

32. American Academy of Child and Adolescent Psychiatry. Practice parameters for the psychiatric assessment of children and adolescents. J Am Acad Child Adolesc Psychiatry 1995;31:1386–402.

33. American Academy of Child and Adolescent Psychiatry. Practice parameter on child and adolescent mental health care in community systems of care. J Am Acad Child Adolesc Psychiatry 2007;46:284–99.

34. American Academy of Child and Adolescent Psychiatry. Practice parameter on the use of psychotropic medication in children and adolescents. J Am Acad Child Adolesc Psychiatry 2009;48:961–73.

35. Myers K, Cain S. Telepsychiatry. In: Dulcan MK, editor. Dulcan's textbook of child and adolescent psychiatry. Arlington (VA): American Psychiatric Publishing, Inc; 2010. p. 649–63.

36. American Psychological Association. Available at: http://apa.org/about/index.aspx. Accessed October 2, 2011.

37. National Association of Social Workers. Available at: www.naswdc.org. Accessed October 2, 2011.

38. American Association for Marriage and Family Therapy. Available at: http://www.aamft.org/iMIS15/AAMFT/Home/AAMFT/Default.asp. Accessed October 2, 2011.

39. American Association of Pastoral Counselors. Available at: www.aapc.org. Accessed October 2, 2011.

40. Dell ML. Religious professionals and institutions: untapped resources for clinical care. Child Adolesc Psychiatr Clin N Am 2004;13:85–110.

41. Walter HJ. School-based interventions. In: Dulcan MK, editor. Dulcan's textbook of child and adolescent psychiatry. Arlington (VA): American Psychiatric Publishing, Inc; 2010. p. 957–76.

42. Diala CC, Mentaner C, Walrath C, et al. Racial/ethnic differences in attitudes toward seeing professional mental health services. Am J Public Health 2002;91:805–7.

43. Nabors LA, Reynolds MW. Program evaluation activities: outcomes related to treatment for adolescents receiving school-based mental health services. Children's Services: Social Policy, Research, and Practice 2000;3:175–89.

44. Walter HJ, Vaighan RD, Armstrong B, et al. Characteristics of users and non-users of health clinics in inner-city junior high schools. J Adolesc Health 1996;18:344–8.

45. Jennings J, Pearson G, Harris M. Implementing and maintaining school-based mental health services in a large, urban school district. J Sch Health 2000;70:201–5.

46. Bostic JQ, Stein B, Schwab-Stone M. Schools. In: Martin A, Volkmar FR, editors. Lewis's child and adolescent psychiatry: a comprehensive textbook. Fourth edition. Philadelphia: Lippincott, Williams & Wilkins; 2007. p. 981–8.

47. Terr L. Individual psychotherapy. In: Dulcan MK, editor. Dulcan's textbook of child and adolescent psychiatry. Arlington (VA): American Psychiatric Publishing, Inc; 2010. p. 807–24.

48. Lewinsohn P, Clarke G, Hops H, et al. Cognitive-behavioral treatment for depressed adolescents. Behav Ther 1990;21:385–401.

49. Lewinsohn P, Clarke G. Psychosocial treatments for adolescent depression. Clin Psychol Rev 1999;19:329–42.

50. Reinecke MA, Ryan NE, DuBois DL. Cognitive-behavioral therapy of depression and depressive symptoms during adolescence: a review and meta-analysis. J Am Acad Child Adolesc Psychiatry 1990;37:26–34.

51. Weisz JR, McCarty CA, Valeri SM. Effects of psychotherapy for depression in children and adolescents: a meta-analysis. Psychol Bull 2006;132:132–49.

52. McCarthy M, Abenojar J, Anders TF. Child and adolescent psychiatry for the future: challenges and opportunities. Psychiatr Clin N Am 2009;32:213–26.

53. Compton SN, March JS, Brent DA, et al. Cognitive-behavioral psychotherapy for anxiety and depressive disorders in children and adolescents: an evidence-based medicine review. J Am Acad Child Adolesc Psychiatry 2004;43:930–59.

54. Weersing VR, Weisz JR. Community clinic treatment of depressed youth: benchmarking usual care against CBT clinical trials. J Consult Clin Psychol 2002;70:299–310.

55. Weersing VR, Brent DA. Cognitive behavioral therapy for depression in youth. Child Adolesc Psychiatric Clin N Am 2006;15:939–57.

56. Kennard BD, Emslie GJ, Mayes TL, et al. Relapse and recurrence in pediatric depression. Child Adolesc Psychiatric Clin N Am 2006;15:1057–79.

57. The TADS Team. The treatment for adolescents with depression study (TADS): long-term effectiveness and safety outcomes. Arch Gen Psychiatry 2007;64: 1132–44.
58. Curry J, Rohde P, Simons A, et al. Predictors and moderators of acute outcome in the treatment for adolescents with depression study (TADS). J Am Acad Child Adolesc Psychiatry 2006;45:1427–39.
59. Kratochvil CJ, Wells K, March JS. Combining pharmacotherapy and psychotherapy: an evidence-based approach. In: Martin A, Scahill L, Kratochvil CJ, editors. Pediatric psychopharmacology: principles and practice. Second edition. New York: Oxford University Press; 2010. p. 407–21.
60. Gunlicks-Stoessel ML, Mufson L. Interpersonal psychotherapy for depressed adolescents. In: Dulcan MK, editor. Dulcan's textbook of child and adolescent psychiatry. Arlington (VA): American Psychiatric Publishing, Inc; 2010. p. 887–95.
61. Mufson L, Dorta KP, Wickramaratne P, et al. A randomized effectiveness trial of interpersonal psychotherapy for depressed adolescents. Arch Gen Psychiatry 2004; 61:577–84.
62. Mufson L, Fairbanks J. Interpersonal psychotherapy for depressed adolescents: a one-year naturalistic follow-up study. J Am Acad Child Adolesc Psychiatry 1996;35: 1145–55.
63. Mufson L, Moreau D, Weissman MM, et al. Modification of interpersonal psychotherapy with depressed adolescents (IPT-A): phase I and II studies. J Am Acad Child Adolesc Psychiatry 1994;33:695–705.
64. Mufson L, Weissman MM, Moreau D, et al. Efficacy of interpersonal psychotherapy for depressed adolescents. Arch Gen Psychiatry 1999;56:573–9.
65. Brent DA, Poling K, McCain B, et al. A psychoeducational program for families of affectively ill children and adolescents. J Am Acad Child Adolesc Psychiatry 1993; 32:770–4.
66. Sanford M, Boyle M, McCleary L, et al. A pilot study of adjunctive family psychoeducation in adolescent major depression: feasibility and treatment effect. J Am Acad Child Adolesc Psychiatry 2006;45:386–95.
67. Lukens EP, McFarlane WR. Psychoeducation as evidence-based practice: considerations for practice, research, and policy. Brief Treat Crisis Interv 2004;4:205–25.
68. Lofthouse N, Fristad MA. Psychosocial interventions for children with early onset bipolar spectrum disorder. Clin Child Fam Psychol Rev 2004;7:71–88.
69. Minuchin S, Fishman HC. Family therapy techniques. Cambridge (MA): Harvard University Press; 1981.
70. Wendel R, Gouze KR. Family therapy. In: Dulcan MK, editor. Dulcan's textbook of child and adolescent psychiatry. Arlington (VA): American Psychiatric Publishing, Inc; 2010. p. 869–86.
71. Buehler C, Gerard JM. Marital conflict, ineffective parenting, and children's and adolescents' maladjustment. J Marriage Fam 2002;64:78–92.
72. Breunlin DC, Schwartz RC, MacKune-Karrer B. Metaframeworks: transcending the models of family therapy. San Francisco: Jossey-Bass; 1992.
73. Wendel R, Gouze KR, Lake M. Integrative module-based family therapy: a model for training and treatment in a multidisciplinary mental health setting. J Marital Fam Ther 2005;31:357–70.
74. Henggeler SW, Rodick JD, Borduin CM, et al. Multisystemic treatment of juvenile offenders: effects on adolescent behavior and family interaction. Dev Psychol 1986;22:132–41.

75. Henggeler SW, Melton GB, Smith LA. Family preservation using multisystemic therapy: an effective alternative to incarcerating juvenile offenders. J Consul Clin Psychol 1992;60:953–61.
76. Pinsof WM, Wynne LC. Toward progress research: closing the gap between family therapy practice and research. J Marital Fam Ther 2000;26:1–8.
77. Dell ML, Vaughan BS, Kratochvil CJ. Ethics and the prescription pad. Child Adolesc Psychiatr Clin N Am 2008;17:93–111.
78. Malik M, Lake J, Lawson WB, et al. Culturally adapted pharmacotherapy and the integrative formulation. Child Adolesc Psychiatric Clin N Am 2010;19:791–814.
79. Pruett KD, Joshi SV, Martin A. Thinking about prescribing: the psychology of psychopharmacology. In: Martin A, Scahill L, Kratochvil CJ, editors. Pediatric psychopharmacology: principles and practice. Second edition. New York: Oxford University Press; 2010. p. 422–33.
80. Dell ML, Kinlaw K. Theory can be relevant: an overview of bioethics for the practicing child and adolescent psychiatrist. Child Adolesc Psychiatr Clin N Am 2008;17:1–19.
81. Hoop JG, Smyth AC, Roberts LW. Ethical issues in psychiatric research on children and adolescents. Child Adolesc Psychiatric Clin N Am 2008;17:127–48.
82. Schetky DH. Ethics. In: Martin A, Volkmar FR, editors. Lewis's child and adolescent psychiatry: a comprehensive textbook. Fourth edition. Philadelphia: Lippincott, Williams and Wilkins; 2007. p. 17–22.
83. Sondheimer A, Jensen P. Ethics and child and adolescent psychiatry. In: Bloch S, Green SA, editors. Psychiatric ethics, 4th edition. New York: Oxford University Press; 2009. p. 385–407.
84. Lo B. Overview of ethical guidelines. In: Resolving ethical dilemmas: a guide for clinicians. Fourth edition. Philadelphia: Lippincott, Williams, and Wilkins; 2009. p. 11–17.
85. Beauchamp TL, Childress JF. Beneficence. In: Principles of biomedical ethics. New York: Oxford University Press; 2009. p. 197–239.
86. Beauchamp TL, Childress JF. Nonmaleficence. In: Principles of biomedical ethics. New York: Oxford University Press; 2009. p. 149–96.
87. Beauchamp TL, Childress JF. Justice. In: Principles of biomedical ethics. New York: Oxford University Press; 2009. p. 240–87.
88. Burke MD. Commentary by a child psychiatrist practicing in a community setting. J Child Adolesc Psychopharmacol 2007;17:297–9.
89. DeBar LL, Lynch F, Powell J, et al. Use of psychotropic agents in preschool children: associated symptoms, diagnoses, and health care services in a health maintenance organization. Arch Pediatr Adolesc Med 2003;157:17–25.
90. Zito JM, Safer DJ, dosReis S, et al. Trends in the prescribing of psychotropic medications to preschoolers. J Am Med Assoc 2000;283:1025–30.
91. Zito JM, Safer DJ, dosReis S, et al. Psychotropic practice patterns for youth: a 10-year perspective. Arch Pediatr Adolesc Med 2003;157:17–25.
92. Zito JM, Safer DJ, Valluri S, et al. Psychotherapeutic medication prevalence in Medicaid-insured preschoolers. J Child Adolesc Psychopharmacol 2007;17:195–203.
93. Olfson M, Marcus SC, Weissman MM, et al. National trends in the use of psychotropic medications by children. J Am Acad Child Adolesc Psychiatry 2002;41:514–21.
94. Vitiello B, Zuvekas SH, Norquist GS. National estimates of antidepressant use among U.S. children, 1997–2002. J Am Acad Child Adolesc Psychiatry 2006;45: 271–9.

95. Olfson M, Marcus SC. National patterns in antidepressant medication treatment. Arch Gen Psychiatry 2009;66:848–56.

96. Lefever GB, Dawson KV, Morrow AL. The extent of drug therapy for attention deficit-hyperactivity disorder among children in public schools. Am J Public Health 1999;89:1359–64.

97. Olfson M, Blanco C, Liu L, et al. National trends in the outpatient treatment of children and adolescents with psychotropic drugs. Arch Gen Psychiatry 2006;63:679–85.

98. Zito JM, Safer DJ, Sal D, et al. Psychotropic medication patterns among youth in foster care. Pediatrics 2008;121:e157–63.

99. Beauchamp TL, Childress JF. Respect for autonomy. In: Principles of biomedical ethics. New York: Oxford University Press; 2009. p. 99–148.

100. Appelbaum PS, Lidz CW, Meisel A. Informed consent: legal theory and clinical practice. New York: Oxford University Press; 1987.

101. Committee on Bioethics of the American Academy of Pediatrics. Informed consent, parental permission, and assent in pediatric practice. Pediatrics 1995;95:314–7.

102. American Academy of Child and Adolescent Psychiatry. Facts for families. Available at: http//www.aacap.org/cs/root/facts_for_families/facts_for_families. Accessed October 15, 2011.

103. Dulcan MK, editor. Helping parents, youth, and teachers understand medications for behavioral and emotional problems: a resource book of medication information handouts. Washington, DC: American Psychiatric Publishing, Inc; 2007.

104. National Institute of Mental Health. Available at: http://www.nimh.nih.gov/index. shtml. Accessed October 15, 2011.

105. Temple R. Anti-depressant use in pediatric populations. Available at: www.fda.gov/NewsEvents/Testimony/ucm113265.htm. Accessed October 26, 2011.

106. Hammad TA, Laughren T, Racoosin J. Suicidality in pediatric patients treated with antidepressant drugs. Arch Gen Psychiatry 2006;63:332–9.

107. Nemeroff CB, Kalali A, Keller MB, et al. Impact of publicity concerning pediatric suicidality data on physician practice patterns in the United States. Arch Gen Psychiatry 2007;64:466–72.

108. Stone M, Laughren T, Jones ML, et al. Risk of suicidality in clinical trials of antidepressants in adults: analysis of proprietary data submitted for U.S. Food and Drug Administration. BMJ 2009;339:b2880.

109. Gibbons RD, Brown CH, Hur K, et al. Early evidence on the effects of regulators' suicidality warnings on SSRI prescriptions and suicides in children and adolescents. Am J Psychiatry 2007;164:1356–63.

110. Kurian BT, Ray WA, Arbogast PG, et al. Effect of regulatory warnings on antidepressant prescribing for children and adolescents. Arch Pediatr Adolesc Medicine 2007;161:690–6.

111. Libby AM, Orton HD, Valuck RJ. Persisting decline in treatment of pediatric depression after FDA warnings. Arch Gen Psychiatry 2009;66:1122–4.

112. Hamilton JD, Bridge J. Supportive psychotherapy, SSRIs, and MDD. J Am Acad Child Adolesc Psychiatry 2006;45:6–7.

113. Kratochvil CJ, Vitiello B, Walkup J, et al. Selective serotonin reuptake inhibitors in pediatric depression: is the balance between benefits and risks favorable? J Child Adolesc Psychopharmacol 2006;16:11–24.

114. Miller NL, Findling RL. Principles of psychopharmacology. In: Dulcan MK, editor. Dulcan's textbook of child and adolescent psychiatry. Arlington (VA): American Psychiatric Publishing, Inc; 2010. p. 667–80.

Depression in Later Life: An Overview with Treatment Recommendations

James M. Ellison, MD, MPH, DFAPA[a],*, Helen H. Kyomen, MD, MS, DFAPA[b],
David G. Harper, PhD[c]

KEYWORDS

- Depression • Elderly • Geriatric • Assessment • Treatment
- Differential Diagnosis

Among older adults, depressive symptoms and syndromes can present differently than in younger populations. Their demographics, phenomenology, assessment, comorbidity pattern, treatment approach, and typical locus of treatment are discussed here with emphasis on the special characteristics of depression as it presents in later life. Discussion of bipolar disorder, bipolar depression, and more extensive reviews of major depressive disorder can be found in several comprehensive recent texts.[1–3]

A focus on the disorders older adults has never been more timely because of the rapid worldwide increase in numbers among members of this age group. In the United States, adults age 65 and older comprised 12.8% of the population in 2010. By 2050, an estimated 20.2% of the population will be 65 and older.[4]

The debilitating effects of depression in later life have been well documented. Depression is a major source of disability among the elderly, responsible for 5.2% of years lived with disability, a degree of morbidity exceeded only by that associated with age-related vision disorders, cataracts, dementias, adult-onset hearing loss, cerebrovascular disease, or osteoarthritis.[5] Furthermore, depression in the elderly is associated with a significant increment in health care costs. In one study, even after adjustment for chronic medical illness, the total ambulatory costs were 43% to 52% higher, and total ambulatory and inpatient costs were 47% to 51% higher in depressed compared with nondepressed elderly patients.[6]

The authors have nothing to disclose.
[a] Geriatric Psychiatry Program, SB322, McLean Hospital, 115 Mill Street, Belmont, MA 02478, USA
[b] Research Administration 2, Mail Stop 317, McLean Hospital, 115 Mill Street, Belmont, MA 02478, USA
[c] Geriatric Psychiatry Program, SB307, McLean Hospital, 115 Mill Street, Belmont, MA 02478, USA
* Corresponding author.
E-mail address: jellison1@partners.org

Psychiatr Clin N Am 35 (2012) 203–229
doi:10.1016/j.psc.2012.01.003
0193-953X/12/$ – see front matter © 2012 Elsevier Inc. All rights reserved.

CHARACTERIZING LATE-LIFE DEPRESSION

Depressive symptoms affect 8% to 16% of community-dwelling elders and higher numbers in long-term care settings,[7] but the 1-year prevalence of major depressive disorder in community-dwelling older adults appears to be consistently lower than in younger adult populations. The Epidemiologic Catchment Area Study, a community-based structured survey in 5 US catchment areas, detected major depression in 1.4% to 3.7% of its 5723 elderly respondents.[8] Although subsequent studies have reported higher 1-year prevalence rates ranging from 2.3% to 4.3%,[9,10] the prevalence in older populations nonetheless is consistently exceeded by that in younger populations.

Depression in older adults can represent chronic, recurrent, or new-onset symptomatology. In many cases, the onset of depression occurs after age 60. Some evidence suggests that major depression's prevalence, although relatively low in the early 60s, begins to increase after age 65.[5,11] Although depression in younger adults and the younger elderly is more prevalent in women, gender disparities in psychological measures of distress associated with depression and anxiety subside by age 80.[12] The existence of ethnic and racial variations in depression's manifestations among the elderly is supported by evidence that US African-Americans are at risk for more severe depressive symptomatology as well as greater likelihood of misdiagnosis and undertreatment.[13]

A variety of socioeconomic, psychiatric, and medical risk factors for depressive symptoms and disorders have been identified and confirmed. Unmarried status, living alone, lack of social support, negative life events including bereavement, and lower socioeconomic status[5,14] are each significant contributors to the risk for late-life depression. Positive family history, female sex, substance abuse, prior depressive episodes, and prior suicide attempts are additional factors that increase risk.[15] Lower household income has been associated with depression in the elderly,[16] and the care giving role confers risk as well, as evidenced by the finding that some 25% to 50% of family caregivers experience depression.[17]

Among older adults with major depression, comorbid psychiatric and medical disorders are frequent. In the Amsterdam study of the elderly, 14.5% of depressed subjects were found to have generalized anxiety, and high rates of depression were noted in subjects with social phobia, panic disorder, and obsessive-compulsive disorder.[18] Chronic comorbid medical illness and cognitive impairment also increase the risk for depression.[14] Among the specific medical disorders that have been linked with an increased risk for depression, current evidence implicates cardiovascular disease, cancer, Parkinson's disease, stroke, lung disease, arthritis, loss of hearing, and dementia.[5,19]

Depressive states that fail to meet to the criteria for diagnosis of major depressive disorder can nonetheless exert debilitating psychosocial effects on older adults. The "geriatric nonmajor depressive syndromes" include such conditions as:

- Major depressive episode in partial remission
- Minor depressive disorder
- Mood disorder caused by a general medical condition
- Dementia with depressed mood
- Adjustment disorder with depressed mood
- Substance- or medication-induced mood disorder
- Anxiety disorder with depressive features
- Dysthymic disorder.

Nonmajor depressive disorders have been found in up to 15% of community-dwelling elders, 25% of elders assessed in primary care, and 50% to 70% of elders residing in long-term care settings.[20]

Depression in later life can present with symptoms that differ from those of depression in younger adults. Elderly depressed patients are more likely to report poor appetite and loss of interest in sex and are less likely to endorse crying spells, sadness, feeling fearful, being bothered, or feeling that life is a failure, compared with younger adults. Overall, older patients have a later age of onset of depressive illness, fewer lifetime episodes, and less frequent concurrent anxiety, and they are more likely to have received electroconvulsive therapy (ECT) at some point in their illness.[21] Some older depressed adults manifest irritability or withdrawal more prominently than sad or depressed mood,[22] whereas others focus on bodily disturbances. The presence of depression with psychotic features, typically characterized by the co-occurrence of mood-congruent delusions with major depressive symptoms, is more common in older than younger adults.

In the elderly, depression may be underreported by older adults who harbor a stigmatized view of mental illness. Clinicians may miss late-life depression as a result of ageist bias that misperceives the presence of depressive symptoms as a normal reaction to aging.[23] In addition, the identification of depression can be impeded in older adults by a variant presentation that emphasizes somatic or cognitive concerns, resulting in an emphasis on co-existing medical problems or a review of medications rather than attention to the patient's mood disorder. The elderly may present with fewer symptoms or a different syndrome of symptoms than is delineated in the Diagnostic and Statistical Manual of Mental Disorders IV text revision (DSM-IV-TR) when diagnosing major depression in younger adults. Patients may have difficulties in reporting appropriate symptoms because of the presence of cognitive deficits. Even after being identified, accessing care for depression in the elderly may be more complex because of fragmentation of care, expensive insurance copayments, and deductible sums that obstruct access to services and medications.[7] Access to specialty assessment and care, when needed, may be impeded by a scarcity of geriatric psychiatrists and limited transportation options. Despite the obstacles to recognition and treatment, however, late-life depression's serious consequences and eminent treatability make it an important condition to identify and treat aggressively in many cases.

DIFFERENTIAL DIAGNOSIS

In evaluating older adults with mood symptoms, formulation of an individualized assessment of alternative diagnostic explanations is of critical value in developing a suitable plan for further assessment and intervention. The differential diagnosis of late-life depression is extensive and includes, among other possibilities, depressive symptoms associated with normative sadness; primary mood disorders (unipolar and bipolar, major and nonmajor); depression secondary to another psychiatric disorder, such as adjustment disorders, bereavement, or schizophrenia; pharmacologically induced depressive symptoms resulting from substance use or medications; and depression associated with a broad range of medical illnesses.

Primary mood disorders include not only major depressive disorder, but also a number of other syndromes characterized by depressive symptoms, including bipolar disorder and dysthymic disorder. Early onset of symptoms and positive family history for major depressive disorder support that diagnosis, although many cases of major depressive disorder present with late-life onset and a negative family history. Assessment of symptoms and severity is aided by the use of the diagnostic criteria listed in the DSM-IV-TR, but these symptoms may be less specific and excessively sensitive in the older population. The DSM-IV-TR criteria for major depression require the presence of either a depressed mood or markedly diminished interest or pleasure in usually pleasurable activities almost daily for a 2-week period. In addition, the patient must experience at least 4 of the following: significant weight loss or gain; insomnia or hypersomnia; psychomotor agitation or retardation; fatigue or loss of energy; feelings of worthlessness or excessive or inappropriate guilt; diminished ability to think or to concentrate; indecisiveness; or recurrent thoughts of death, suicidal ideation, suicide attempt, or a specific plan for suicide.[24] A diagnosis of major depressive disorder is made only when the symptoms are not attributable to drugs, a general medical condition, or recent bereavement.

Assessment can be aided by using scales validated in older adult populations, including the *Geriatric Depression Scale (GDS, 15- and 30-item versions),*[25,26] *the Cornell Scale for Depression in Dementia (CSDD),*[27] *the Patient Health Questionnaire-9 (PHQ-9),*[28] *the Hamilton Depression Scale (HDS),*[29] *and the Beck Depression Inventory.*[30] These instruments help to identify depressed patients who may need further clinical and laboratory assessment.

Geriatric Depression Scale

The GDS takes 5 to 7 minutes to complete, can be self-administered, has 84% sensitivity and 95% specificity, and correlated well with the HDS. Its validity has been seen in inpatients and outpatients with comorbid medical illnesses or mild to moderate cognitive impairment. The original 30-item scale and 15-item short form are each sensitive and specific. The strength of the GDS lies in its focus on aspects of depression that are cognitive and affective rather than targeted to identify neuroveg-etative symptoms, because instruments that identify depression in the elderly on the basis of such vegetative symptoms as insomnia and low energy risk low specificity (too many false-positive results) because of the relative nonspecificity of these symptoms in later life.

Cornell Scale for Depression in Dementia

The CSDD is a psychometrically validated rating scale that was designed specifically for the clinical assessment of depression in patients whose cognitive impairment interferes with accurate response to questions about depressive symptoms. It consists of 19 caregiver- and clinician-rated items. It has high interrater reliability (k=0.67) and internal consistency (alpha coefficient=0.84). Total CSDD scales are correlated highly (0.83) with depressive subtypes of varying intensity classified according to Research Diagnostic Criteria.

Patient Health Questionnaire

The PHQ-9 is a 9-item depression scale, designed to assist primary care clinicians in diagnosing and monitoring treatment. It is based on the DSM-IV diagnostic criteria for major depressive disorder. Of the PHQ-9's 2 parts, the first assesses the patient's symptoms and functional impairment to make a tentative diagnosis of depression. Another part derives a severity score that can be used to help select and monitor treatment.

Hamilton Depression Scale

The HDS is an interviewer-administered survey of symptoms that can be used in patients of any age to derive an index of depression severity. Because it is long, complex, and must be administered by a clinician, it is used more typically in research than in clinical settings. It was designed to monitor depressive symptoms and treatment outcomes, rather than to screen for depression.

Beck Depression Inventory

The Beck Depression Inventory, with 2 iterations following its original version published in 1961, is a 21-item test covering various symptoms of depression. It requires administration by a clinician. Although it was not developed for specific use in the elderly, still, its questions can be helpful in elucidating mood and somatic concerns related to depression.

Beyond identifying depressive symptoms, a comprehensive depression evaluation includes a history and physical examination with special attention to stressors such as functional limitations or disability, chronic and new medical symptoms and illnesses, losses, stressors, and self-assessment of health status. To rule out medical conditions that may simulate or exacerbate depression, the laboratory assessment can include a chemistry profile with liver function tests, blood urea nitrogen, creatinine, thyroid function tests, vitamin B12 and folate levels, complete blood count, clean-catch urinalysis, chest x-ray, electrocardiogram, and neuroimaging study.

Because many older adults are prescribed multiple concurrent medications, it is imperative to rule out depression that is secondary to the use of pharmacologic agents. Antihypertensive agents such as reserpine, methyldopa, beta-blockers, clonidine, calcium channel blockers, and angiotensin-converting enzyme inhibitors have been associated with inducing depressed states.[31] Because patients who are on these medications are likely to have cardiovascular disease independently associated with depression,[32] there is controversy about whether these medications or the conditions they treat are more relevant to the induction of depressive symptoms. Systemic corticosteroids such as prednisone have also been associated with depression as well as with mania and psychosis.[24,31] Lipid-lowering agents, selective estrogen receptor modulators, nonsteroidal anti-inflammatory drugs, interferon, histamine-2 receptor antagonists, sedative-hypnotics such as benzodiazepines or barbiturates, and opioids have also been reported to affect mood in some patients.[31,33] If medication-induced depression is suspected, elimination of these medications from the patient's treatment regimen or their replacement with medications less likely to affect the central nervous system may be helpful. If this is not possible or successful, initiation of specific treatment of depression is indicated. Preventive approaches, in which exposure to these medications or similar derivatives is avoided, are also important, especially if there is a history of sensitivities to these medications.

Addictive substances capable of inducing depressive symptoms include sedative-hypnotics, opioids, and alcohol. Alcohol is the most commonly reported substance of abuse in elderly.[34] Depressive symptoms in the elderly that are associated with the use of sedative-hypnotics or opioids are often iatrogenic. Treatment of substance-induced depression in the elderly relies upon identification, detoxification and withdrawal, and relapse prevention. Substance abuse may mask the presence of a psychiatric disorder such as depression or anxiety, and clinicians should attempt to address needs or symptoms that the patient may be managing through the misuse of substances. Involvement of the patient's support system and treating clinicians, especially any who are facilitating the misuse of substances, increases the likelihood of a successful outcome. Brief but frequent counseling sessions that include motivation-for-change strategies, patient and family education and evaluation with direct feedback, contracting and goal setting, behavioral modification techniques, and the use of written materials such as self-help manuals may be useful.[35] Twelve-step groups such as Alcoholics Anonymous may provide additional peer support, and groups focused on the needs of older adults are found in some locations.

Certain chronic and acute medical disorders can increase the risk of depressive symptoms and major depressive disorder in later life. Major depressive disorder is estimated to occur in 4% of those with 1 or more medical conditions compared with 2.8% of those without.[36] Medical illnesses may exacerbate or cause depressive signs or symptoms through effects on mood, neuroendocrine and immune function, self-care abilities, and social interaction, which are mediated through the patient's premorbid personality, ego defenses, and coping style.[37] Higher rates of major depression have been reported in patients with myocardial infarction, diabetes mellitus, human immunodeficiency virus–related illness, cancer, stroke, and Parkinson's disease[38] as well as in dementia[39] and mild cognitive impairment (MCI).[40]

The concept of vascular depression was developed after observations that depression was common in patients with vascular and cerebrovascular disease. Alexopoulos and colleagues[41] proposed a working clinical definition of vascular depression involving 2 cardinal features: (1) depression with onset after 65 years of age or change in the course of depression after the onset of vascular disease in patients with earlier onset depression, and (2) clinical or laboratory evidence of vascular disease or vascular risk factors such as strokes, transient ischemic attacks, atrial fibrillation, angina pectoris, myocardial infarction, carotid stenosis, hypertension, or hyperlipidemia.[41,42]

Depression associated with medical illness is probably best addressed from a preventive perspective with amelioration of modifiable risk factors that may increase the risk of these illnesses. In some cases, treatment of a medical disorder relieves depressive symptoms as well; in others, initiation of specific treatment for depression is necessary. In general, identification of depression associated with a medical disorder should elicit consideration of independent concurrent treatment of depressive symptoms.

TREATMENT OF DEPRESSION IN LATER LIFE

Beyond recognition and treatment of medical conditions resulting in depressive symptoms, the treatment of primary depression in later life can involve nonpharmacologic, pharmacologic, or neurotherapeutic approaches shown efficacious. Individual psychotherapeutic approaches that have been found to be effective in elderly with depression include brief psychodynamic psychotherapy, cognitive behavior therapy, interpersonal psychotherapy, and problem-solving therapy.[43] Group, couple, and family psychotherapeutic approaches using supportive, insight-oriented, cognitive behavior and interactive therapies and provision of a structured and supportive milieu with attention to functional and safety assessments and concerns can serve helpful adjunctive roles in stabilizing and promoting the well being of elderly depressed patients.

Pharmacologic Treatment

Pharmacologic interventions have been shown to be safe and effective in treating older adults, especially when the depression is severe and the patient is experiencing more debilitating symptoms such as intense anxiety; neurovegetative signs such as anhedonia, insomnia, poor concentration, appetite disturbances, or psychomotor retardation or agitation; guilty ruminations or delusions; or suicidal ideation. The choice of antidepressant is influenced by clinical factors such as the patient's symptoms, concurrent medical problems, medications currently taken, and antidepressant side-effect profile and also in some cases by the practical issues of medication cost and insurance coverage.

The ideal antidepressant for an elderly person would be effective in all patients, alleviating symptoms completely and rapidly and maintaining therapeutic benefits over an extended time period. The ideal antidepressant would produce no adverse effects or drug interactions, have no toxicity in overdose, enhance functionality and quality of life, and be affordable. It would have a predictable dose-effect response and meaningful blood level parameters with reference ranges validated in elderly patients. Its metabolism would not be affected by compromised renal or hepatic function. Its elimination half-life would be suitable for convenient once-a-day dosing.[44] Although no current medication is blessed with all of these properties, we are fortunate to be able to choose among a range of generic, affordable antidepressants with validated effectiveness in the elderly and relative safety and tolerability.

Pharmacologic Treatment Phases: Acute, Continuation, Maintenance

The treatment of depression may be divided into acute, continuation, and maintenance phases. In general, the dose of antidepressant for an elderly patient is generally one-third to one-half of that recommended for a younger adult patient because of the anticipated effects of aging on the pharmacodynamic effects of antidepressants and on pharmacokinetic parameters including drug distribution, metabolism, and elimination. Although an initial partial response may be seen within 1 to 3 weeks, older patients may take up to 6 to 8 weeks to respond to a therapeutic antidepressant dose. Expert consensus guidelines endorse waiting a minimum of 2 to 3 weeks and as long as 7.5 weeks before deeming an antidepressant trial to have failed.[45] Thus, it is important to encourage patients to continue antidepressant medications even when they are unable to note change or improvement early in their treatment. It is often worthwhile to point out that a patient's subjective sense of improvement and well being is typically one of the final symptoms to improve during recovery from depression. Of note, improvement within the first 4 to 6 weeks of treatment is associated with an increased likelihood of continued benefit from maintenance treatment. In contrast, a change in treatment regimen should be considered for those without improvement during this period.[46]

After the acute response or remission of depression, a continuation treatment phase begins. Monitoring for ongoing effectiveness, side effects, and treatment adherence is suggested for 6 to 12 months, with the objectives of consolidating gains and preventing relapse. A consensus of experts has recommended that patients be continued on the dose of antidepressant that achieved the acute response or remission.[45]

After the continuation phase, many patients are advised to enter a maintenance phase of treatment to prevent illness recurrence. Factors such as the number and severity of depressive episodes, response to treatment, concomitant anxiety symptoms,[45] and delayed response to treatment during the first episode[47] may be important considerations when planning maintenance treatment duration. Expert consensus guidelines recommend that treatment extend for 1 or more years after a severe first episode and for 3 or more years after a third or subsequent episode.[45]

Pharmacologic Agent Classes

Currently available antidepressant medications represent several classes of agents with similar antidepressant efficacy. Differences in side effect profile, interactions, and out-of-pocket cost are important determinants in the choice of medication for an elderly patient. The classes of heterocyclic antidepressants (HCAs), monoamine oxidase inhibitors (MAOIs), selective serotonin reuptake inhibitors (SSRIs), serotonin norepinephrine reuptake inhibitors (SNRIs), and serotonin antagonist/reuptake inhibitors (SARIs) each have multiple members (**Table 1**).

Single agents currently represent the classes of noradrenergic and specific serotonergic antidepressant (NaSSA), norepinephrine and dopamine reuptake

Table 1
Summary of antidepressant medications

Pharmacologic Classes	Proposed Method of Action	Side Effects/Adverse Effects	Cautions/Contraindications
Heterocyclic antidepressants:	Inhibition of presynaptic reuptake of the monoamine neurotransmitters serotonin and norepinephrine	Sedation	History of cardiac disease
Tricyclic antidepressants (TCAs):		Confusion	QTc interval of over 450 ms
Tertiary amines:		Orthostatic hypotension	Bundle branch block
Amitriptyline		Cardiovascular events	Recent myocardial infarction
Imipramine		Dry mouth	Closed-angle glaucoma
Trimipramine		Increased appetite	Monoamine oxidase inhibitor use
Doxepin		Constipation/impaction	Can be highly toxic in overdosage
Clomipramine[a]		Urinary hesitancy or retention	
Amoxapine		Erectile dysfunction	
Secondary amines:		Mydriasis	
Nortriptyline		Blurry vision	
Desipramine		Falls	
Protriptyline			
Tetracyclic antidepressant:		Seizures	(TCA cautions/contraindications also apply to maprotiline)
Maprotiline		Skin rash	
		(TCA adverse effects also apply to maprotiline)	
MAOIs:	Inhibition of the monoamine oxidase enzymes	Hypertensive crises	Interactions with concurrent medications—consider psychopharmacologic consultation
Phenelzine		Increased appetite with weight gain	
Tranylcypromine		Induction of mania or hypomania	Interactions with tyramine rich foods—consider dietary consultation
Isocarboxazid		Orthostatic hypotension	
Selegiline (skin patch)		Sexual dysfunction	
Moclobemide[b]		Swelling of the ankles or feet	
		Increased sweating	
		Skin rash	
		Constipation	
		Drowsiness	
		Dry mouth	
		Insomnia	
		Nightmares	
		Fatigue	
		Hepatic transaminase elevations	

SSRIs: Fluoxetine Sertraline Paroxetine Fluvoxamine Citalopram Escitalopram Vilazodone	Inhibition of presynaptic reuptake of the monoamine neurotransmitter serotonin	Bruising Bleeding Anorexia Nausea Increased appetite Diarrhea Weight changes Anxiety Lightheadedness Headache Bruxism Insomnia Sleep fragmentation Somnolence Libido reduction Orgasmic dysfunction Hyponatremia Akathisia Falls Bradycardia Hypotension	Cardiac conduction delay MAOI use Discontinuation syndrome with abrupt withdrawal
SNRIs: Venlafaxine Milnacipran[a] Duloxetine Desvenlafaxine	Inhibition of presynaptic reuptake of the monoamine neurotransmitters serotonin, norepinephrine, and dopamine	SSRI adverse effects also apply to SNRIs	MAOI use Discontinuation syndrome with abrupt withdrawal
SARI: Nefazodone Trazodone	Weak inhibition of presynaptic reuptake of the monoamine neurotransmitter serotonin with potent postsynaptic 5HT2A receptor antagonism	Sedation Orthostatic hypotension Hepatic failure (nefazodone) Priapism (trazodone)	MAOI use

(continued on next page)

Table 1
(continued)

Pharmacologic Classes	Proposed Method of Action	Side Effects/Adverse Effects	Cautions/Contraindications
NaSSA: Mirtazapine	Antagonism of presynaptic noradrenergic alpha-2 autoreceptors and heteroreceptors and H1, 5HT2, and 5HT3 receptors	Sedation Confusion Dizziness Anxiety Appetite enhancement with weight gain Dry mouth Nausea Vomiting Constipation Flulike symptoms Chest pain Tachycardia Seizures	History of cardiac disease QTc interval of over 450 ms Bundle branch block Recent myocardial infarction Monamine oxidase inhibitor use
NDRI: Bupropion	Inhibition of presynaptic reuptake of the monoamine neurotransmitters, norepinephrine and dopamine	Seizures Headache Somnolence Insomnia Agitation Dizziness Diarrhea Dry mouth Nausea	History of seizures MAOI use
NRI: Reboxetine[b]	Inhibition of presynaptic reuptake of the monoamine neurotransmitter, norepinephrine	Dry mouth Constipation Urinary hesitancy or retention Agitation Anxiety Somnolence Sexual dysfunction	Hypotension MAOI use Seizure disorder Glaucoma

	Mechanism	Side effects	Contraindications
SRE: Tianeptine[b]	Enhancement of presynaptic reuptake of the monoamine neurotransmitter serotonin	Dry mouth Constipation Dizziness Somnolence	Monoamine oxidase inhibitor use
Stimulants: Methylphenidate[a] Dextroamphetamine[a] Modafinil[a] Armodafinil[a]	Methylphenidate inhibits presynaptic reuptake of dopamine, resulting in increased synaptic dopamine levels. Amphetamine inhibits presynaptic reuptake of dopamine, norepinephrine, and serotonin while also increasing the release of these neurotransmitters into the synapse. The mechanism of action of modafinil/armodafinil is complex and not fully understood but may involve inhibition of presynaptic reuptake of dopamine and an increase in the presynaptic release of norepinephrine and dopamine, as well as an elevation of hypothalamic histamine levels.	Tachycardia Elevated blood pressure Anxiety Induction of mania Insomnia Exacerbation of psychosis Appetite suppression	Acute coronary disease Seizure disorder MAOI use Methyldopa use

a Not indicated for depressive disorders.
b Not available in the United States.

inhibitor (NDRI), norepinephrine reuptake inhibitor (NRI), and serotonin reuptake enhancer (SRE). The class of stimulants are also discussed, although data for their monotherapeutic antidepressant effects are limited.[48]

The HCAs, comprising tricyclic antidepressants (TCAs) and the sole tetracyclic agent, maprotiline, are believed to achieve an antidepressant effect through inhibition of presynaptic reuptake of the monoamine neurotransmitters, serotonin and norepinephrine. Tricyclic antidepressant anti-alpha-1-adrenergic side effects include sedation and orthostatic hypotension. Reviewing the patient's electrocardiogram (ECG) is recommended before beginning TCA treatment in patients with a history of heart disease or who are older than 45 years of age. Quinidine-like cardiac conduction abnormalities with potentially hazardous prolongation of the PR, QRS or QTc intervals can occur, so routine ECG monitoring is recommended. There is an increased risk of sudden death with TCAs in patients who have a QTc interval of more than 450 milliseconds. When a bundle branch block is present, TCAs may increase the risk of second- or third-degree block. In addition, TCAs should not generally be used within 2 weeks of an acute myocardial infarction. Antihistaminic side effects of some TCAs include sedation and increased appetite. Anticholinergic side effects include dry mouth, constipation, urinary hesitancy or retention, erectile dysfunction, and mydriasis. Tricyclic antidepressants should be avoided in patients with closed-angle glaucoma. If the patient is in a depressed phase of bipolar illness, treatment must proceed with caution (and concurrent mood stabilizer use is recommended) because of the risk of triggering manic symptoms. In those who are at high risk of suicide, it is not advisable to prescribe large quantities of TCAs at one time because of potential overdose toxicity of TCAs. Tricyclic antidepressants are characterized as tertiary or secondary amines. The tertiary amines include amitriptyline, imipramine, trimipramine, doxepin, clomipramine, and amoxapine. The tertiary amines are more typically sedating, anticholinergic, and associated with postural hypotension. They may especially predispose elderly patients to increased confusion, blurry vision, constipation, impaction, urinary retention, falls, and cardiovascular effects and are used infrequently in aged patients. The secondary amines include nortriptyline, desipramine, and protriptyline, which are considered relatively safer for use in elderly patients. Nortriptyline and desipramine are the TCAs that are most often used. They have less severe anticholinergic and orthostatic effects than the tertiary amine TCAs, and standards have been established to guide dosing, including clinically relevant plasma reference levels. Nortriptyline has been found to have especially good outcomes when its use is accompanied by plasma level monitoring; expert consensus guidelines recommend starting nortriptyline at doses of 10 to 30 mg/d with target plasma levels between 50 and 150 ng/mL[45]; in the elderly, plasma levels in the lower range can be therapeutic. Desipramine is often effective as doses of 25 to 100 mg/d. Doses greater than 150 mg/d are not recommended. Tricyclic antidepressants are inexpensive, can be given once daily, and may be preferred in patients who are anorexic or have chronic pain. Maprotiline is used infrequently in elderly because of its long half-life and association with seizures and a relatively higher frequency of a reversible skin rash.

Monoamine Oxidase Inhibitors

Monoamine oxidase inhibitors competitively bind the monoamine oxidase enzyme, which breaks down catecholamines and indoleamines in presynaptic neurons and neuronal synapses and ingested tyramine, a neurotransmitterlike chemical, in the intestines. Phenelzine, tranylcypromine, isocarboxazid, selegiline, and moclobemide (not available in the United States) are MAOIs. This class of medications has no anticholinergic activity, is relatively well tolerated, and may be helpful in patients who have not responded to other antidepressants or who have an atypical depression, concurrent panic attacks, or social phobia. Despite their availability, the MAOIs are used sparingly in the elderly because of concerns regarding adverse effects such as hypertensive crises that can be initiated by intake of tyramine-rich foods or medications that are metabolized primarily by MAO, such as sympathomimetics contained in decongestants; meperidine; dextromethorphan; monoamines, such as l-dopa, l-tryptophan, l-tyrosine, and phenylalanine; some antihypertensives; and antidepressants that inhibit synaptic reuptake of monoamines. Psychopharmacologic consultation is suggested before initiating MAOI treatment to assess the safety of concurrently prescribed medications and for education about the tyramine-restricted diet that is required for all the MAOI antidepressants except for transdermal selegiline in its lowest dose of 6 mg/d.[48]

Selective Serotonin Reuptake Inhibitors

Selective serotonin reuptake inhibitors include fluoxetine, sertraline, paroxetine, fluvoxamine, citalopram, escitalopram, and vilazodone. These antidepressants are considered to be as efficacious as HCAs and MAOIs. Because of their more restricted receptor selectivity, the SSRIs lack the anti-alpha-1-adrenergic, antihistaminic and anticholinergic (with the exception of paroxetine) side effects of the HCAs. At therapeutic doses, cardiovascular toxicity is minimal, and overdoses with SSRIs are consequently less dangerous than with HCAs or MAOIs. Despite their cardiac safety, however, the serotonin reuptake inhibitors are not without side effects. The most frequent side effects are nausea, anxiety, anorexia, diarrhea, dizziness, nervousness, headache, insomnia, libido reduction, and sexual function impairment. Hyponatremia caused by SSRIs is seen more often in the elderly and rarely in younger adults.[49] Extrapyramidal side effects such as akathisia are occasionally observed. Weight loss with fluoxetine has been associated with pretreatment high body mass index.[50] In the elderly, an expert consensus group suggested initiating treatment of late-life depression with citalopram or sertraline, starting at 10 to 20 mg/d and 25 to 50 mg/d, respectively.[51] A subsequent US Food and Drug Administration warning that citalopram can interfere with cardiac conduction and that this effect is more likely to become hazardous at doses greater than 40 mg/d (or 20 mg/d for the elderly) might lead clinicians to favor sertraline or to verify cardiac safety of the citalopram dose with pre- and posttreatment ECGs. Paroxetine and fluoxetine were rated by expert consensus as less desirable treatments for depressed older adults.[51] Paroxetine is perhaps the least preferred SSRI for elderly patients because of its anticholinergic effects, drug-drug interactions, nonlinear kinetics, and strong association with an unpleasant discontinuation syndrome.

Serotonin-Norepinephrine Reuptake Inhibitors

SNRIs inhibit serotonin, norepinephrine, and dopamine presynaptic reuptake and include venlafaxine, milnacipran (indicated for fibromyalgia treatment rather than antidepressant use in the United States), duloxetine, and desvenlafaxine. All except desvenlafaxine have been studied in the elderly. Unlike the TCAs, these medications lack anti-alpha-1-adrenergic effects and do not significantly antagonize histaminic or cholinergic neurotransmission. Venlafaxine acts more selectively on serotonin reuptake, similarly to an SSRI, at lower doses; at higher doses, it exerts greater dual reuptake inhibition. Duloxetine, milnacipran, and desvenlafaxine exert dual reuptake inhibition even at lower doses. Although not dictated by evidence, the SNRIs are often used as a treatment for patients who have not responded to an SSRI trial. Duloxetine, which carries indications for the treatment of several pain-associated syndromes as well as depression, has been shown to reduce not only depressive symptoms but also self-rated pain measures in comparison with placebo.[52,53]

Abrupt discontinuation of an SSRI or SNRI may lead to a discontinuation syndrome characterized by uncomfortable symptoms of dizziness, nausea, headache, irritability, insomnia, anxiety, depression, fatigue, diarrhea, abnormal dreams, hyperhidrosis, and paresthesiae (described as "buzzing" or "shocklike" sensations). Discontinuation syndrome is more likely to occur with cessation of those agents with shorter elimination half-lives. It often can be prevented by educating patients and caregivers of the problems associated with sudden discontinuation of SSRIs and SNRIs. In some cases, the substitution of an SSRI or SNRI with longer elimination half-life for a shorter-acting agent facilitates gradual dose reduction and discontinuation.[48]

Serotonin Antagonist/Reuptake Inhibitors

SARIs combine a weak serotonin reuptake inhibition effect with potent postsynaptic 5HT2A receptor antagonism. Nefazodone and trazodone are SARIs. Nefazodone also has weak norepinephrine reuptake inhibition and weak alpha-1 receptor blocking effects, whereas trazodone has alpha-1 and histamine receptor blocking properties. Trazodone use as an antidepressant is limited by sedative and orthostatic side effects and rare but serious priapism.[54] Nefazodone has not been studied in the elderly; because it has been linked with infrequent but serious cases of liver failure, it is no longer considered a first-line choice for aged patients.

Mirtazapine

Mirtazapine, the sole available NaSSA in the United States, antagonizes presynaptic noradrenergic alpha-2 autoreceptors and heteroreceptors and H1, 5HT2, and 5HT3 receptors. Clinically, this results in a reduction of depression mediated by increased synaptic norepinephrine levels accompanied by sedation, appetite enhancement, and minimal nausea. Mirtazapine is considered by many clinicians to be very helpful in treating those depressed older adults with anxiety, insomnia, and loss of appetite. In studies with elderly subjects, mirtazapine was reported to be no less effective than amitriptyline, trazodone, or paroxetine[55–57] and to have an earlier onset of action than paroxetine.[57] Doses of mirtazapine less than 15 mg/d may facilitate a predominantly sedating, antihistaminic effect; higher doses are less sedating.[1–3,48]

Bupropion

Bupropion is the sole NDRI available for clinical use in the United States. Bupropion is available in immediate release (IR), slow release (SR) and extended release (XL) forms. It is typically nonsedating, has minimal effects on weight gain or sexual function, and has no anticholinergic side effects. The XL form can be given on a once-daily schedule. The most common side effects are headache, somnolence, insomnia, agitation, dizziness, diarrhea, dry mouth, and nausea. Seizures were a concern after bupropion's initial marketing, but its seizure-inducing rate, and especially that of the slower-release forms, is considered acceptably low among patients with no history of seizures, co-administered seizure-facilitating drugs, eating disorder, or other risk factors. To further reduce seizure risk, it is recommended that the IR form be given on a 3-times-daily regimen or the SR form be given on a twice-daily regimen, with no greater than 450 mg/d total IR dose or 400 mg/d total SR dose and no single dose over 200 mg, except with XL forms, which may be given up to 300 mg at a single dose and up to 450 mg/d.

Reboxetine

Reboxetine, available in Europe but not in the United States, is the only clinically available NRI. In a study of late-life depression, it was reported to be as effective as imipramine.[58] Compared with imipramine, there were fewer reported cardiac side effects, less hypotension, and more insomnia.

Tianeptine

Tianeptine, also available in Europe but not the United States, is the only clinically available SRE. It decreases the expression of serotonin mRNA and reduces the number of serotonin transporter binding sites.[59,60] It enhances serotonin reuptake in the cortex and hippocampus and may alter the norepinephrine system indirectly by its action on the serotonin system. Tianeptine's most common side effects include nausea, constipation, abdominal pain, headache, dizziness, and altered dreaming.

Stimulants

Stimulants, such as methylphenidate, dextroamphetamine, and the atypical stimulant, modafinil, have been suggested as adjunctive antidepressant agents in withdrawn and apathetic elderly patients on the basis of very limited evidence. The elimination half-life of methylphenidate is about 4 hours, and of dextroamphetamine, about 12 hours. Methylphenidate often is preferred because of its shorter half-life because it may be less likely to induce insomnia or prolonged appetite suppression. These medications have a relatively rapid onset of action and can be used alone or in combination with other antidepressants. Side effects range from tachycardia and increased anxiety to appetite suppression. Contraindications to this class of medications include acute coronary disease, seizure disorder, monoamine oxidase inhibitor use, and methyldopa use.

Electroconvulsive Therapy

ECT can be used to treat depression and is especially helpful for depression with psychosis. It is a fast-acting and efficacious treatment for depression with safety on a par with that of antidepressant treatment in many cases. The rate of response to ECT ranges from about 70% to more than 80%.[61] The duration of response can be lasting. When brief, effectiveness may require a maintenance treatment schedule. ECT is generally recommended for patients who cannot tolerate or do not respond to antidepressant medications, exhibit significant psychotic or severe self-destructive behaviors, or have previously responded well to ECT. Relative contraindications to ECT include uncontrolled hypertension, recent myocardial infarction, or increased intracranial pressure. The presence of these factors suggests that the treatments be delivered in a "high-risk" setting in which cardiovascular parameters can be monitored intensively. Electroconvulsive therapy may have the adverse effects of acute, transient anterograde and retrograde amnesia. Infrequently, patients may experience a more persistent sense of memory disturbance, the nature of which is poorly understood.

Repetitive Transcranial Magnetic Stimulation

Repetitive transcranial magnetic stimulation has recently become available as a clinical intervention for treating depression. Evaluation of its efficacy suggests beneficial effects in the elderly with clinically defined vascular depression at a total cumulative dose of 12,000 pulses, with response rate of 33%. A higher dose of repetitive transcranial magnetic stimulation was reported to produce more significant results. A total cumulative dose of 18,000 pulses has been reported to yield a response rate of about 39%.[62] Repetitive transcranial magnetic stimulation seems to offer a potentially efficacious treatment that is not associated with significant cognitive or cardiac complications. The most common side effects have been headache and neck pain, with rare occurrence of seizures.

RELATIONSHIP OF COGNITIVE IMPAIRMENT TO LATE-LIFE DEPRESSION

The frequent concurrent appearance of cognitive impairment and depressive symptoms in older adults has led clinicians and researchers to explore possible relationships between these 2 symptom clusters. In an early effort to understand cognitive impairment as a concomitant of depression, pseudodementia, a term that was initially introduced by Wernicke to designate hysterical psychoses, was used by Madden and colleagues[63] in the early 1950s to describe patients with symptoms of cognitive impairment that resolved with treatment of a psychotic disorder. Kiloh[64] emphasized the link between depression and potentially reversible cognitive symptoms. In the 1970s, the concept of a pseudodementia syndrome associated with depression was expanded by Charles Wells,[65] who explored the role of cognitive symptoms as a defense against overwhelming depressive affect. Later, recognition of the relationship between pseudodementia symptoms and increased risk for subsequent true cognitive deterioration resulted in new designations for cognitive disturbance in depressed individuals. *Depression-induced organic mental disorder,*[66] *four ideal types of depression and dementia syndromes,*[67] *depression-related cognitive dysfunction,*[68] and the currently favored term, *dementia syndrome of depression,*[69] describe this relationship. In each case, however, these terms suggest a reversible cognitive deterioration in the context of a late-life mood episode.[70]

It is now recognized that patients diagnosed with late-life mood disorders can experience cognitive deficits in several neuropsychological domains. Information processing speed, verbal and nonverbal memory, and executive functioning are particularly affected.[71–74] These cognitive symptoms do not always respond fully to effective antidepressant treatment, and cognitive impairment in some domains can persist even in euthymic patients whose depressive symptoms have remitted with treatment.[75,76]

The persistence of cognitive symptoms beyond the duration of a depressive episode suggests that a deeper pathological process may be associated with the occurrence of cognitive deterioration in late-life mood disorders. It is still unclear, however, what role depression may be playing in the context of continuing cognitive impairment. Is depression a symptom of dementia? Does a history of mood disorder constitute a risk factor for later dementia diagnosis? Can depression be a prodromal symptom of an incipient dementia?

Depression as a Symptom of Dementia

Depression has been noted to occur in patients with a previously diagnosed dementia[39,77–79] or MCI[80,81] suggesting that depression could be considered one of the many "behavioral and psychological symptoms of dementia" (BPSD).[82] Depressive symptoms in patients with dementia have been linked with frontal[83] and parietal[84] white matter hyperintensities. Apathy, a common and significant BPSD, which can be confused with depression, has also been linked with frontal white matter hyperintensities.[84] Positron emission tomography studies using (18)F-fluorodeoxyglucose have shown frontal hypometabolism in the dorsolateral prefrontal cortex and apathy associated with hypometabolism in the orbitofrontal cortex.[85]

Depression as a Risk Factor for Dementia

Several studies have shown an association between late-life depression and an increased risk for the development of dementia of Alzheimer's, mixed, or vascular types.[86–92] Other studies, however, have disputed this suggestion with negative findings.[93–95] Reviewing the many studies reported during the last several years, it may be possible to speculate on the reasons behind these disparate findings. One important feature of the positive studies is that they pursue either a dose-response design,[88,91] include a large number of subjects to provide adequate power to see effects of severe depression,[86,89,96] have a high threshold severity cutoff,[91] or use a combination of these strategies.[92] Dose in this context is analogous to the severity of depressive symptoms whether associated with dysthymic or major depressive disorders and has been used to arrive at hazard ratios or odds ratios.

Depression as a Prodrome for Dementia

Based on the epidemiologic evidence, it seems reasonable to consider late-life depression to be either a possible risk factor for the development of dementia or a possible prodromal symptom of dementia. Distinguishing between these 2 scenarios, however, requires further evidence. Depression seen as a prodromal manifestation of dementia implies the involvement of linked or shared neurologic substrates. Therefore, the onset of mood symptoms should predictably lead to cognitive disturbance. Depression as a risk factor for later dementia, however, would likely include not only late onset but also early depressive episodes. Similarly, there would likely be a dose-response function from depression to dementia risk. Several studies have addressed these issues by finding an increased risk of dementia in subjects with a history of depression[97,98] as well as prospectively examining risk of dementia in those with depression at various time lags[96,99] or by examining a number of depressive episodes using a dose-response methodology during follow-up.[100] The evidence, therefore, supports the idea that depression and number of depressive episodes are independent risk factors for the subsequent development of dementia.

The fact that depression is an independent risk factor for dementia as demonstrated by time lag studies does not clarify the relationship between depression and dementia when the 2 occur coincidentally or sequentially. Indeed, identifying depression as an independent risk factor for incident dementia is not mutually exclusive of depressive symptomatology being a prodrome of cognitive impairment or dementia.[101,102] It is quite possible that different mechanisms may explain the occurrence of depression in either situation[103] given the different cognitive domains in which initial deficits may be expressed in either situation.

Competing and Complementary Hypotheses

Dysregulation of hypothalamic–pituitary–adrenal axis

One explanation of the relationship between late-life depression and cognitive impairment has arisen from the observation of decreased hippocampal volume in depressed patients. Major depression is associated with dysregulation of the hypothalamic–pituitary–adrenal axis resulting in increased 24-hour cortisol levels and loss of suppression of cortisol secretion through negative feedback mechanisms. This loss of control appears to be mediated both by increased hypothalamic secretion of corticotropin-releasing factor and by impaired negative feedback as demonstrated by loss of inhibitory effects on cortisol secretion by the glucocorticoid analogue, dexamethasone. Together, these influences result in increased levels of cortisol throughout the diurnal cycle, a dysregulated condition shared by chronic stress[104] and aging.[105] In animals[106] as well as in humans,[107,108] elevated glucocorticoid levels have been linked to hippocampal atrophy. Longitudinal studies suggest that cumulative exposure to excessive glucocorticoids results in memory impairment and reduced hippocampal volume.[109] These findings are very similar to studies of hippocampal volumes in aging and depression, which show a strong dose-response relationship between depression history severity and reduction of hippocampal volume. Various measures of depression intensity have all shown that they impact hippocampal volume, including total days depressed, total days of untreated depression, duration since first depressive episode, and early-onset as opposed to late-onset depression.[110]

Cerebrovascular disease

A second hypothesized relationship between late-life depression and cognitive impairment proposes that this link is mediated by the effects of cerebrovascular disease. There is substantial evidence that the relative risk of coronary artery disease,[111] stroke,[112] and possibly diabetes[113] is increased by a history of depression. Cerebrovascular ischemic white matter lesions[114] characterized by reduced fractional anisotropy, as measured by diffusion tensor imaging,[115] have also been observed in patients with late-life depression. Magnetic resonance imaging findings show that white matter lesions influence the later development of depression and particularly late-onset, late-life depression.[116,117] The volume of these ischemic lesions in patients with late-life depression correlates significantly and negatively with cognitive performance.[118] Depression and vascular disease, therefore, appear to have a bidirectional relationship, each increasing the other's risk[119] and each increasing the risk of cognitive impairment.

Inflammation

Recently, an additional hypothesis has drawn attention to the relationship between late-life depression, cognitive decline, and inflammation. Inflammation in the central nervous system is mediated through a specialized system that is separate, though in communication with, the peripheral inflammatory system.[120] Peripheral and central inflammation have been shown to increase with age,[121,122] and, in the central nervous system, inflammation is characterized by increasing levels of activated and primed microglia, continuous production of pro-inflammatory cytokines, and a decrease in anti-inflammatory molecules.[51] Depression has been linked with activation of cell-mediated immunity since the early 1990s[123] linking together the observations of increased hypothalamic–pituitary–adrenal activation and increased inflammatory response in depression.[124,125] In the most recent epidemiologic study, interleukin (IL)-1ra levels were found to significantly predict the development of depressive symptoms at 3- and 6-year follow-up[126] suggesting a causal role of inflammation in the development of late-life depression. A recent finding has since confirmed that reduced gray matter volume in hippocampus is associated with high levels of IL-6 in young adults.[127] Several large epidemiologic studies, in fact, have found increased IL-6 levels to be a strong predictor of depression.[128–131] The observation of a relationship between hippocampal atrophy and high levels of IL-6[127] suggests an inflammatory mechanism for hippocampal volume loss in depression. An association between systemic inflammation and the development of cognitive decline has also been explored and supported.

LOCUS OF CARE

Late-life depression is pervasive, debilitating, and intimately linked with the presence and development of medical disorders. Many cases of late-life depression, however, go undetected or untreated despite the patient's ongoing involvement with a primary care clinician who recognizes the importance of this condition.[132] Older adults often prefer to receive treatment for depression, along with care for medical conditions, in primary care settings.[15,133] Yet, the adequacy of primary care clinicians' preparation for the treatment of mental disorders in older adults is variable and in many cases quite limited.[134]

It is by no means necessary to refer all depressed older adults to behavioral or mental health specialists or specialty settings for assessment and treatment. Effective detection and treatment of depression in primary care settings have been reported in a series of demonstration projects that enhance usual treatment practices in cost-effective and practical ways to improve outcomes. These modified primary care treatment models include the Prevention of Suicide in Primary Care Elderly: Collaborative Trial (PROSPECT) and Primary Care Research in Substance Abuse and Mental Health for the Elderly (PRISM). PROSPECT[135] was designed to prevent suicide among older primary care patients by reducing suicidal ideation and depression. The interventions consisted of recognition of depression and suicide ideation by primary care physicians, application of a treatment algorithm for geriatric depression in the primary care setting, and treatment management by health specialists such as nurses, social workers, and psychologists. In PRISM,[136] clinical outcomes were compared for patients who were randomly assigned to integrated care or enhanced specialty care. Integrated care was comprised of mental health services colocated in primary care with primary care physician collaboration. Enhanced specialty care included referral to physically separate mental health or substance abuse clinics. Although comprehensive and effective, the enhancements to usual primary care approaches that were incorporated into these demonstration projects may be difficult to accomplish in many primary care settings.

Some patients with late-life depression should be referred for specialty care to a psychiatrist (or clinical nurse specialist) or geriatric psychiatrist. General psychiatry residencies prepare their trainees to some extent to treat late-life depression by including a geriatric training experience, and some psychiatrists subsequently receive additional specialized training in the form of a geriatric psychiatry fellowship that permits the psychiatrist to be examined and certified as a geriatric psychiatry specialist. Geriatric psychiatry fellowship typically includes advanced training and supervision in the cognitive, behavioral, and emotional conditions that affect the elderly. Psychiatrists with expertise in the treatment of older adults can support the work of primary care clinicians who treat late-life depressive disorder patients. Unfortunately, because the 80 new geriatric psychiatrists graduated each year barely compensate for the annual attrition among these specialists, it is estimated that there will be only 2,640 geriatric psychiatrists by the year 2030, or only 1 per 5,682 older adults with a psychiatric disorder.[137] This is only half the number estimated to be necessary to serve the older population.[138] Because the limited number of geriatric psychiatrists is inadequate to provide care to all mentally ill older adults, it is critical that primary care physicians, geriatricians, psychologists, social workers, and advanced practice nurses sharpen their skills in caring for this vulnerable and affected population. Fortunately, primary care clinicians have identified the desirability of training in the recognition and treatment of late-life depression.[139] If routine care of depressed elders can be managed effectively in primary care settings, geriatric psychiatrists are thereby more available to assume the care of more complex, treatment-resistant, or clinically risky patients such as those who have failed prior adequate depression treatments; those who are at significant acute risk for self-harm or suicide; those who abuse alcohol or other substances; those who suffer from complicating comorbid psychiatric conditions such as personality disorders, psychoses, or dementias; or those in need of technically specialized psychiatric services such as electroconvulsive therapy or repetitive transcranial magnetic stimulation.

SUMMARY

We have already entered a new, more exciting, and hopeful era in the treatment of late-life depression. The increasing numbers of older adults who are surviving to more advanced ages and the greater recognition of late-life depression's prevalence and impact on quality of life emphasize how important it is to detect and treat this disorder. Our increasing repertoire of evidence-based psychotherapeutic, pharmacologic, and neurotherapeutic treatment interventions offers many treatment alternatives, allowing substantial individualization of treatment approach. Demonstration of the effectiveness of depression treatment in primary care suggests the feasibility of increasing our patients' access to care. Growing appreciation of the pathophysiology of depression and its interrelationships with cognitive impairment may increase our ability to limit or delay certain aspects of cognitive impairment through more aggressive treatment of depression. Improved recognition and treatment of late-life depression holds great potential for improving physical and mental health in later life, reducing disability in later years, and improving quality of life.

REFERENCES

1. Roose SP, Sackeim HA, editors. Late-life depression. New York: Oxford University Press; 2004.
2. Ellison JM, Kyomen HH, Verma S, editors. Mood disorders in later life. 2 edition. New York: Informa Healthcare; 2008.
3. Katona C. Depression in old age. Chichester: John Wiley & Sons, Ltd; 1994.
4. Bureau USC. Statistical abstract of the United States. 2011. Available at: http://www.census.gov/compendia/statab/cats/population.html. Accessed August 14, 2011.
5. Kohn R, Gum AM, King-Kallimanis B. The epidemiology of major depression in geriatric populations. In: Ellison JM, Kyomen H, Verma S, editors. Mood disorders in later life. 2 edition. New York: Informa Healthcare; 2008. p. 37–64.
6. Katon WJ, Lin E, Russo J, et al. Increased medical costs of a population-based sample of depressed elderly patients. Arch General Psychiatry 2003;60(9):897–903.
7. Kyomen HH, Gottlieb GL. Financial issues in the delivery of geraitric psychiatric care. In: Sadock BJ, Sadock VA, Ruiz P, editors. Comprehensive textbook of psychiatry IX. Philadelphia: Lippincott Williams and Wilkins; 2009. p. 4185–93.
8. Weissman MM, Bruce ML, Leaf PJ, et al. Affective disorders. In: Robins LN, Regier DA, editors. Psychiatric disorders in America: The Epidemiologic Catchment Study. New York: Free Press; 1991. p. 53–80.
9. Robins LN, Wing J, Wittchen HU, et al. The Composite International Diagnostic Interview. An epidemiologic instrument suitable for use in conjunction with different diagnostic systems and in different cultures. Arch Gen Psychiatry 1988;45(12):1069–77.
10. Steffens DC, Skoog I, Norton MC, et al. Prevalence of depression and its treatment in an elderly population: the Cache County study. Arch Gen Psychiatry 2000;57(6):601–7.

11. Solhaug HI, Romuld EB, Romild U, et al. Increased prevalence of depression in cohorts of the elderly: an 11-year follow-up in the general population—the HUNT study. Int Psychogeriat 2012;24(1):151–8.
12. Pachana NA, McLaughlin D, Leung J, et al. Anxiety and depression in adults in their eighties: do gender differences remain? Int Psychogeriat 2012;24(1):145–50.
13. Shellman J, Granara C, Rosengarten G. Barriers to depression care for black older adults. Practice and policy implication. J Gerontol Nurs 2011;37(6):13–7.
14. Barua A, Ghosh MK, Kar N, et al. Socio-demographic factors of geriatric depression. Indian J Psychol Med 2010;32(2):87–92.
15. Cole MG, Dendukuri N. Risk factors for depression among elderly community subjects: a systematic review and meta-analysis. Am J Psychiatry 2003;160(6): 1147–56.
16. Glaesmer H, Riedel-Heller S, Braehler E, et al. Age- and gender-specific prevalence and risk factors for depressive symptoms in the elderly: a population-based study. Int Psychogeriat 2011;23(8):1294–300.
17. Clark MC, Nicholas JM, Wassira LN, et al. Psychosocial and biological indicators of depression in the caregiving population. Biol Res Nurs 2011. [Epub ahead of print].
18. Beekman AT, de Beurs E, van Balkom AJ, et al. Anxiety and depression in later life: Co-occurrence and communality of risk factors. Am J Psychiatry 2000; 157(1):89–95.
19. Winter Y, Korchounov A, Zhukova TV, et al. Depression in elderly patients with Alzheimer dementia or vascular dementia and its influence on their quality of life. J Neurosci Rural Pract 2011;2(1):27–32.
20. Lavretsky H, Lyness JM. Geriatric nonmajor depressive syndromes: minor depression, dysthymia, and subsyndromal depression. In: Ellison JM, Kyomen H, Verma S, editors. Mood disorders in later life. 2 edition. New York: Informa Healthcare; 2008. p. 15–36.
21. Hybels CF, Landerman LR, Blazer DG. Age differences in symptom expression in patients with major depression. Int J Geriatr Psychiatry 2011. DOI: 10.1002/gps.2759. [Epub ahead of print].
22. Gallo JJ, Rabins PV, Lyketsos CG, et al. Depression without sadness: functional outcomes of nondysphoric depression in later life. J Am Geriatr Soc 1997;45(5): 570–8.
23. Silton NR, Flannelly KJ, Milstein G, et al. Stigma in America: has anything changed? Impact of perceptions of mental illness and dangerousness on the desire for social distance: 1996 and 2006. J Nerv Ment Dis 2011;199(6):361–6.
24. American Psychiatric Association. Diagnostic and statistical manual of mental disorders (4th ed., text rev.). Washington, DC: Author; 2000.
25. Yesavage JA, Brink TL, Rose TL, et al. Development and validation of a geriatric depression screening scale: a preliminary report. J Psychiatr Res 1982;17(1):37–49.
26. Sheikh JI, Yesavage JA. Geriatric depression scale (GDS): recent evidence and development of a shorter version. In: Brink TL, editor. Clinical gerontology: a guide to assessment and intervention. New York: The Haworth Press; 1986. p. 165–73.
27. Alexopoulos GS, Abrams RC, Young RC, et al. Cornell scale for depression in dementia. Biol Psychiatry 1988;23(3):271–84.
28. Kroenke K, Spitzer RL, Williams JB. The PHQ-9: validity of a brief depression severity measure. J Gen Intern Med 2001;16(9):606–13.
29. Hamilton M. A rating scale for depression. J Neurol Neurosurg Psychiatry 1960;23: 56–62.
30. Beck AT, Ward CH, Mendelson M,et al. An inventory for measuring depression. Arch Gen Psychiatry 1961;4:561–71.

31. Kotlyar M, Dysken M, Adson DE. Update on drug-induced depression in the elderly. Am J Geriatr Pharmacother 2005;3(4):288–300.

32. Rudisch B, Nemeroff CB. Epidemiology of comorbid coronary artery disease and depression. Biol Psychiatry 2003;54(3):227–40.

33. Rosen D, Smith ML, Reynolds CF 3rd. The prevalence of mental and physical health disorders among older methadone patients. Am J Geriatr Psychiatry 2008;16(6): 488–97.

34. Ward EN. Substance use disorders and late-life depression. In: Ellison JM, Kyomen H, Verma S, editors. Mood disorders in later life. 2nd edition. New York: Informa Healthcare; 2008. p. 197–208.

35. Menninger JA. Assessment and treatment of alcoholism and substance-related disorders in the elderly. Bull Menning Clin 2002;66(2):166–83.

36. Patten SB. Long-term medical conditions and major depression in a Canadian population study at waves 1 and 2. J Affect Disord 2001;63(1–3):35–41.

37. Blazer DG 2nd, Hybels CF. Origins of depression in later life. Psychol Med 2005; 35(9):1241–52.

38. Katon WJ. Clinical and health services relationships between major depression, depressive symptoms, and general medical illness. Biol Psychiatry 2003;54(3): 216–26.

39. Lyketsos CG, Lopez O, Jones B, et al. Prevalence of neuropsychiatric symptoms in dementia and mild cognitive impairment: results from the cardiovascular health study. JAMA 2002;288(12):1475–83.

40. Barnes DE, Alexopoulos GS, Lopez OL, et al. Depressive symptoms, vascular disease, and mild cognitive impairment: findings from the Cardiovascular Health Study. Arch Gen Psychiatry 2006;63(3):273–9.

41. Alexopoulos GS, Meyers BS, Young RC, et al. 'Vascular depression' hypothesis. Arch Gen Psychiatry 1997;54(10):915–22.

42. Kelly RE, Alexopoulos GS. The vascular depression concept and its implications. In: Ellison JM, Kyomen H, Verma S, editors. Mood disorders in later life. 2 edition. New York: Informa Healthcare; 2008. p. 161–77.

43. Antognini FC, Liptzin B. Psychotherapy for late-life mood disorders. In: Ellison JM, Kyomen H, Verma S, editors. Mood disorders in later life. 2 edition. New York: Informa Healthcare; 2008. p. 315–37.

44. DeVane CL. Pharmacologic characteristics of ideal antidepressants in the 21st century. J Clin Psychiatry 2000;61 (Suppl 1)1:4–8.

45. Alexopoulos GS, Katz IR, Reynolds CF 3rd, et al. The expert consensus guideline series. Pharmacotherapy of depressive disorders in older patients. Postgrad Med 2001;Spec No Pharmacotherapy:1–86.

46. Sackeim HA, Roose SP, Burt T. Optimal length of antidepressant trials in late-life depression. J Clin Psychopharmacol 2005;25(4 Suppl 1):S34–7.

47. Flint AJ, Rifat SL. The effect of treatment on the two-year course of late-life depression. Br J Psychiatry 1997;170:268–72.

48. Ellison JM, Sivrioglu EY, Salzman C. Pharmacotherapy of late-life depression: evidence-based recommendations. In: Ellison JM, Kyomen H, Verma S, editors. Mood disorders in later life. 2 edition. New York: Informa Healthcare; 2008. p. 239–90.

49. Jacob S, Spinler SA. Hyponatremia associated with selective serotonin-reuptake inhibitors in older adults. Annals Pharmacother 2006;40(9):1618–22.

50. Goldstein DJ, Hamilton SH, Masica DN, et al. Fluoxetine in medically stable, depressed geriatric patients: effects on weight. J Clin Psychopharmacol 1997;17(5): 365–9.

51. Alexopoulos GS, Morimoto SS. The inflammation hypothesis in geriatric depression. Int J Geriatr Psychiatry 2011. DOI: 10.1002/gps.2672. [Epub ahead of print].

52. Nelson JC, Wohlreich MM, Mallinckrodt CH, et al. Duloxetine for the treatment of major depressive disorder in older patients. Am J Geriatr Psychiatry 2005;13(3): 227–35.

53. Raskin J, Wiltse CG, Siegal A, et al. Efficacy of duloxetine on cognition, depression, and pain in elderly patients with major depressive disorder: an 8-week, double-blind, placebo-controlled trial. Am J Psychiatry 2007;164(6):900–9.

54. Rothschild AJ. The diagnosis and treatment of late-life depression. J Clin Psychiatry 1996;57 (Suppl 5):5–11.

55. Halikas J. Org 3770 (mirtazapine) versus trazodone: a placebo controlled trial in depressed elderly patients. Hum Psychopharmacol 1995;10:S125–33.

56. Hoyberg OJ, Maragakis B, Mullin J, et al. A double-blind multicentre comparison of mirtazapine and amitriptyline in elderly depressed patients. Acta psychiatrica Scand 1996;93(3):184–90.

57. Schatzberg AF, Kremer C, Rodrigues HE, et al. Double-blind, randomized comparison of mirtazapine and paroxetine in elderly depressed patients. Am J Geriatr Psychiatry 2002;10(5):541–50.

58. Katona C, Bercoff E, Chiu E, et al. Reboxetine versus imipramine in the treatment of elderly patients with depressive disorders: a double-blind randomised trial. J Affect Disord 1999;55(2–3):203–13.

59. Kuroda Y, Watanabe Y, McEwen BS. Tianeptine decreases both serotonin transporter mRNA and binding sites in rat brain. Eur J Pharmacol 1994;268(1):R3–5.

60. Watanabe Y, Sakai RR, McEwen BS, et al. Stress and antidepressant effects on hippocampal and cortical 5-HT1A and 5-HT2 receptors and transport sites for serotonin. Brain Res 1993;615(1):87–94.

61. Seiner S, Burke A. Electroconvulsive therapy and neurotherapeutic treatments for late-life mood disorders. In: Ellison JM, Kyomen H, Verma S, editors. Mood disorders in later life. 2nd edition. New York: Informa Healthcare; 2008. p. 291–313.

62. Jorge RE, Moser DJ, Acion L, et al. Treatment of vascular depression using repetitive transcranial magnetic stimulation. Arch Gen Psychiatry 2008;65(3):268–76.

63. Madden JJ, Luhan JA, Kaplan LA, et al. Nondementing psychoses in older persons. JAMA 1952;150(16):1567–70.

64. Kiloh LG. Pseudo-dementia. Acta psychiatrica Scand 1961;37:336–51.

65. Wells CE. Pseudodementia. Am J Psychiatry 1979;136(7):895–900.

66. McAllister TW. Overview: pseudodementia. Am J Psychiatry 1983;140(5):528–33.

67. Feinberg T, Goodman B. Affective illness, dementia, and pseudodementia. J Clin Psychiatry 1984;45(3):99–103.

68. Stoudemire A, Hill C, Gulley LR, et al. Neuropsychological and biomedical assessment of depression-dementia syndromes. J Neuropsychiatry Clin Neurosci. 1989; 1(4):347–61.

69. Folstein MF, McHugh PR. Dementia syndrome of depression. In: Katzman R, Terry RD, Bick LD, editors. Alzheimer's disease, senile dementia and related disorders. New York: Raven; 1978. p. 281–9.

70. Nussbaum PD. Pseudodementia: a slow death. Neuropsychol Rev 1994;4(2): 71–90.

71. Boone KB, Lesser IM, Miller BL, et al. Cognitive functioning in older depressed putpatients: relationship of presence and severity of depression to neuropsychological test scores. Neuropsychology 1995;9(3):390–8.

72. Butters MA, Whyte EM, Nebes RD, et al. The nature and determinants of neuropsychological functioning in late-life depression. Arch Gen Psychiatry 2004;61(6):587–95.

73. Hart RP, Kwentus JA, Taylor JR, et al. Rate of forgetting in dementia and depression. J Consult Clin Psychol 1987;55(1):101–5.

74. Sheline YI, Barch DM, Garcia K, et al. Cognitive function in late life depression: relationships to depression severity, cerebrovascular risk factors and processing speed. Biol Psychiatry 2006;60(1):58–65.

75. Butters MA, Becker JT, Nebes RD, et al. Changes in cognitive functioning following treatment of late-life depression. Am J Psychiatry 2000;157(12):1949–54.

76. Nebes RD, Pollock BG, Houck PR, et al. Persistence of cognitive impairment in geriatric patients following antidepressant treatment: a randomized, double-blind clinical trial with nortriptyline and paroxetine. J Psychiatr Res 2003;37(2):99–108.

77. Ballard C, Bannister C, Solis M, et al. The prevalence, associations and symptoms of depression amongst dementia sufferers. J Affect Dis 1996;36(3–4):135–44.

78. Migliorelli R, Teson A, Sabe L, et al. Prevalence and correlates of dysthymia and major depression among patients with Alzheimer's disease. Am J Psychiatry 1995; 152(1):37–44.

79. Park JH, Lee SB, Lee TJ, et al. Depression in vascular dementia is quantitatively and qualitatively different from depression in Alzheimer's disease. Dementia and geriatric cognitive disorders. 2007;23(2):67–73.

80. Ellison JM, Harper DG, Berlow Y, et al. Beyond the "C" in MCI: noncognitive symptoms in amnestic and non-amnestic mild cognitive impairment. CNS Spectr 2008;13(1):66–72.

81. Ritchie K. Mild cognitive impairment: an epidemiological perspective. Dialogues Clin Neurosci 2004;6(4):401–8.

82. Casanova MF, Starkstein SE, Jellinger KA. Clinicopathological correlates of behavioral and psychological symptoms of dementia. Acta neuropathologica 2011;122(2): 117–35.

83. Barber R, Scheltens P, Gholkar A, et al. White matter lesions on magnetic resonance imaging in dementia with Lewy bodies, Alzheimer's disease, vascular dementia, and normal aging. J Neurol Neurosurg Psychiatry 1999;67(1):66–72.

84. Starkstein SE, Mizrahi R, Capizzano AA, et al. Neuroimaging correlates of apathy and depression in Alzheimer's disease. J neuropsychiatr clin neurosci 2009; 21(3):259–65.

85. Holthoff VA, Beuthien-Baumann B, Kalbe E, et al. Regional cerebral metabolism in early Alzheimer's disease with clinically significant apathy or depression. Biol Psychiatry 2005;57(4):412–21.

86. Buntinx F, Kester A, Bergers J, et al. Is depression in elderly people followed by dementia? A retrospective cohort study based in general practice. Age Ageing 1996;25(3):231–3.

87. Gatz JL, Tyas SL, St John P, et al. Do depressive symptoms predict Alzheimer's disease and dementia? J Gerontol A Biol Sci Med Sci. 2005;60(6):744–7.

88. Chen R, Hu Z, Wei L, et al. Severity of depression and risk for subsequent dementia: cohort studies in China and the UK. Br J Psychiatry 2008;193(5):373–7.

89. Cankurtaran M, Yavuz BB, Cankurtaran ES, et al. Risk factors and type of dementia: vascular or Alzheimer? Arch Gerontol Geriatr 2008;47(1):25–34.

90. Irie F, Masaki KH, Petrovitch H, et al. Apolipoprotein E epsilon4 allele genotype and the effect of depressive symptoms on the risk of dementia in men: the Honolulu-Asia Aging Study. Arch Gen Psychiatry 2008;65(8):906–12.

91. Saczynski JS, Beiser A, Seshadri S, et al. Depressive symptoms and risk of dementia: the Framingham Heart Study. Neurology 2010;75(1):35–41.

92. Byers AL, Covinsky KE, Barnes DE, et al. Dysthymia and depression increase risk of dementia and mortality among older veterans. Am J Geriatr Psychiatry 2011. [Epub ahead of print].

93. Chen P, Ganguli M, Mulsant BH, et al. The temporal relationship between depressive symptoms and dementia: a community-based prospective study. Arch Gen Psychiatry 1999;56(3):261–6.

94. Ganguli M, Du Y, Dodge HH, et al. Depressive symptoms and cognitive decline in late life: a prospective epidemiological study. Arch Gen Psychiatry 2006;63(2): 153–60.

95. Becker JT, Chang YF, Lopez OL, et al. Depressed mood is not a risk factor for incident dementia in a community-based cohort. Am J Geriatr Psychiatry 2009; 17(8):653–63.

96. Green RC, Cupples LA, Kurz A, et al. Depression as a risk factor for Alzheimer disease: the MIRAGE Study. Archives Neurol 2003;60(5):753–9.

97. Speck CE, Kukull WA, Brenner DE, et al. History of depression as a risk factor for Alzheimer's disease. Epidemiology 1995;6(4):366–9.

98. Geerlings MI, den Heijer T, Koudstaal PJ, et al. History of depression, depressive symptoms, and medial temporal lobe atrophy and the risk of Alzheimer disease. Neurology 2008;70(15):1258–64.

99. Dal Forno G, Palermo MT, Donohue JE, et al. Depressive symptoms, sex, and risk for Alzheimer's disease. Ann Neurol 2005;57(3):381–7.

100. Dotson VM, Beydoun MA, Zonderman AB. Recurrent depressive symptoms and the incidence of dementia and mild cognitive impairment. Neurology 2010;75(1):27–34.

101. Brommelhoff JA, Gatz M, Johansson B, et al. Depression as a risk factor or prodromal feature for dementia? Findings in a population-based sample of Swedish twins. Psychol Aging 2009;24(2):373–84.

102. Bhalla RK, Butters MA, Mulsant BH, et al. Persistence of neuropsychologic deficits in the remitted state of late-life depression. Am J Geriatr Psychiatry 2006;14(5):419–27.

103. Rapp MA, Dahlman K, Sano M, et al. Neuropsychological differences between late-onset and recurrent geriatric major depression. Am J Psychiatry 2005;162(4): 691–8.

104. Checkley S. The neuroendocrinology of depression and chronic stress. Br Med Bull 1996;52(3):597–617.

105. McEwen BS. Stress and the aging hippocampus. Frontiers in neuroendocrinology. 1999;20(1):49–70.

106. McEwen BS, Magarinos AM. Stress effects on morphology and function of the hippocampus. Ann NY Acad Sci. 1997;821:271–84.

107. Woon FL, Sood S, Hedges DW. Hippocampal volume deficits associated with exposure to psychological trauma and posttraumatic stress disorder in adults: a meta-analysis. Prog Neuropsychopharmacol Biol Psychiatry 2010;34(7):1181–8.

108. Starkman MN, Giordani B, Gebarski SS, et al. Decrease in cortisol reverses human hippocampal atrophy following treatment of Cushing's disease. Biol Psychiatry 1999;46(12):1595–602.

109. Lupien SJ, Fiocco A, Wan N, et al. Stress hormones and human memory function across the lifespan. Psychoneuroendocrinology 2005;30(3):225–42.

110. Butters MA, Young JB, Lopez O, et al. Pathways linking late-life depression to persistent cognitive impairment and dementia. Dialogue Clin Neurosci 2008;10(3): 345–57.

111. Ariyo AA, Haan M, Tangen CM, et al. Depressive symptoms and risks of coronary heart disease and mortality in elderly Americans. Cardiovascular Health Study Collaborative Research Group. Circulation 2000;102(15):1773–9.

112. Larson SL, Owens PL, Ford D, et al. Depressive disorder, dysthymia, and risk of stroke: thirteen-year follow-up from the Baltimore epidemiologic catchment area study. Stroke 2001;32(9):1979–83.

113. Eaton WW, Armenian H, Gallo J, et al. Depression and risk for onset of type II diabetes. A prospective population-based study. Diabetes Care 1996;19(10):1097–102.

114. Thomas AJ, O'Brien JT, Davis S, et al. Ischemic basis for deep white matter hyperintensities in major depression: a neuropathological study. Arch Gen Psychiatry 2002;59(9):785–92.

115. Shimony JS, Sheline YI, D'Angelo G, et al. Diffuse microstructural abnormalities of normal-appearing white matter in late life depression: a diffusion tensor imaging study. Biol Psychiatry 2009;66(3):245–52.

116. Krishnan KR, Hays JC, Blazer DG. MRI-defined vascular depression. Am J Psychiatry 1997;154(4):497–501.

117. Steffens DC, Krishnan KR, Crump C, et al. Cerebrovascular disease and evolution of depressive symptoms in the cardiovascular health study. Stroke 2002;33(6):1636–44.

118. Sheline YI, Price JL, Vaishnavi SN, et al. Regional white matter hyperintensity burden in automated segmentation distinguishes late-life depressed subjects from comparison subjects matched for vascular risk factors. Am J Psychiatry 2008;165(4):524–32.

119. Thomas AJ, Kalaria RN, O'Brien JT. Depression and vascular disease: what is the relationship? J Affect Dis 2004;79(1–3):81–95.

120. Quan N, Banks WA. Brain-immune communication pathways. Brain Behav Immun 2007;21(6):727–35.

121. Gruver AL, Hudson LL, Sempowski GD. Immunosenescence of ageing. J Pathol 2007;211(2):144–56.

122. Sparkman NL, Johnson RW. Neuroinflammation associated with aging sensitizes the brain to the effects of infection or stress. Neuroimmunomodulation 2008;15(4–6):323–30.

123. Maes M. Depression is an inflammatory disease, but cell-mediated immune activation is the key component of depression. Prog Neuropsychopharmacol Biol Psychiatry 2011;35(3):664–75.

124. Maes M, Bosmans E, Meltzer HY, et al. Interleukin-1 beta: a putative mediator of HPA axis hyperactivity in major depression? Am J Psychiatry 1993;150(8):1189–93.

125. Maes M, Scharpe S, Meltzer HY, et al. Relationships between interleukin-6 activity, acute phase proteins, and function of the hypothalamic-pituitary-adrenal axis in severe depression. Psychiatry Res 1993;49(1):11–27.

126. Milaneschi Y, Corsi AM, Penninx BW, et al. Interleukin-1 receptor antagonist and incident depressive symptoms over 6 years in older persons: the InCHIANTI study. Biol Psychiatry 2009;65(11):973–8.

127. Marsland AL, Gianaros PJ, Abramowitch SM, et al. Interleukin-6 covaries inversely with hippocampal grey matter volume in middle-aged adults. Biol Psychiatry 2008;64(6):484–90.

128. Dentino AN, Pieper CF, Rao MK, et al. Association of interleukin-6 and other biologic variables with depression in older people living in the community. J Am Geriatr Soc 1999;47(1):6–11.

129. Penninx BW, Kritchevsky SB, Yaffe K, et al. Inflammatory markers and depressed mood in older persons: results from the Health, Aging and Body Composition study. Biol Psychiatry 2003;54(5):566–72.

130. Tiemeier H, Hofman A, van Tuijl HR, et al. Inflammatory proteins and depression in the elderly. Epidemiology 2003;14(1):103–7.

131. Bremmer MA, Beekman AT, Deeg DJ, et al. Inflammatory markers in late-life depression: results from a population-based study. J Affect Disord 2008;106(3): 249–55.

132. Harman JS, Brown EL, Have TT, et al. Primary care physicians attitude toward diagnosis and treatment of late-life depression. CNS Spectr 2002;7(11):784–90.

133. Bushnell J, McLeod D, Dowell A, et al. Do patients want to disclose psychological problems to GPs? Family Pract 2005;22(6):631–7.

134. Committee on the Future Health Care Workforce for Older Americans, Institute of Medicine. Retooling for an aging America: building the health care workforce. Washington, DC: The National Academies Press; 2008.

135. Alexopoulos GS, Reynolds CF 3rd, Bruce ML, et al. Reducing suicidal ideation and depression in older primary care patients: 24-month outcomes of the PROSPECT study. Am J Psychiatry 2009;166(8):882–90.

136. Krahn DD, Bartels SJ, Coakley E, et al. PRISM-E: comparison of integrated care and enhanced specialty referral models in depression outcomes. Psychiatr Serv 2006; 57(7):946–53.

137. DeLauro HRL. Congressional Record, June 27, 2005. Available at: http://books.google.com/books?id=XVm35w7gi6QC&pg=PA761&lpg=PA761& dq=2640+geriatric+psychiatrist+5000_2030&source=bl&ots=pGAoLklTkp& sig=cKywsEh68dfrU3JvRy9R4y9xzUk&hl=en&ei=KEtlTpvsHIXZgAf25YjFBg&sa= X&oi=book_result&ct=result&resnum=3&ved=OCCsQ6AEwAg#v=onepage& q=2640&f=false. Accessed August 8, 2011.

138. Bartels SJ. Improving system of care for older adults with mental illness in the United States. Findings and recommendations for the President's New Freedom Commission on Mental Health. Am J Geriatr Psychiatry 2003;11(5):486–97.

139. Sussman T, Yaffe M, McCusker J, et al. Improving the management of late-life depression in primary care: barriers and facilitators. Depression Res Treat 2011; 2011:326307.

Depression in Medically Ill Patients

Sandra Rackley, MD[a,b], J. Michael Bostwick, MD[c,*]

KEYWORDS
- Depression • Adjustment disorder • Differential diagnosis
- Medical illness • Antidepressant medication
- Psychotherapy

"Depression" in medically ill patients is first and foremost a phenotype. Many underlying etiologies may take a final common pathway of producing such a phenotype, but have divergent implications for prognosis and management. Thus appropriate management requires first establishing the most likely diagnosis that has caused depression to be considered. This article reviews common etiologies for a "depressed" appearance in medically ill patients and proposes management strategies in each sphere of the bio-psycho-social-spiritual model.

UNIQUE CHALLENGES IN ASSESSING DEPRESSION IN MEDICALLY ILL PATIENTS

Working with medically ill patients routinely poses pragmatic challenges not typically encountered in general psychiatric practice. Hospitalized patients are rarely afforded rest and privacy. Many evaluations are conducted with no more privacy than a curtain between patients and their roommates. Interruptions are common from nursing staff, other consulting services, technicians performing bedside tests, and transporters trying to whisk patients off to remote procedures. Illness-related fatigue or medication side effects may challenge the patient's ability to tolerate a standard diagnostic interview, with the result that evaluations may need to be broken up into several brief sessions rather than a single extended one. Many medical illnesses and medications can impair cognition on physiologic grounds, and the psychological impact of facing a life-limiting illness can dim patients' memory of less emotionally salient information. Astute clinicians will be mindful of these factors during assessment and modify their approaches as indicated—by abbreviating an interview and returning later, gently

The authors have nothing to disclose.
[a] Departments of Psychiatry and Pediatrics, The George Washington University School of Medicine, 2300 I Street NW, Washington, DC 20037, USA
[b] Psychiatry Consultation-Liaison and Emergency Department Services, Children's National Medical Center, 111 Michigan Avenue NW, Washington, DC 20010, USA
[c] Department of Psychiatry and Psychology, Mayo Clinic College of Medicine, 200 1st Street SW, Rochester, MN 55905, USA
* Corresponding author.
E-mail address: bostwick.john@mayo.edu

Psychiatr Clin N Am 35 (2012) 231–247
doi:10.1016/j.psc.2011.11.001
0193-953X/12/$ – see front matter © 2012 Elsevier Inc. All rights reserved.

assisting a patient with recall, acknowledging the difficulty of discussing sensitive topics under less-than-ideal conditions, or simply offering to adjust the angle of a bed, add a blanket, or bring a glass of water. They may find their alliance improved through these simple nods to shared humanity in the midst of what can be the dehumanizing experience of hospitalization.

"DEPRESSION" AS A RESULT OF THE PSYCHOLOGICAL IMPACT OF ILLNESS

Emotional ups and downs are a normal part of human experience, and they can be particularly intense during the course of a medical illness. Transition points in illness—diagnosis, initiation or change of treatment, relapse/recurrence, change in prognosis, or a move into a chronic or terminal phase—may be times of particular vulnerability to distress, but like any other life experience, medical illness brings unpredictable emotional reactions as well.

When does emotional upset in the context of illness move from normal to pathologic? As in any other experience, a patient's emotional state exists on a continuum that progresses from distressing, to maladaptive, to pathologic. When applied to being "down" in the context of medical illness, this continuum might roughly correspond to a hierarchy of expected responses, starting with demoralization and hopelessness, ramping up to adjustment disorder, and culminating in one of the depressive disorders.

Much work has been done clarifying the difference between each of these intensities. Clinically, the distinction is made based on intensity, duration, and burden of symptoms. True depression is a syndrome that consists of mood change or anhedonia accompanied by several other emotional, somatic, and cognitive symptoms, persisting for several weeks.[1] Conceptually, this reflects suffering that has "taken on a life of its own" and no longer exists solely in reaction to a given stressor. In general clinical practice, nonaffective symptoms are often used to help make this distinction, but as noted previously, medical illness causes somatic and cognitive symptoms of its own that can make this distinction challenging. Several rating scales of depression in medically ill patients have been studied and may aid diagnosis.[2,3] However, the most powerful method of distinction may be the easiest: simply asking a medically ill patient "are you depressed?" had higher sensitivity and specificity for major depressive disorder than many more complex screening instruments.[4]

In medically ill patients, a distinction is made between depression and demoralization. In the former, anhedonia predominates; in the latter, helplessness.[5] Underpinning the helplessness of demoralization are disempowerment and futility: Nothing can change. Nothing will ever change.[6] In addition to the emotional distress wrought by demoralization, several studies have associated demoralization with lower quality of life and intensified desire for hastened death in terminally ill patients[7–9] who do not otherwise meet criteria for a diagnosis of major depression.

Adjustment disorders are also associated with significant impairment in functioning, so much so that they are often confused with depression and treated pharmacologically.[10] An important driver of these emotional states in medically ill patients can be poorly managed physical symptoms. Undertreated pain or nausea are among the most distressing symptoms that accompany illnesses such as cancer and acquired immunodeficiency syndrome (AIDS), and the patient's distress may prompt a consultation for depression. Simply clarifying with the patient whether there are any physical factors that, if removed, would brighten his or her mood often can bring these to the fore and suggest an easy intervention.

The distinction of "normal" from distressing or maladaptive emotional reactions is often as much a cultural and existential distinction as it is a clinical one, and this line is often in the eye of the beholder (the patient). Exploring with patients how they reacted to stressors in the past, what they would have expected themselves to feel in the midst of their experience, and how they have seen others in their social and cultural milieu react to illness may help physicians and patients to clarify together whether there are concerns, and if so, where they lie. Consulting with someone who shares the patient's culture—a staff member, for example, or an interpreter—can help to contextualize the patient's behavior and symptomatology against a standard that may be unfamiliar to the provider.

"DEPRESSION" AS A RESULT OF THE PHYSIOLOGIC IMPACT OF ILLNESS OR TREATMENT

Medical illness can induce symptoms suggestive of depression through physiologic as well as psychological pathways. At times, the intensity and range of symptomatology that last for an extended period of time can meet full criteria for a depressive episode with the *Diagnostic and Statistical Manual of Mental Disorders*, 4th edition, Text Revision (DSM-IV-TR) specifier that it is a depressive episode in the context of a medical illness. At other times, some symptoms may be present, such as irritability or disturbed sleep, but not enough to meet criteria for a full depressive syndrome. **Box 1** lists several medications commonly implicated in the onset of depressive symptoms. Almost every medical condition has been associated with depression in the literature, but sorting through which links are more physiologic than psychological represents fertile ground for further study. Depression arising in the context of medical illness and treatment has contributed much to several current hypotheses

---

Box 1
Medications commonly associated with depressive symptoms

Antiepileptics

Angiotensin-converting enzyme inhibitors

Antihypertensives (especially clonidine, methyldopa, thiazides)

Antimicrobials (amphotericin, ethionamide, metronidazole)

Antineoplastics (procarbazine, vincristine, vinblastine, asparaginase)

Benzodiazepines

Beta-blockers

Calcium channel blockers

Corticosteroids

Endocrine modifiers (especially estrogens, leuprolide)

Interferon

Isotretinoin

Metoclopramide

Nonsteroidal anti-inflammatory drugs (especially indomethacin)

Opiates

Sedative–hypnotic agents

Statins

of depression pathogenesis and our understanding of the interconnectedness of psyche and soma. For example, mood symptoms after certain localized strokes gave rise to anatomic suggestions correlating depression with lesions in the left frontal lobe and also helped broaden the understanding of mechanisms of neurologic injury in stroke.[11] The ubiquity of depressive symptomatology in patients receiving alpha interferon puts the focus on potential psychoneuroimmunologic mechanisms.[12]

Establishing a timeframe for the onset of depressive symptoms in relation to the appearance of the medical illness may help distinguish those secondary to medical illness from primary depressive episodes stemming from endogenous vulnerability or associated with psychological factors. In the former situation, depression emerges after the medical illness. In the latter situation, the depressive situation is already established, with the medical illness superimposed upon it. In many cases, the patient has not made these connections, and the clinician will have to review records or walk the patient through a timeline of illness exacerbations and treatment to see if the emergence of depressive symptoms correlates with the patient being given a new diagnosis or initiating medications such as corticosteroids. When important medical treatments are the etiology of depressive symptoms, such as with levetiracetam for epilepsy or alpha interferon for hepatitis, the medical team should discuss with the patient the risks and benefits of continuing the offending treatment protocol. Adjunctive antidepressant pharmacotherapy may help when medical treatments cannot be discontinued, but can also fail to dispatch symptoms while imposing drug–drug interactions of its own.

DEPRESSION AS A CAUSE OF MEDICAL ILLNESS

A growing literature points to depression as a risk factor either for induction of certain medical illnesses or for poorer prognosis once the illness is established.[13,14] This suggests that the links between psyche and soma are bidirectional. Some of these links are simply behavioral: depression robs a person of psychic energy that they then cannot expend on eating well, exercising regularly, and attending to appropriate preventive care. Depressed patients may also be more prone to using substances such as tobacco, illicit drugs, and alcohol as a way of ameliorating depressed mood while simultaneously increasing the risk for secondary medical issues.[15] Once patients are medically ill, it is well established that adherence to treatment recommendations is more challenging for depressed patients.[16–18]

Perhaps more intriguing are the suggestions that depression itself may modify the body. Hypothalamic–pituitary–adrenal (HPA) axis dysfunction in the context of depression may be a consequence of long-term maladaptation to psychological and physiologic stressors.[19] Lower survival in depressed patients with coronary artery disease may be a consequence of poor self-care behaviors,[20] but there is also suggestion of greater platelet activation via serotonin pathways and bidirectional links between depression and coronary health.[21] A study of interferon use in patients with hepatitis suggested that viral response to treatment directly correlated with level of depressive symptomatology: that is, the patients whose viral loads dropped the most were the ones who became most severely depressed, again underscoring the possibility that depression and inflammation regulation may be linked.[22] Several studies have suggested that depressed patients have shorter telomeres than age-matched controls,[23,24] suggesting a relationship between depression and more rapid cellular aging.

MASKED PRESENTATIONS OF DEPRESSION

Depression can also underlie medical complaints, and some estimates place depression as the most common illness presenting to primary care providers.[25] In "pseudodementia" cognitive complaints come to the fore, but careful inquiry can establish that prominent memory and decision-making difficulties are undergirded by the attentional problems, indecisiveness, and anhedonia that points to a major depressive disorder. This presentation can be particularly common in elderly patients, but depression should be carefully considered in the differential of cognitive concerns presenting in younger patients.

Pain out of proportion to physical findings or other difficulties in managing physical symptoms of illness is another common initial presentation of depression in medically ill patients. In these patients, depressive illness may rob them of the psychological energy that typically facilitates resilience and cognitive flexibility for managing physical symptoms, leading to intensified pain complaints. Downstream consequences of depression may affect pain: Sleep disturbance can affect the intensity with which pain is perceived. Diminished physical activity as a result of depression can contribute to a cycle of deconditioning and intensified pain, and decreased appetite and oral intake can lead to slowed gastrointestinal motility that may itself be experienced as increased abdominal pain. Depression may also intensify pain perception through physiologic changes in top-down nociceptive processing: a growing body of evidence suggests that changes in stress response, intracellular signalling, and emotional and cognitive regulation associated with depression may increase central and peripheral sensitivity to pain signaling.[26]

A patient may emphasize the physical complaints of major depressive disorder to the exclusion of cognitive or affective symptoms. Fatigue, sleep disruption, weight loss, and cognitive dulling are core symptoms of a major depressive disorder but mood changes may go unnoticed or be understood by both patients and their doctors as secondary to the physical symptoms. This may be particularly true for patients from cultures or communities that emphasize somatic rather than psychological expressions of distress.[27,28] An appropriate evaluation to rule out common physiologic etiologies of such symptoms is important, but particularly if the physiologic symptoms are accompanied by symptoms such as mood changes, anhedonia, and depressive cognitions, it may be reasonable to proceed with a closely monitored trial of depression treatment before embarking on a search for more esoteric etiologies of vague physical complaints.

WHEN "DEPRESSION" IS NOT DEPRESSION AT ALL

Other illnesses can lead to the appearance of "depression" without this being the appropriate diagnosis. Hypoactive delirium is a common mimic of depression in medically ill patients, as its presenting symptoms—behavioral withdrawal, sleep disturbance, affective flattening, and amotivation—overlap closely with a depressive "phenotype." Delirium can be distinguished from depression, however, by fluctuations in cognition throughout the day as well as acute onset. A bedside cognitive examination of such a patient may reveal abnormalities of thought process behind the patient's bland or inappropriately reactive affect. Medication, infection, metabolic derangements, and hypoxia are common culprits leading to delirium. When these symptoms arise it is prudent to review a patient's recent medication changes, any new physical symptoms or changes in vital signs, and changes in laboratory values. It is also crucial to remember the possibility of substance withdrawal leading to delirium, particularly in acutely medically ill patients who may have been hospitalized for an emergent issue and not disclosed their ongoing substance use at home.

Similarly, dementia can cause a patient to appear amotivated, withdrawn, and affectively blunted. Subtle cognitive impairments may initially be missed by a busy medical service focused on managing acute medical issues, until the patient's distress, disorientation, or difficulty with adherence prompts concerns about mood issues. Using a structured mental status examination to evaluate for cognitive impairment and obtaining collateral history from family, friends, and primary care providers about the patient's recent baseline can help establish the proper diagnosis, thus making it possible to tailor treatments that acknowledge the patient's cognitive limitations.

Substance intoxication (whether with alcohol, illicit substances, or prescribed medications) can produce a behavioral syndrome that appears consistent with a depressive episode, including suicidal ideation and dramatic emotional posturing, but it resolves quickly when the effect of the substance wears off. Although mood and substance use disorders are commonly comorbid, it is essentially impossible to accurately assess for ongoing mood issues until the patient is no longer intoxicated.

Pain itself can conjure the phenotype of depression when it is untreated or inadequately managed. Particularly when pain is acute, as after surgery or in the wake of major traumatic injury, it is a mistake to minimize analgesia out of concern for inducing or feeding addiction. Those already tolerant to narcotics will need even higher doses to rein in "pain-on-pain." When it vanquishes anguish in an individual who has reason to be hurting, morphine assumes the guise of an antidepressant and will of course prove more effective in this setting than an actual antidepressant.

MIXED PICTURES

What makes psychosomatic medicine so interesting and challenging is the recognition that psyche and soma are intimately intertwined and the Cartesian duality that drives a wedge between objective signs and subjective symptoms does not reflect our patients' reality. A biopsychosociospiritual formulation—and of course the tools relevant to each realm—is indispensable in creating a coherent explanation of a patient's experience and formulating integrated treatment goals.

SPECIAL CONSIDERATIONS WHEN TREATING DEPRESSION IN MEDICALLY ILL PATIENTS
Biological Interventions

In general, the guidelines for pharmacologic treatment of depression in medically ill patients mirror those for general populations, with extra sensitivity to side effects and drug–drug interactions. Medications should be chosen to take advantage of beneficial side effects while avoiding undesirable ones and minimizing polypharmacy. In a depressed medically ill patient with significant sleep issues, mirtazapine may be a first choice to address both issues. When depression accompanies neuropathic pain or migraine, a tricyclic antidepressant (TCA) or duloxetine may be a good initial step. Both selective serotonin reuptake inhibitors (SSRIs) and TCAs have been successfully used to treat functional abdominal pain in patients with and without comorbid depressive symptoms (**Box 2**).

A common consultation question regards alternate routes of antidepressant administration for patients unable to take pills because of swallowing difficulties (eg, secondary to mucositis or esophageal lesions), malabsorption issues, gastrointestinal obstruction, or NPO status for surgery or other concerns. Unfortunately, most Food and Drug Administration (FDA)-approved antidepressants in the United States are

---

Box 2
Suggested medications for depression comorbid with prominent physical symptoms

Pain

  TCAs

  Duloxetine

  SSRIs (for abdominal pain)

Insomnia

  TCAs

  Mirtazapine

Fatigue

  Bupropion

  Stimulants (methylphenidate, amphetamines)

---

available only in oral form. The monoamine oxidiase inhibitor (MAO-I) selegiline is available in a transdermal patch, but the rare but real risk of hypertensive crisis and drug–drug interactions, as well as the need for tyramine restriction at all but the lowest dose, makes this a particularly challenging medication to use in medically ill patients.[29] If mechanical swallowing difficulties are the primary issue, patients may be able to successfully take a liquid formulation of their antidepressant or an orally disintegrating tablet such as mirtazapine. The atypical antipsychotics olanzapine, aripiprazole, and risperidone also come in an orally disintegrating tablet, and data and FDA indication support their use in depression at least as adjunctive treatments.[30] Some atypical and typical antipsychotics are available for intramuscular injection, but the data for these is only available for management of acute agitation and not for adjunctive or primary depression treatment and the half-lives and need for intramuscular injection limit ongoing use. Emerging depression treatments such as ketamine may eventually be particularly useful in these situations, but for now remain experimental. Hospital pharmacists should be consulted for possible alternate routes of medication. In some cases they can compound enemas or liquid draughts that are not commercially available.

Somatic treatments other than antidepressants have value in depressed medically ill patients. Though studies proving antidepressant efficacy are inconsistent, stimulant medications such as methylphenidate or amphetamine-based products are frequently employed rapidly to improve motivation, energy, and appetite in medically ill patients who are debilitated more than depressed.[31] Stimulants can potentiate narcotic analgesics, and may be of particular use in the palliative care population.[32] Electroconvulsive therapy (ECT) has been safely and successfully used in patients with a variety of severe medical illnesses including those in terminal phases.[33–36] One advantage is that it acts quickly when the patient's condition does not permit waiting the weeks that may be required for antidepressants to take effect.[37] ECT can be considered for patients with treatment-resistant depression, unremitting suicidality, intolerance to oral medications, or neuromuscular emergencies such as neuroleptic malignant syndrome. Other neuromodulatory therapies may also be useful in similar situations, but have a less established evidence base. Transcranial magnetic stimulation (TMS) has shown promise in improving depressive symptoms in patients with various neurologic disorders including Parkinson's disease, epilepsy, and stroke[38] and has been used safely in pregnant patients.[39] In contrast, studies of vagal nerve stimulation (VNS) in patients with epilepsy have shown mixed benefit for mood symptoms[40,41] and one study of deep brain stimulation (DBS) in patients with Parkinson's disease actually indicated that mood worsened despite improvement in movement symtpoms.[42] Further study of these therapies in medically ill patients is needed.

Medically ill patients may be particularly vulnerable to adverse effects of antidepressant medications. Medical illness and its treatment can affect peak serum drug levels through fluid shifts and weight changes, and in certain situations a patient's volume of distribution can change dramatically from day to day. Hepatic and renal impairment can affect the metabolism and elimination of antidepressants. If a patient is on a mood stabilizer or an antidepressant with a narrow therapeutic index such as lithium or one of the TCAs, it is important to start with lower doses than usual, monitor closely for side effects suggestive of supratherapeutic blood levels, and continue frequently monitoring serum drug levels until fluctuations have subsided. One of the newer medications may be safer in settings of rapid fluid shifts, compromised metabolism, or impaired excretion.

For patients with cardiac disease or those on medications such as methadone that may lead to QTc prolongation, it is important to be sensitive to the potential for further QTc prolongation with many of the antidepressants. Information about prolongation of the QTc can be found in the prescribing information and many electronic drug references. Cumulative anticholinergic burden of medications is another consideration, particularly when a patient is particularly susceptible to delirium. The TCAs have more anticholinergic effect than most of the SSRIs, but paroxetine, in particular, also has significant anticholinergic properties. Sedative/hypnotic agents can also precipitate or perpetuate delirium in vulnerable patients.

Metabolic interactions mediated through the cytochrome P450 system are increasingly recognized as significant. Patients can have a genetic polymorphism leading to slowed metabolism by one or more of the P450 enzymes. Many medications including psychotropics can also affect various P450 enzymes, which are crucial in metabolism of several antiepileptic agents, antibiotics, and antiretrovirals, among others. In combination with an intermediate or slow metabolizer phenotype these interactions can dramatically change typical pharmacokinetics. Side effects can appear at relatively low doses when unmetabolized drug accumulates, or conversely, slow metabolizers may not respond as expected when prodrugs must be converted to active agent. One such agent is codeine, which fails in standard doses to provide effective analgesia to slow 2D6 metabolizers who cannot convert it to its active metabolite, morphine.[43] In one of the more stunning examples of P450 interactions, paroxetine and fluoxetine were commonly prescribed to women receiving tamoxifen as a way of treating depression and hot flashes, until it was discovered that such patients had poorer long-term survival than tamoxifen-treated women not receiving these medications. Tamoxifen is actually a prodrug, converted through 3A4 and 2D6 to endoxifen, the active anti-estrogen. As potent 2D6 inhibitors, paroxetine and fluoxetine slowed this conversion, inhibiting the therapeutic effect of the tamoxifen.[44,45] P450-based drug–drug interaction guidance is increasingly incorporated into electronic drug reference databases and electronic prescribing applications.

Serotonin syndrome is another concern in medically ill patients. The typical triad includes mental status changes (including agitation, confusion, disorientation, anxiety), autonomic instability (hypertension, hyperpyrexia, tachycardia, nausea, diarrhea), and neuromuscular hyperactivity (hyperreflexia, clonus, tremor, myoclonus). In medically ill patients, this constellation of symptoms may go unrecognized or misidentified as sepsis or anxiety, delaying appropriate intervention. Medically ill patients may be on several serotonergic medications. Slowed metabolism and drug–drug interactions may result in toxic accumulation of drugs and their metabolites, causing a serotonin syndrome. Of particular concern is linezolid, an antibiotic commonly used in critically ill patients with treatment-resistant bacterial infections, which is also a reversible MAO-I.[46] Linezolid's product labeling recommends that patients have a washout of their antidepressant before starting linezolid; in certain patients for whom future linezolid treatment is likely, it may be advisable to either use an SSRI with a shorter half-life (such as sertraline) that could be rapidly discontinued, or a nonserotonergic antidepressant such as bupropion, though the latter has also been associated with serotonin syndrome when given in conjunction with linezolid.[47] Antidepressants should be started with caution in patients already on the antibiotic.

Emerging data suggests intravenous ketamine, an N-methyl-D-aspartate (NMDA) modulator with dissociative effects, can be useful in rapidly ameliorating treatment-resistant depression in otherwise healthy patients.[48,49] It is being used experimentally in emergency rooms with impressive success in obliterating acute suicidality for up to a week.[50] Ketamine may also augment analgesia and improve mood in medically ill patients. A study of patients undergoing cholecystectomy found that ketamine administered during operative anesthesia induction both reduced postoperative opiate need and improved postoperative mood symptoms in patients depressed preoperatively.[51] Low-dose ketamine is increasingly used as an analgesic adjunct in patients with nociceptive and neuropathic pain issues, leading to improved pain control and lower overall opiate use, and has shown benefit in "resetting" opiate-induced hyperalgesia.[52] Recent case reports suggest a role for ketamine in alleviating depression in the palliative care population, improving mood within hours of first dose.[53]

There has also been renewed interest in the use of psilocybin, a compound found in several species of mushrooms that is rapidly metabolized to psilocin, a potent serotonin agonist with hallucinogenic activity. A recent small open-label study suggested psilocybin can alleviate dysphoria and anxiety in terminally ill cancer patients.[54]

Psychotherapeutic Interventions

Medical illness can lead to social isolation, challenge patients' autonomy and sense of self-efficacy, threaten physical and psychological integrity, and overwhelm typical mechanisms of coping. To address these aspects of the illness experience, supportive and problem-solving approaches are useful in psychotherapy with depressed medically ill patients. The ego strength required to maintain integrity in the face of medical illness may limit tolerance for regression induced by more exploratory and dynamic therapies. For many patients, it is sufficient to have the psychiatrist help them discover how to adapt their typical coping mechanisms to deal with the new and often unfamiliar situation in which they find themselves. The psychiatrist may be aware of resources such as support groups or hospital services available to the patient, and can also serve as a liaison between patient, team, and institution, as needed, to help facilitate identifying and properly addressing patient concerns.

Simple changes to the hospital environment and routines can be vitally important to patients with persistent illness. Minimizing unnecessary nocturnal interruptions for laboratory tests or vital sign measurements and maintaining a quiet environment at night can promote good sleep and go a long way toward enhancing patient coping. Helping patients use the phone or access the Internet to remain in contact with friends and family; making available a patient library with books and videos for distraction; educating patients and their support network about illnesses, procedures, and management strategies through written literature or in-hospital video on demand; or consulting chaplaincy services to provide support through conversation, prayers, and sacraments can shore up flagging coping strategies. Hospitals are increasingly incorporating complementary and alternative therapies such as massage, acupuncture, aromatherapy, and other mind–body modalities to encourage relaxation and improve pain management.

A growing pediatric literature suggests the importance of developmentally appropriate interventions to help children cope with illness and hospitalizations.[55] Many childrens' hospitals have shifted from the traditional "ward" to a "sleep-in" model encouraging parents to remain with their children "24-7" throughout their children's hospitalizations. Child Life Specialists prepare children for procedures by giving them tours of surgical suites and demonstrating what will happen to them on stuffed animals. They coach children on how to manage anxiety during procedures, and offer activities such as "ouch-free" playrooms and social functions free of any painful medical interventions.

Evidence-based psychotherapies have frequently been adapted for patients with medical illness. Interpersonal psychotherapy (IPT) can be readily used in depressed medically ill patients, with a focus on the role transitions and role disputes that invariably accompany chronic illness.[56] Cognitive–behavioral therapy (CBT) can help patients recognize thought distortions that accompany illness, and can also encourage behavioral activation that is so vitally important to recovery, particularly in medically ill individuals.[57–59]

Narrative and existential therapies can be particularly useful at the bedside as patients struggle to understand this new version of themselves and come to terms with physical losses in the midst of life-changing circumstances.[60,61] Serious illness may affect multiple domains, including how patients view themselves, how they relate to others, and how they envision their spirituality. Illness may alter how patients perceive the hospital environment in which they currently reside and how they imagine the world outside will respond to them and they to it when they reenter it, potentially disfigured, disabled, or both by their disease.[62,63] Griffith and Gaby describe what they call "existential postures" rooted in the vulnerability that serious disease inflicts on sufferers, causing usual goal-directed coping strategies to collapse.[5] These fundamentally passive states include confusion, isolation, despair, helplessness, meaningless, cowardice, and resentment. In a crisis the patient regresses into one of these stances—"a withdrawal from active engagement with living"—and it becomes the physician's task to identify which of these states are in play.

Griffith and Gaby encourage the provider to engage the patient in brief psychotherapy at the bedside, eliciting the illness-related themes to which they are vulnerable and the dimensions in which these vulnerabilities are playing out.[5] Drawing on a life narrative approach, physicians seek to normalize their patients' distress and help them perceive the significant challenges the illness represents to their beliefs about how their lives should have unfolded.[64] Having done this diagnostic work collaboratively, the physician and patient together problem-solve and tailor an active strategy for confronting the situation with the goal of restoring morale. Each of Griffith and Gaby's vulnerabilities is paired with a resilient posture. As brief therapy progresses, confusion morphs into coherence, isolation into communion, despair into hope, helplessness into self-agency, meaninglessness into purpose, cowardice into courage, and resentment into gratitude.[5] The practical result of confronting and overcoming sources of existential angst is improved coping skills. Through the process of collaborative problem-solving, the physician helps the patient achieve "relief, reward, quiescence, equilibrium."[62]

Social Interventions

The interpersonal environment of support groups reduces isolation and provides non-threatening environments in which patients can voice fears, ask questions, and receive suggestions from fellow sufferers for management of issues that arise during the course of illness. Some studies suggested that support-group participation might prolong survival in women with advanced cancer.[65] Although later studies were unable to replicate these findings,[66] many patients find that having this support adds "life to years" even when it does not add "years to life." Illness-specific foundations and organizations often have local chapters that offer support groups or other ways to connect, educational resources, financial support, advocacy resources, and the ability to channel energy into fundraisers that support research or social services. In medically ill patients, self-image can painfully be injured. The cosmetics industry sponsors the "Look Good, Feel Better" program, which provides online and in-person seminars on hair and skin care for both women and men facing cancer, and a partner program called "2bMe" for teens. Ronald McDonald houses for parents of ill children and other sponsored lodgings for patient families during transplant and cancer treatment provide social events and support group meetings as well as economical places to stay during extended treatment protocols. Social workers in subspecialty clinics can be an invaluable resource for matching patients with programs to help them through their treatments.

Adolescents, in particular, are at an intensely social developmental stage, and patient support networks can be vitally important for putting them in touch with others with the same disease when illness has created undesired distinctions from healthy peers. Illness-specific weekend gatherings, summer camps, and support groups can both reduce isolation and enhance treatment adherence during these challenging years. Foundations such as "Make-a-Wish" can provide an opportunity for a child and family to share an experience they might not otherwise be able to afford, and these trips can provide hope and motivation for the child who eagerly anticipates a diversion from the rigors of treatment.

Family members or a medical team may ask a psychiatrist to assess the medically ill patient for depression when the driving concern is actually depression, hopelessness, exhaustion, or frustration in someone in the patient's support network, projected on to the patient. Higher depression risk among family caregivers of medically ill patients is clearly established, and these caregivers often are so focused on the needs of their loved one that they minimize or deny their own stress. The consultant may need to give family members permission to care for themselves during a difficult time, perhaps by reminding them that if they are emotionally healthier, they will be better equipped to care for their loved one. Hospital staff such as social workers and chaplains may be particularly helpful in this regard, and some programs—especially cancer centers, dementia programs, and hospices—may specifically incorporate caregiver support programs. Particular attention may need to be given to children of a sick parent or siblings of a sick child, who often get lost in the shuffle as the healthy parents focus on caring for their partners or sick children. Gentle inquiry about how the other children in the family are faring may invite a parent to explore such concerns.

Caring for severely ill patients takes its toll on physicians and nurses. The palliative care and oncology literature is replete with studies of burnout and depression in these professionals, but all areas of medicine can require work with severely ill patients, and burnout is not restricted to cancer workers alone. The art of psychiatric liaison includes being aware of undercurrents of hopelessness and frustration among care team members. Simply acknowledging to frontline providers that the care of these patients is challenging may be all that is needed, but at times more comprehensive support with team leaders modeling good self-care may be indicated if a team is struggling through a particularly trying time.

A growing trend in treating depression in medically ill patients focuses on managing it in the "medical home," the setting in which the patient's primary illness is addressed. Particularly emphasized in the care of chronically ill children, the medical home model encourages health care professionals to collaborate in a single location with the goal of providing more integrated and timely care for complex conditions. Various approaches that integrate depression treatment in the medical home have been studied. The first, enhanced education of primary care physicians in screening for and appropriate treatment of depression, has shown only limited efficacy in improving depression outcomes.[67] Models of "co-location," in which a mental health professional, either a psychiatrist or a therapist, practices in the primary care office in hopes of facilitating rapid assessment and treatment while minimizing stigma, have shown some benefit.[25] Collaborative models, in which a psychiatrist either provides real-time case consultation to primary care physicians or supervises clinic-based care managers, have generated enthusiasm because of studies demonstrating both improved patient outcomes and cost-effective allocation of limited subspecialty resources.[68–70]

Spiritual Interventions

Spirituality, or the personal experience of connection with the transcendent, and religiosity, or the practices and rituals associated with corporate belief and membership, often assume a prominent role in patients' mental lives as they face severe illness.

For some, this connection with spirituality and religion supports coping and recovery.[71] Several studies demonstrate improved medical and mental health outcomes with spiritual and religious activities such as prayer or meditation, attendance at religious gatherings, or a sense of existential well-being.[72–74] Patients' spiritual practices can be supported and encouraged as a way of coping during their medical illness. Members of a patient's religious community can be invaluable in providing support—through physical presence and prayer, and often through concrete assistance such as transport or bringing meals to a home during extended recovery. Thus,

---

Box 3
The FICA assessment

F—Faith or belief: "Do you consider yourself spiritual or religious?" or "Do you have spiritual beliefs that help you cope with stress?" If the patient responds "No," the health care provider might ask, "What gives your life meaning?" Sometimes patients respond with answers such as family, career, or nature.

I—Importance: "What importance does your faith or belief have in your life? Have your beliefs influenced how you take care of yourself in this illness? What role do your beliefs play in regaining your health?"

C—Community: "Are you part of a spiritual or religious community? Is this of support to you and how? Is there a group of people you really love or who are important to you?" Communities such as churches, temples, and mosques, or a group of like-minded friends can serve as strong support systems for some patients.

A—Address in Care: "How would you like me, your healthcare provider, to address these issues in your healthcare?"

From The George Washington Institute for Spirituality and Health (GWish). FICA spiritual history tool. Available at: http://www.gwumc.edu/gwish/clinical/fica.cfm.

inquiry about the patient's spiritual life and religious community can be an important piece of psychosocial assessment. Puchalski and colleagues suggest the use of the FICA questions (**Box 3**) as a brief, belief-neutral means of assessing the potential import of faith in coping with illness.[75]

For other patients, religion or spirituality may be a source of distress when facing medical illness. Personal or institutional beliefs may suggest that a patient's lack of faith is preventing healing. Patients often find themselves angry with their deity about their illness, and depending on their belief system, may also be frightened or guilty about the implications of that anger. For some, facing serious illness raises distressing questions about the afterlife. Cognitive and physical limitations brought on by illness may make it challenging for a patient to engage in their typical spiritual and religious activities and lead to downstream distress. Finally, the presence of depression can distort one's relationship with the transcendent as it distorts many other relationships in a patient's life.[76] Inquiry about how a patient's spiritual beliefs or practices have changed in the context of illness can bring some of these issues to the fore.

Hospital chaplains can be invaluable partners in addressing spiritual and religious concerns with patients. Chaplains are often highly trained professionals: to be certified as a chaplain, most need to have graduate-level theological education and a minimum of a year of supervised residency in chaplaincy, an experience not unlike a psychiatry residency that includes individual and group supervision, self-reflection, and exposure to patients facing a variety of illnesses. Chaplains typically take an ecumenical approach to spiritual and religious concerns and can both support patients in using their spirituality to cope with illness and help address spiritual and religious concerns. When particular patients require a member of their own particular religious group, many chaplains' offices will have a list of local religious leaders who are available to hospital patients.

SUMMARY

In medically ill patients, given the many entities the phenotype of depression may represent, clinicians must be prepared to cast their diagnostic nets widely, not settling for the obvious but frequently incorrect choice of major depressive episode and throwing antidepressants at it willy nilly. Having chosen the correct diagnosis from among a broad differential of depression "look-alikes," clinicians can draw upon a broad swath of treatment modalities including medications, psychotherapy, social supports, and spiritual interventions. Working as a psychiatrist in the medical arena requires the curiosity and analytic skills of a detective and the breadth of knowledge of a polymath adapting therapeutic tools from across the biopsychosociospiritual spectrum to the specific needs of the patient.

REFERENCES

1. American Psychiatric Association. Diagnostic and statistical manual of mental disorders: DSM-IV-TR. 4th edition. Washington, DC: American Psychiatric Publishing; 2000.
2. Lloyd-Williams M, Dennis M, Taylor F. A prospective study to compare three depression screening tools in patients who are terminally ill. Gen Hosp Psychiatry 2004;26(5): 384–9.
3. Nease DE Jr, Maloin JM. Depression screening: a practical strategy. J Fam Pract. 2003;52(2):118–24.
4. Chochinov HM, Wilson KG, Enns M, et al. "Are you depressed?" Screening for depression in the terminally ill. Am J Psychiatry 1997;154(5):674–6.

5. Griffith JL, Gaby L. Brief psychotherapy at the bedside: countering demoralization from medical illness. Psychosomatics 2005;46(2):109–16.

6. Sansone RA, Sansone LA. Demoralization in patients with medical illness. Psychiatry (Edgmont) 2010;7(8):42–5.

7. Breitbart W, Rosenfeld B, Pessin H, et al. Depression, hopelessness, and desire for hastened death in terminally ill patients with cancer. JAMA 2000;284(22):2907–11.

8. Rosenfeld B, Breitbart W, Gibson C, et al. Desire for hastened death among patients with advanced AIDS. Psychosomatics 2006;47(6):504–12.

9. Rosenfeld B, Gibson C, Kramer M, et al. Hopelessness and terminal illness: the construct of hopelessness in patients with advanced AIDS. Palliat Support Care 2004;2(1):43–53.

10. Strain JJ, Smith GC, Hammer JS, et al. Adjustment disorder: a multisite study of its utilization and interventions in the consultation-liaison psychiatry setting. Gen Hosp Psychiatry 1998;20(3):139–49.

11. Fang J, Cheng Q. Etiological mechanisms of post-stroke depression: a review. Neurol Res 2009;31(9):904–9.

12. Maes M, Yirmyia R, Noraberg J, et al. The inflammatory & neurodegenerative (I&ND) hypothesis of depression: leads for future research and new drug developments in depression. Metab Brain Dis 2009;24(1):27–53.

13. Hoen PW, Whooley MA, Martens EJ, et al. Differential associations between specific depressive symptoms and cardiovascular prognosis in patients with stable coronary heart disease. J Am Coll Cardiol 2010;56(11):838–44.

14. Pan A, Okereke OI, Sun Q, et al. Depression and incident stroke in women. Stroke 2011. Available at: http://www.ncbi.nlm.nih.gov/pubmed/21836097. Accessed August 14, 2011.

15. Duivis HE, de Jonge P, Penninx BW, et al. Depressive symptoms, health behaviors, and subsequent inflammation in patients with coronary heart disease: prospective findings from the heart and soul study. Am J Psychiatry 2011;168(9):913–20.

16. Krousel-Wood M, Islam T, Muntner P, et al. Association of depression with antihypertensive medication adherence in older adults: cross-sectional and longitudinal findings from CoSMO. Ann Behav Med 2010;40(3):248–57.

17. Gonzalez JS, Batchelder AW, Psaros C, et al. Depression and HIV/AIDS treatment nonadherence: a review and meta-analysis. JAIDS 2011;58(2):181.

18. Hood KK, Rausch JR, Dolan LM. Depressive symptoms predict change in glycemic control in adolescents with type 1 diabetes: rates, magnitude, and moderators of change. Pediatr Diabetes 2011. Available at: http://www.ncbi.nlm.nih.gov/pubmed/21564454. Accessed September 20, 2011.

19. Bremne JD, Vermetten E. Stress and development: behavioral and biological consequences. Dev Psychopathol 2001;13(3):473–89.

20. Whooley MA, de Jonge P, Vittinghoff E, et al. Depressive symptoms, health behaviors, and risk of cardiovascular events in patients with coronary heart disease. JAMA 2008;300(20):2379–88.

21. Serrano CV Jr, Setani KT, Sakamoto E, et al. Association between depression and development of coronary artery disease: pathophysiologic and diagnostic implications. Vasc Health Risk Manag. 2011;7:159–64.

22. Loftis JM, Socherman RE, Howell CD, et al. Association of interferon-alpha-induced depression and improved treatment response in patients with hepatitis C. Neurosci Lett 2004;365(2):87–91.

23. Hartmann N, Boehner M, Groenen F, et al. Telomere length of patients with major depression is shortened but independent from therapy and severity of the disease. Depress Anxiety 2010;27(12):1111–6.

24. Simon NM, Smoller JW, McNamara KL, et al. Telomere shortening and mood disorders: preliminary support for a chronic stress model of accelerated aging. Biol Psychiatry 2006;60(5):432–5.

25. Katon W, Schulberg H. Epidemiology of depression in primary care. Gen Hosp Psychiatry 1992;14(4):237–47.

26. Maletic V, Raison CL. Neurobiology of depression, fibromyalgia and neuropathic pain. Front Biosci 2009;14:5291–338.

27. Kleinman A. Culture and depression. N Engl J Med 2004;351(10):951–3.

28. Kirmayer LJ. Cultural variations in the clinical presentation of depression and anxiety: implications for diagnosis and treatment. J Clin Psychiatry 2001;62(Suppl 13):22–8 [discussion: 29–30].

29. Nandagopal JJ, DelBello MP. Selegiline transdermal system: a novel treatment option for major depressive disorder. Expert Opin Pharmacother 2009;10(10):1665–73.

30. Komossa K, Depping AM, Gaudchau A, et al. Second-generation antipsychotics for major depressive disorder and dysthymia. Cochrane Database Syst Rev 2010;12: CD008121.

31. Hardy SE. Methylphenidate for the treatment of depressive symptoms, including fatigue and apathy, in medically ill older adults and terminally ill adults. Am J Geriatr Pharmacother 2009;7(1):34–59.

32. Dalal S, Melzack R. Potentiation of opioid analgesia by psychostimulant drugs: a review. J Pain Symptom Manage 1998;16(4):245–53.

33. Rasmussen KG, Rummans TA, Richardson JW. Electroconvulsive therapy in the medically ill. Psychiatr Clin North Am 2002;25(1):177–93.

34. Schak KM, Mueller PS, Barnes RD, et al. The safety of ECT in patients with chronic obstructive pulmonary disease. Psychosomatics 2008;49(3):208–11.

35. Rasmussen KG, Keegan BM. Electroconvulsive therapy in patients with multiple sclerosis. J ECT 2007;23(3):179–80.

36. Mueller PS, Albin SM, Barnes RD, et al. Safety of electroconvulsive therapy in patients with unrepaired abdominal aortic aneurysm: report of 8 patients. J ECT 2009;25(3):165–9.

37. Rasmussen KG, Richardson JW. Electroconvulsive therapy in palliative care. Am J Hosp Palliat Care 2011;28(5):375–7.

38. Fregni F, Pascual-Leone A. Transcranial magnetic stimulation for the treatment of depression in neurologic disorders. Curr Psychiatry Rep 2005;7(5):381–90.

39. Kim DR, Epperson N, Paré E, et al. An open label pilot study of transcranial magnetic stimulation for pregnant women with major depressive disorder. J Womens Health (Larchmt) 2011;20(2):255–61.

40. Levy ML, Levy KM, Hoff D, et al. Vagus nerve stimulation therapy in patients with autism spectrum disorder and intractable epilepsy: results from the vagus nerve stimulation therapy patient outcome registry. J Neurosurg Pediatr 2010;5(6):595–602.

41. Noe KH, Locke DEC, Sirven JI. Treatment of depression in patients with epilepsy. Curr Treat Options Neurol 2011;13(4):371–9.

42. Strutt AM, Simpson R, Jankovic J, et al. Changes in cognitive-emotional and physiological symptoms of depression following STN-DBS for the treatment of Parkinson's disease. Eur J Neurol 2011. Available at: http://www.ncbi.nlm.nih.gov/pubmed/21668586. Accessed October 16, 2011.

43. Leppert W. CYP2D6 in the metabolism of opioids for mild to moderate pain. Pharmacology 2011;87(5–6):274–85.

44. Stearns V. Active tamoxifen metabolite plasma concentrations after coadministration of tamoxifen and the selective serotonin reuptake inhibitor paroxetine. Cancer Spectrum Knowl Environ 2003;95:1758–64.

45. Sideras K, Ingle JN, Ames MM, et al. Coprescription of tamoxifen and medications that inhibit CYP2D6. J Clin Oncol 2010;28(16):2768–76.

46. Sola CL, Bostwick JM, Hart DA, et al. Anticipating potential linezolid-SSRI interactions in the general hospital setting: an MAOI in disguise. Mayo Clin Proc 2006;81(3): 330–4.

47. Marcucci C, Sandson NB, Dunlap JA. Linezolid-bupropion interaction as possible etiology of severe intermittent intraoperative hypertension? Anesthesiology 2004; 101(6):1487–8.

48. DiazGranados N, Ibrahim LA, Brutsche NE, et al. Rapid resolution of suicidal ideation after a single infusion of an N-methyl-D-aspartate antagonist in patients with treatment-resistant major depressive disorder. J Clin Psychiatry 2010;71(12):1605–11.

49. Ibrahim L, Diazgranados N, Luckenbaugh DA, et al. Rapid decrease in depressive symptoms with an N-methyl-D-aspartate antagonist in ECT-resistant major depression. Prog Neuropsychopharmacol Biol Psychiatry 2011;35(4):1155–9.

50. Larkin GL, Beautrais AL. A preliminary naturalistic study of low-dose ketamine for depression and suicide ideation in the emergency department. Int J Neuropsychopharmacol 2011;14(8):1127–31.

51. Kudoh A, Takahira Y, Katagai H, et al. Small-dose ketamine improves the postoperative state of depressed patients. Anesth Analg 2002;95(1):114–8.

52. Cohen SP, Liao W, Gupta A, et al. Ketamine in pain management. Adv Psychosom Med 2011;30:139–61.

53. Stefanczyk-Sapieha L, Oneschuk D, Demas M. Intravenous ketamine "burst" for refractory depression in a patient with advanced cancer. J Palliat Med 2008;11(9): 1268–71.

54. Grob CS, Danforth AL, Chopra GS, et al. Pilot study of psilocybin treatment for anxiety in patients with advanced-stage cancer. Arch Gen Psychiatry 2011;68(1):71–8.

55. Pao M, Ballard ED, Rosenstein DL. Growing up in the hospital. JAMA 2007;297(24): 2752–5.

56. Poleshuck EL, Talbot NE, Zlotnick C, et al. Interpersonal psychotherapy for women with comorbid depression and chronic pain. J Nerv Ment Dis 2010;198(8):597–600.

57. Dobkin RD, Menza M, Bienfait KL. CBT for the treatment of depression in Parkinson's disease: a promising nonpharmacological approach. Expert Rev Neurother 2008; 8(1):27–35.

58. Hopko DR, Bell JL, Armento M, et al. Cognitive-behavior therapy for depressed cancer patients in a medical care setting. Behav Ther 2008;39(2):126–36.

59. O'Hea E, Houseman J, Bedek K, et al. The use of cognitive behavioral therapy in the treatment of depression for individuals with CHF. Heart Fail Rev 2009;14(1):13–20.

60. Chochinov HM, Kristjanson LJ, Breitbart W, et al. Effect of dignity therapy on distress and end-of-life experience in terminally ill patients: a randomised controlled trial. Lancet Oncol 2011;12(8):753–62.

61. Breitbart W, Gibson C, Poppito SR, et al. Psychotherapeutic interventions at the end of life: a focus on meaning and spirituality. Can J Psychiatry 2004;49(6):366–72.

62. Schlozman SC. An approach to the psychosocial treatment of the medically ill patient. Med Clin North Am 2010;94(6):1161-7, x.

63. Kissane DW, Clarke DM, Street AF. Demoralization syndrome—a relevant psychiatric diagnosis for palliative care. J Palliat Care 2001;17(1):12–21.

64. Viederman M. The psychodynamic life narrative: a psychotherapeutic intervention useful in crisis situations. Psychiatry 1983;46(3):236–46.

65. Spiegel D, Bloom JR, Kraemer HC, et al. Effect of psychosocial treatment on survival of patients with metastatic breast cancer. Lancet 1989;2(8668):888–91.

66. Edwards AG, Hulbert-Williams N, Neal RD. Psychological interventions for women with metastatic breast cancer. Cochrane Database Syst Rev 2008;3:CD004253.
67. Asarnow JR, Jaycox LH, Anderson M. Depression among youth in primary care models for delivering mental health services. Child Adolesc Psychiatr Clin North Am 2002;11(3):477–97, viii.
68. Pyne JM, Fortney JC, Curran GM, et al. Effectiveness of collaborative care for depression in human immunodeficiency virus clinics. Arch Intern Med 2011;171(1): 23–31.
69. Katon W, Unützer J, Wells K, et al. Collaborative depression care: history, evolution and ways to enhance dissemination and sustainability. Gen Hosp Psychiatry 2010; 32(5):456–64.
70. Gilbody S, Bower P, Fletcher J, et al. Collaborative care for depression: a cumulative meta-analysis and review of longer-term outcomes. Arch Intern Med 2006;166(21): 2314–21.
71. Mueller PS, Plevak DJ, Rummans TA. Religious involvement, spirituality, and medicine: implications for clinical practice. Mayo Clin Proc 2001;76(12):1225–35.
72. Koenig HG, George LK, Titus P. Religion, spirituality, and health in medically ill hospitalized older patients. J Am Geriatr Soc 2004;52(4):554–62.
73. Nelson CJ, Rosenfeld BJ, Breitbart W, et al. Spirituality, religion, and depression in the terminally ill. Psychosomatics 2002;43(3):213.
74. Ai AL, Ladd KL, Peterson C, et al. Long-term adjustment after surviving open heart surgery: the effect of using prayer for coping replicated in a prospective design. Gerontologist 2010;50(6):798–809.
75. The George Washington Institute for Spirituality and Health (GWish). FICA Spiritual History Tool. Available at: http://www.gwumc.edu/gwish/clinical/fica.cfm. Accessed September 21, 2011.
76. Griffith JL. Religion that heals, religion that harms: a guide for clinical practice. 1st edition. New York: Guilford Press; 2010.

Management of Treatment-Resistant Depression

Gabor I. Keitner, MD[a,b,c,*], Abigail K. Mansfield, PhD[a,b]

KEYWORDS

- Depression • Treatment • Treatment resistance
- Disease management

The effectiveness of treatments for depression is suboptimal for a significant portion of individuals diagnosed with depressive illnesses.[1] At least 20% do not respond satisfactorily and approximately 50% will experience a chronic or recurrent course of illness.[2,3] Patients who have not responded adequately to evidence-based treatments after receiving adequate doses for an appropriate duration are said to have treatment-resistant depression (TRD). Many definitions of treatment resistance have been proposed. Eleven terms and six criteria have been used to describe resistance/refractoriness to treatment.[4]

Further refinement of the understanding of TRD has occurred through staging the degree of resistance to treatment based on increasing failure to respond to increasing numbers of treatment trials.[5–8] An assumption underlying staging models is that further treatment trials should lead to greater numbers of patients responding. In reality, in medicine, the failure to respond to an effective treatment usually indicates a lower probability of responding to other treatments.[2] Another significant shortcoming of various definitions of TRD and staging methods is that they all focus exclusively on symptom reduction as the outcome measure. They do not include consideration of change in functioning, quality of life, or social relationships. They also focus on response to medication trials and ignore the potential benefit that could be derived from psychosocial treatments.

In general, depression is considered resistant when at least two appropriate antidepressant trials from two different pharmacologic classes fail to produce significant improvement.[9] It is important to ensure that the medications have been taken at an optimal dose for a sufficient period of time before assuming that the patient has TRD.

The authors have nothing to disclose.
[a] Department of Psychiatry and Human Behavior, The Warren Alpert Medical School of Brown University, 222 Richmond Street, Providence, RI 02912, USA
[b] Department of Psychiatry, Rhode Island Hospital, 593 Eddy Street, Providence, RI 02903, USA
[c] Department of Psychiatry, The Miriam Hospital, 164 Summit Avenue, Providence, RI 02906, USA
* Corresponding author. Department of Psychiatry, Rhode Island Hospital, 593 Eddy Street, Providence, RI 02903.
E-mail address: Gkeitner@lifespan.org

Psychiatr Clin N Am 35 (2012) 249–265
doi:10.1016/j.psc.2011.11.004
0193-953X/12/$ – see front matter © 2012 Elsevier Inc. All rights reserved.

BURDEN/IMPACT OF TRD

Major depression generates one of the greatest burdens of all diseases worldwide.[10] It is the second most costly disorder in the United States, with cost figures estimated at $80 to $130 billion annually. Up to 40% of these costs can be attributed to TRD.[11]

A number of contributors to the morbidity burden for TRD have been identified, including early age at onset, adverse events, frequent recurrences, possible suppression of brain neurogenesis, neuronal atrophy, and hippocampal dysfunction.[12] Patients with TRD are twice as likely to be hospitalized, have more outpatient visits, use more psychotropic medications, and have 19 times the depression-related costs ($28,000 vs $1455) compared to patients with depressions that respond to treatment.[3]

COURSE

By definition, patients with TRD are expected to have a more difficult course of illness. Patients with TRD who continued to receive a variety of treatments in routine clinical practice, including switching and augmenting pharmacologic trials as well as electroconvulsive therapy (ECT), continued to have significant symptoms and functional disability over a 24-month period. The response rate during this time was 18.4% and the remission rate was 7.8%. Despite the use of a wide range of treatments, patients with TRD had a very low rate of sustained treatment response.[13]

A systematic review of nine outcome studies that involved 1279 subjects and a follow-up duration between 1 and 10 years reported similar conclusions. Remission rates at 1 year were less than 20% while up to 80% relapsed within 1 year of treatment. TRD was associated with poor quality of life and increased mortality.[14]

The STAR*D study of 3671 patients treated at 41 different clinical sites also found the likelihood of remission decreased substantially after failing two aggressive medication trials. Rates of relapse increased with each new treatment trial, as did intolerance of side effects, leading to treatment attrition.[15]

An interesting report of long-term inpatient treatment of patients with TRD in England provides a more optimistic perspective.[16] Of 225 patients admitted to a special inpatient program for refractory affective disorders, 69% showed a 75% reduction of depressive symptoms. Patients were treated with milieu therapy, high-dose medications, psychotherapy, family work, and gradual discharge. Patients stayed in the hospital for up to 72 weeks, with maximum improvement not occurring until, on average, 40 weeks of treatment. This was an observational study without a control group and results were reported only for symptoms at time of discharge from the unit without any follow-up data. Nonetheless, this suggests that some patients with TRD may benefit from more long-term, intensive treatment in inpatient or residential settings.

A worrisome trend relating to the long-term use of antidepressant drugs has been identified.[17,18] The long-term use of antidepressants may contribute not only to tolerance of the therapeutic effect of the drugs but also to increasing resistance to its actions, leading to worse long-term outcomes. Tolerance refers to a pharmacodynamic process that changes sensitivity to a drug, leading to progressive loss of effect. Resistance is used to describe refractoriness to the action of a previously effective drug that has been discontinued and is less effective when readministered. A meta-analysis suggests that patients who use antidepressants are more likely to relapse (42%) when discontinuing the antidepressant than the patients who did not receive an antidepressant.[19] An oppositional model of tolerance to the effects of antidepressants has been proposed as an explanation.[20] Psychotropic drugs alter neurotransmitter functions in the brain. The brain in response attempts a series of compensatory adaptations to reestablish homeostasis. Over time, however, the medications override and exhaust these compensatory mechanisms, leading to long-lasting changes in neurotransmitter and receptor functions.[21] The net effect may be to increase the likelihood of developing TRD. These findings suggest that patients with typical depression may develop TRD as a result of using psychotropic medications.

RISK FACTORS

A variety of attempts have been undertaken to identify potential risk factors and predictors of chronicity of depression and resistance to treatment. Eleven clinical variables that differentiated 356 patients with TRD from 346 depressed patients with good response to treatment have been identified.[22] They include anxiety comorbidity, panic disorder, social phobia, personality disorder, suicidality, melancholia, number of hospitalizations, recurrent episodes, early age at onset, and nonresponse to the first antidepressant ever tried. The most powerful associated factor in this population was a comorbid anxiety disorder.

The presence of a comorbid personality disorder has also been found to be associated with poor response to treatment in a sample of more than 8000 outpatients treated for major depression.[23]

Chronic forms of depression (dysthymia, chronic major depression, recurrent major depression with incomplete remission, double depression) may be forms of TRD. Chronic depressions are also associated with increased health care utilization, hospitalizations, and disease burden. A systematic review of 25 studies with 5192 patients with chronic forms of depression was undertaken to identify risk factors for chronicity.[24] The following risk factors were found to be definitively linked to chronicity: anxiety and personality disorders, comorbid substance abuse, low social integration, low social support, and negative social interactions. Inconsistent results were found for: low socioeconomic status, older age, low educational status, marital status, life events, female gender, and number of depressive episodes.

Patients who continue to have residual symptoms of depression at the end of acute treatment are at higher risk of recurrence, relapse and TRD.[25,26] This observation has led to a call for "pushing" treatment to achieve full remission and not being satisfied with partial response.[27–29] Incomplete response to antidepressant treatment with persistence of residual symptoms, however, may be one marker of TRD.[30] If that is the case, overly aggressive pharmacologic treatments will unlikely be of further benefit and may cause more side effects, treatment attrition, and demoralization due to repeated failure to respond to treatment.

As noted previously, treatment with antidepressant medications may itself be another risk factor for TRD.[18,31] Continued drug treatment may induce processes that oppose the initial acute effects of a drug, lead to receptor alteration, and contribute to a treatment-resistant long-term course.

ASSESSMENT OF TRD

A comprehensive biopsychosocial assessment should always be undertaken when evaluating a new patient for treatment. This perspective is even more important in the assessment of patients with TRD given the broad range of factors associated with its presentation and its poor response to pharmacotherapy.

Biological assessment should include a thorough medical and laboratory evaluation. Comorbid medical conditions such as hypothyroidism, cancer, diabetes, chronic pain, hypertension, sleep apnea, arthritis, and many others should be ruled out or, if present, their appropriate management should be coordinated with the patient's primary care physician. Comorbid anxiety disorders and substance abuse disorders should also be assessed and treated if present.

Psychological assessment should evaluate the patient's temperament and personality style, including frustration tolerance and coping skills. It is important to determine the meaning of the patient's illness and symptoms and overall satisfaction with his or her life. What are the patient's goals in life and what is preventing him or her from achieving them? Is the patient religious? Issues of spirituality should be reviewed. The assessment should involve a determination of the presence or absence of a personality disorder. Borderline personality disorders in patients with a history of physical or sexual abuse along with problems of attachment in early years need to be addressed.

A psychological assessment is important because temperament,[32] personality style,[33-35] and the meaning the patient attributes to his or her illness[36-39] all impact how the patient adjusts to his or her illness. For example, if a patient has always had difficulty tolerating distress, distress tolerance skills will need to be addressed in treatment, given the persistent nature of TRD and the chronicity of its symptoms. If a patient views depression as a life-destroying force, attention will need to be given to identifying and directing energy toward valued goals even as depressive symptoms persist. If a patient is religious, his or her spirituality may serve as a pillar of strength during difficult times.[40] By contrast, if a patient is not religious, identifying other sources of meaning can be helpful. If a patient has borderline personality disorder, particularly with a history of physical, emotional, or sexual abuse, creating a strong therapeutic alliance with well delineated boundaries is especially important, given that issues of emptiness, abandonment, and interpersonal turmoil are likely to surface over the course of treatment.

Social assessment should include evaluation of the patient's social support network. Does the patient have friends, involved family members? A patient's significant others are likely to have a significant impact (both positive and negative) on his or her depression.[40,41] Supportive relationships can buffer the impact of the depression whereas critical, conflicted, and turbulent relationships can impede improvement. Information should be solicited about patients' work situations and presence or absence of structure in their lives. If the patient has a family, a meeting should be held with all interested family members to evaluate and assess their functioning, their understanding of the depression, and ways in which they may be helping or hindering the patient's response to treatment.[42]

PHARMACOLOGIC TREATMENT OPTIONS

A number of reviews have outlined pharmacologic treatment options for patients with TRD[11,43,44] and have come to similar conclusions. There are two main pharmacologic treatment options: switching and augmenting. Switching can occur within or between classes of compounds. Augmenting can be tried with a wide range of psychoactive agents. The advantages of switching include avoidance of polypharmacy and side effects as well as lower cost. A disadvantage is that partial response of a first agent may be lost if the agent is discontinued. The advantage of augmenting is that a partial response can be built on, but with more side effects and greater cost.

There is hope that biomarkers will be found to guide treatment selection. At this time, however, there is not enough evidence to justify routine genotyping for patients with TRD.[45] Pharmacogenetic testing for genetic variants of metabolizing enzymes may be considered for patients who do not respond to pharmacotherapy. However, there is at present no reliable basis for recommending such testing for any given patient.

Switching Options

Overall there is no firm evidence of better outcome when switching within class, for example, one selective serotonin reuptake inhibitor (SSRI) to another, over switching to another class of compounds, for example, to a non-SSRI, for SSRI nonresponders. Souery and colleagues[46] found that switching to a different class of antidepressants was not associated with a better response or remission rate. There is also very little evidence to guide how such switching should be done. Given lack of solid evidence to guide clinical practice, common sense suggests that if a switching strategy is chosen, an agent from a different chemical class may make more sense than giving a different agent from the same class as, if one class did not work, other drugs in the same class probably will not work either because the mechanisms of action are the same.

Augmenting Options

Augmenting options have been more extensively studied but conclusions are still limited by small sample sizes and lack of placebo controls.[44] A review of 10 studies of augmentation of antidepressants with lithium in 269 patients found that lithium was significantly more effective than placebo.[47] Patients with TRD were augmented with lithium or triiodothyronine (T3) in the STAR*D study. Both groups showed only modest remission rates (lithium, 15.9% and T3, 24.7%) that were not significantly different from each other.[48] It is worth noting that patients with recurrent major depression treated with lithium had an 88.5% lower risk for suicide or suicide attempts over time than those not treated with lithium.[49]

Augmentation with atypical antipsychotics has also been shown to be effective in improving at least short-term outcome. A meta-analysis of 16 placebo-controlled trials of 3480 patients concluded that atypical antipsychotics were significantly more effective than placebo in leading to remission.[50] The number needed to treat to achieve one remission was nine patients. The overall pooled response rate for treatment with an atypical antipsychotic was 44.2% compared with 29.9% for placebo. The use of atypical antipsychotics was associated with a significantly higher rate of attrition due to side effects including weight gain and metabolic syndrome, as well as extrapyramidal symptoms. There were no significant differences in efficacy among the atypical agents, including olanzapine, risperidone, quetiapine, and aripiprazole. At this time there are no data to guide the clinical use of these agents. We do not know what the optimal doses are for each compound for TRD, how long to give them before expecting positive results, or how long to continue them regardless of whether patients respond to them.

The use of T3 as an augmenting agent with tricyclic antidepressants has some research support, although a recent review questions its efficacy in augmenting SSRIs.[51] As previously noted, the use of T3 in the STAR*D study led to a 24.7% remission rate. T3 is well tolerated at low doses.

The use of other antidepressants such as buproprion, mirtazapine, and tricyclic or heterocyclic antidepressants as augmenting agents has also been suggested. There is very little quality evidence to support their use. Most reports are based on small sample sizes or open-label studies. There is also a possibility that concurrent use of multiple psychotropic agents may increase monoaminergic perturbations, leading to oppositional tolerance and a greater risk of relapse if they are discontinued.[19]

A whole host of other augmenting agents have also been suggested. These include buspirone, amantadine, pramipexole, ripinirol, pindolol, inositol, melatonin, omega-3 fatty acids, S-adenosyl-L-methionine, folic acid, lamotrigine, modafinil, riluzole, and topiramate.[43] There is no good research support for the routine use of any of these agents as effective treatments for TRD.

Although it is understandable that considerable effort has gone into the search for some effective agent to help in the treatment of TRD, the fact that so many agents have been tried with so little benefit suggests that there are very few effective pharmacologic options that bring about remission or even response. This reality also suggests that there needs to be a shift from over-reliance on pharmacotherapy in the treatment of TRD.

NONPHARMACOLOGIC TREATMENTS FOR TRD

ECT has been in use since the 1930s. It is relatively effective in TRD and may have a rapid onset of action.[52,53] There does not appear to be a difference in effectiveness based on unilateral or bilateral electrode placement.[54] Relapse rates after ECT are, unfortunately, high.[53] Common side effects include memory loss and headaches.

Vagus nerve stimulation (VNS) has been approved by the U.S. Food and Drug Administration (FDA) as an adjunctive treatment for use in TRD since 2005. VNS requires the implantation of a pacemaker in the chest with electrodes connected to the vagus nerve. Stimulation parameters can be programmed remotely. There is much controversy about its effectiveness even as it continues to be advocated for use in TRD.[43,55–58] The Centers for Medicare and Medicaid Services and Blue-Cross Blue Shield refuse to cover payment for VNS because of lack of scientific evidence of its effectiveness.[59] Further, greater past resistance to pharmacotherapy is associated with a poorer response to VNS.[60,61] The most common side effects to VNS are hoarseness, coughing, dyspnea, and neck pain. Implantation can occur in an outpatient surgical facility, although episodes of arrhythmia, hypertension, bradycardia, and asystole have been reported.[59]

Repetitive transcranial magnetic stimulation (rTMS) involves repeated subconvulsive magnetic stimulation to the brain. It does not have FDA approval for treatment of TRD. Some studies have reported effectiveness[62–64] while others have not.[65–67] Predictors of poor response to rTMS include refractoriness to pharmacotherapy, longer duration of depression, and melancholic features,[68,69] all of which are hallmarks of TRD. A 4- to 6-week course of treatment may be needed to produce a good clinical outcome.[69] The procedure appears to be safe, with relatively mild side effects such as tinnitus, headaches, and facial twitches.[70] Apart from questionable effectiveness, its major drawback is cost.

Psychosurgery and deep brain stimulation (DBS) have been used as measures of last resort for patients at high risk from their untreatable depression. These treatments are considered to be experimental owing to the small numbers of patients studied. They are also considered palliative and risky because of the invasiveness of the procedures.[71,72]

PSYCHOTHERAPY FOR TRD

There is little research examining psychotherapy for TRD. A recent thorough review of randomized trials found only six unique studies of psychotherapy for TRD.[73] One of the studies, the STAR*D study, examined psychotherapy in two treatment arms, augmentation and substitution. Of the six randomized trials of psychotherapy for TRD, all but one found that psychotherapy offered some benefit for TRD. Studies examined whether psychotherapy was efficacious when augmenting pharmacotherapy, and whether it was efficacious when substituted for pharmacotherapy.

Two moderate sized trials showed augmentation of psychopharmacologic treatment with 16 sessions of cognitive psychotherapy to decrease symptoms as much as augmentation with another pharmacologic agent.[74,75] A moderate-sized substitution trial showed psychotherapy to be as effective as pharmacotherapy in reducing symptoms.[74] One small study found that augmenting pharmacologic treatment with dialectical behavior therapy was beneficial,[76] while another small study found that augmenting pharmacologic treatment with cognitive therapy was less effective than augmentation with lithium carbonate.[77] Two studies with very small sample sizes found similar benefit when antidepressant medication was augmented or substituted with cognitive therapy.[78,79] In summary, cognitive therapy and dialectical behavior therapy appear to lead to some decrease in depressive symptoms for patients with TRD, either as stand-alone treatment or in combination with pharmacotherapy.

Although symptom reduction is an important consideration in evaluating treatments, so is treatment retention. In five out of seven studies, psychotherapy had a better retention rate than augmentation or continued pharmacotherapy. This, combined with the finding that psychotherapy appears to be about as effective as pharmacotherapy in reducing depressive symptoms, makes psychotherapy a reasonable treatment option for TRD. A significant challenge for psychotherapists working with patients with TRD may be in finding ways to protect therapists from burnout resulting from the unremitting nature of TRD.

FAMILY THERAPY FOR TRD

Families of depressed patients are significantly impacted by the depression. The ways in which families respond to the depression, in turn, have an influence on the duration of the depressive episode and its likelihood of responding to treatment.[80–82] There have been very few studies investigating the efficacy of family treatments for depression.[83–86] Suggestions for ways of including the family in the treatment of chronic forms of depression have been advanced[87] but there have not been any studies of family treatments for patients with TRD. One study recruited 121 patients who had significant suicide risk, whose depression was severe enough to require hospitalization, and who had psychiatric and medical comorbid conditions to participate in a randomized 24-week treatment subsequent to their discharge from hospital. Patients were assigned to four treatment conditions including pharmacotherapy alone; combined pharmacotherapy and cognitive therapy; combined pharmacotherapy and family therapy; and combined pharmacotherapy, cognitive therapy, and family therapy. Remission (16%) and improvement (29%) rates were low overall, reflecting the severity of depression in these patients. Patients who received additional family therapy had significantly better outcomes than those who did not. Patients receiving family therapy had a significantly faster decrease in depressive symptoms and suicidal ideation, significantly higher rates of improvement, a nonsignificant tendency toward lower self-reported depression, and a greater proportion of patients whose illness remitted. The overall pattern suggested that adding family therapy to pharmacotherapy substantially improved the outcome of severely depressed patients. It was particularly noteworthy that these results were obtained with relatively few (mean = 5) family therapy sessions.[88]

Family approaches have been applied to a wide variety of chronic medical conditions. Given that depression, particularly TRD, is a chronic disorder, the literature evaluating the benefit of family interventions for chronic diseases is of relevance to the management of TRD. Hartmann and colleagues[89] conducted a meta-analysis of randomized clinical trials evaluating the effects of family-based interventions, for adult patients with chronic disease compared to standard treatment.

Family interventions were categorized as either generally psychoeducational or aimed at addressing relationships and improving family functioning directly. Family was defined as any significant person(s) with a close relationship to the patient. This meta-analysis focused on three outcomes: (1) physical health of the patient including level of dependency, clinical symptoms, self-rated physical health status, and disease management; (2) the mental health of the patient including degree of depression, degree of anxiety, quality of life, general mental health, and self-efficacy; and (3) the health of family members including caregiver burden, depression, anxiety, general mental health, and self-efficacy in the family member. Subanalyses were conducted to identify possible moderators such as types of disease, types of interventions, and types of family members involved in the treatment.

Fifty-two randomized clinical trials involving more than 8000 patients of whom 52% were women were chosen from more than 4000 potentially eligible studies. The diseases studied included cardiovascular diseases, stroke, cancer, arthritis, diabetes, AIDS, and systemic lupus erythematosus. All family interventions led to significantly better physical health of patients compared to standard treatment. Both psychoeducational and relationship-focused interventions showed a significant positive effect. The overall effect was greater when the family member involved in the treatment was a spouse rather than any other type of relationship.

Family interventions also led to improved mental health of the patient compared to standard treatment. In this case it did not matter whether the involved family member was a spouse or another type of family member. Again, both psychoeducational and relationship-focused interventions showed similarly significant positive effects. Family members' health such as caregiver burden, depression, anxiety, quality of life, and self-efficacy were all improved by family interventions. Relationship-focused interventions were more effective than those focused on psychoeducation in ameliorating family members' health.

The results of this meta-analysis showed that family-oriented interventions in chronic illnesses were more effective for improving health outcomes and reducing mental health problems in both patient and caregivers than commonly used treatments.[89] Although the effect sizes were small, they were statistically significant. The effects corresponded to an odds ratio of 1.7 to 1.84, meaning that patients receiving the family intervention had a 72% to 84% greater chance of improved health compared to those receiving usual care. Family interventions produced a more sustained improvement than standard care alone. There was also a tendency toward greater benefits from a longer course of family treatment, and from involving spouses in treatment as opposed to other family members. These reviews demonstrate that many different types of family interventions are effective in helping to deal with a wide range of medical illnesses. They do not provide information on what specific interventions may be the most helpful for a given illness at a particular point in time, nor do they specify the mechanisms that lead to change.

DISEASE MANAGEMENT

From the preceding text it should be evident that, although there are many treatment options that have been tried and studied for TRD, none is consistently effective in bringing about sustained remission or even response. One reason for the continued search for the optimal treatment of TRD is the current biomedical etiologic and treatment model. This model emphasizes the cure and eradication of disease, an active medical role for the physician, and an acquiescent passive role for the patient. Depression is a heterogeneous disorder including major and minor variations, acute, chronic and recurrent forms, as well as forms with melancholic, atypical, and psychotic features. In addition, there may be "good responsive" and "poorly responsive" variants of depression. Long-term follow-up studies indicate that 15% to 30% of patients with major depressive disorder have a favorable response to standard therapy, with remission of depressive symptoms and maintenance of a euthymic state. At the other extreme, 10% to 30% of patients experience a chronic course characterized by continuous symptoms and functional impairment despite treatment. The remaining patients have an intermittent course characterized by remissions, subthreshold symptoms, recurrences, and relapses.[30] Patients with "good responsive" forms of depression are likely to do well with a wide range of treatments. Patients with "poorly responsive" forms of depression are very unlikely to achieve remission with any currently available treatment. Providing more and insufficiently tested treatments is likely to make these patients worse due to the burden of the treatments and an increasing sense of helplessness and demoralization in the face of repeated treatment failures. The challenge to the field at this time is to develop ways of distinguishing, a priori, which of these forms of depression a particular patient is suffering from at a given time. The only way to determine this, currently, is through a sequence of treatment trials. Nonresponse to at least two adequate treatment trials with persistent residual symptoms may be the best currently available marker for "poorly responsive" types of depression or TRD. For patients who are diagnosed with TRD, an emphasis on learning to live with ongoing symptoms is likely to be more helpful than continued ineffective attempts to eradicate symptoms.

TRD should be thought of and managed as a chronic disease similar to other chronic conditions such as diabetes, arthritis, asthma, and chronic pain.[30,90] Chronic disease management models have been used successfully in the treatment of a number of chronic medical conditions and have been adapted to the management of depression.[91]

A systematic review of 102 studies of disease management programs for 11 chronic conditions including depression, diabetes, rheumatoid arthritis, back pain, chronic obstructive pulmonary disease, hypertension, and hyperlipidemia showed disease management improved patient satisfaction, patient adherence, and disease control.[92] A systematic review and meta-analysis of 10 randomized controlled trials of disease management programs for depression as compared with usual primary care found that patient satisfaction and adherence to treatment improved significantly with disease management.[93] Another meta-analysis of 37 randomized studies including 12,355 patients with depression receiving collaborative care in a primary care setting showed that depression outcomes were improved at 6 months and there was evidence of longer term benefits for up to 5 years in comparison to patients receiving standard care.[94] A further systematic review of 28 randomized controlled trials of primary care patients receiving multicomponent interventions found strong evidence supporting the short-term benefits of care management for depression.[95] Collaborative care is a process that encourages the coordination and integration of care between mental health and medical/nursing providers and focuses on the whole person and the whole family. Disease management refers to the attitudes and skills that patients and family members can learn to cope more effectively with a chronic illness.

Most of these studies focused on depressed patients in primary care settings and did not include the most difficult to treat patients. One open-label trial tested a short-term adjunctive disease management program for depression for patients who received or were currently receiving, but failed or responded poorly to several trials of adequate antidepressant medications and continued to experience at least moderate levels of depression. The intervention helped patients to set realistic expectations of outcome; focus on well-being in spite of the illness; learn to become aware of the importance of compliance; learn to maintain, change, or create meaningful behaviors and roles; deal with the emotional sequelae of having a chronic condition; and focus less on depressive symptoms and more on functioning and quality of life. Family members were included in the intervention. By the end of the 16 weeks there was significant improvement in quality of life and psychosocial and family functioning. Levels of depression improved but continued to persist at a moderate level, suggesting that patients could perceive improvement in their lives even as their depression persisted.[96]

Components of Disease Management

The elements that are common to most disease management approaches include education, practice guidelines and coordination of care, patient support, outcome measures, and self-management. A core feature of a disease management approach is to help patients to accept the reality of their condition and to focus less on symptoms and more on functioning and quality of life. Therapists are concerned that telling patients about their likely prognosis will cause their depression to worsen. However, by the time most patients have failed a number of treatment trials, they are aware that their illness is not likely to readily remit. They often feel responsible for continuing to feel depressed, and believe that they must not be doing the right things, or that their therapists are not competent enough. Acknowledgment and validation that they are dealing with a difficult form of depressive illness may be perceived as reassuring and may also provide a new way for them to manage their illness. Acceptance of the reality of a chronic illness does not mean the abandonment of hope for improvement. A disease management program also provides reassurance and a framework for therapists allowing them to continue to feel optimistic about treatment without resorting to poorly tested treatment options.

Patients and family members need to be educated about the signs and symptoms of depression and available treatments. They need to understand the course and outcome of depression and its likelihood of relapsing along with prodromal and residual symptoms. Therapists also need to be educated about the available evidence for the effectiveness of different treatments. They should be trained to tolerate their patients' distress while helping them to develop the coping skills necessary to manage their illness.

Evidence-based practice guidelines should be followed for the diagnosis and treatment of the depression. It is important to make sure that patients are receiving an adequate dose and duration of the primary therapeutic agent. It is also important to coordinate care when multiple caretakers are involved. Patients often have a psychopharmacologist, a psychotherapist, and perhaps a family therapist. There is often very little communication between these providers because of time constraints and because time to coordinate care is not reimbursable. An interdisciplinary discussion of case formulation and treatment options can be very useful. A variety of mental health professionals including psychotherapists, social workers, and clinical nurse specialists can all be important providers of disease management programs.

Patients need support to persist in acquiring and maintaining coping skills to deal with their illness. This support can be provided in person, via telephone, or through online computer connections. Such contact can also remind patients to take their medications, keep their appointments, and follow through with action plans. Self-help groups such as the National Alliance on Mental Illness (NAMI) or the Depression and Bipolar Support Alliance (DBSA) can also serve an important role in helping patients accept and deal with their illness.

Outcome measures should be used to monitor change over time. These measures can be obtained at follow-up visits or through telephone or computer contacts.[97]

Outcome measures should focus not only on symptoms of depression but also on quality of life, family and social functioning, general functioning, and compliance with treatment.[98–100]

Self-management skills are central to disease management programs.[97] These skills provide some degree of control to patients in managing their illness. They also provide concrete achievable goals. Patients should be taught the importance of a healthy diet and weight control. A healthy diet can contribute to a general sense of well-being. Physical activity and exercise are particularly helpful in managing depression by improving mood and cardiovascular tone and possibly increasing neurogenesis in various brain regions.[101,102] Sleep hygiene is another important area about which patients can learn. Sleep problems are common in TRD and continuous use of hypnotic agents may exacerbate insomnia. Relaxation training and mindfulness techniques can also help patients feel more in control and focus less on their depression. Spiritual counseling to help patients find meaning in their lives may also be very important for some patients with TRD. Psychotherapy can help patients learn self-management skills such as tolerating feelings, improving relationships, and finding meaning.

SUMMARY

Given the limitations of evidence for treatment options that are consistently effective for TRD and the possibility that TRD is in fact a form of depression that has a low probability of resolving, how can clinicians help patients with TRD? Perhaps the most important conceptual shift that needs to take place before treatment can be helpful is to accept TRD as a chronic illness, an illness similar to many others, one that can be effectively managed but that is not, at our present level of knowledge, likely to be cured. An undue focus on remission or even a 50% diminution of symptoms sets unrealistic goals for both patients and therapists and may lead to overtreatment and demoralization. The focus should be less on eliminating depressive symptoms and more on making sense of and learning to function better in spite of them. It is important to acknowledge the difficult nature of the depressive illness, to remove blame from the patient and clinician for not achieving remission, to set realistic expectations, and to help promote better psychosocial functioning even in the face of persisting symptoms. The critical element when implementing such an approach is a judicious balance between maintaining hope for improvement without setting unrealistic expectations. It is important to reemphasize that following a disease management model with acceptance of the reality of a chronic illness is not nihilistic and does not mean the abandonment of hope for improvement.

The first step in treating a patient with TRD is to perform a comprehensive assessment of the patient's past and current treatment history to ensure that evidence-based treatment trials have in fact been undertaken, and if not, such treatment trials should be implemented. If the patient continues to have significant residual symptoms, it is important to determine the impact is of these symptoms on the patient's quality of life and ability to function. It is also important to evaluate the factors that may be contributing to the persistence of depressive symptoms such as comorbid personality disorders, somatic disorders, substance abuse, and work and interpersonal conflicts. The treatment of patients with TRD needs to move beyond attempts to modify symptoms without taking into consideration and attempting to modify the patient's personality, coping skills, and social system.

Further somatic treatment trials can be undertaken, if desired by the patient and therapist, as a small (5%–15%) percentage of patients may respond and further treatment trials, and this may engender hope. The risk with this approach is that patients and therapists may not work at disease management skills if they believe there may be a resolution of the depression if they could just find the right medication or intervention. Therapists may also feel pressured by patients, families, insurance companies, as well as their own sense of helplessness to escalate treatment in a more and more aggressive manner in an attempt to achieve an elusive remission.

A disease management program can provide the therapist and patient with sufficient structure, skills, and goals to encourage ongoing treatment without resorting to unproven measures that may create more side effects and problems. It is particularly important to include the patient's significant others in the reformulation of the patient's problem and thereby learn how to manage the illness more effectively. Significant others and family members can be invaluable in providing support for dealing with the difficult process of acquiring a new skill set. Indeed, they spend significantly more time with the patient than does any therapist. Family members are likely to provide this kind of support only if they have been part of the assessment and treatment process.

Patients with a wide range of chronic medical illnesses can and do learn to function effectively and to achieve a satisfying quality of life in spite of their illness. There is no reason to think that patients with TRD should not be able to achieve a similar level of illness management, functioning, and quality of life.

REFERENCES

1. Rush AJ, Thase M, Dube S. Research issues in study of difficult-to-treat depression. Biol Psychiatry 2003;53:743–53.
2. Sackeim HA. The definition and meaning of treatment resistant depression. J Clin Psychiatry 2001;62(16):10–7.
3. Crown WH, Finkelstein S, Berndt ER, et al. The impact of treatment-resistant depression on health care utilization and costs. J Clin Psychiatry 2002;63(11): 963–71.
4. Berlim MT, Turecki G. What is the meaning of treatment resistant/refractory major depression (TRD)? A systematic review of current randomized trials. Eur Neuropsychopharmacol 2007;17(11):696–707.
5. Thase M, Rush AJ. What at first you don't succeed: sequential strategies for antidepressant nonresponders. J Clin Psychiatry 1997;58(Suppl 13):23–9.
6. Souery D, Amsterdam J, de Montigny C, et al. Treatment resistant depression: methodological overview and operational criteria. Eur Neuropsychopharmacol 1999; 9(1–2):83–91.
7. Fava M. Diagnosis and definition of treatment-resistant depression. Biol Psychiatry 2003;53:649–59.
8. Fekadu A, Wooderson S, Donaldson C, et al. A multidimensional tool to quantify treatment resistance in depression: the Maudsley staging method. J Clin Psychiatry 2009;70(2):177–84.
9. Berlim MT, Turecki G. Definition, assessment, and staging of treatment-resistant refractory major depression: a review of current concepts and methods. Can J Psychiatry 2007;52(1):46–54.
10. Lopez AD, Mathers CD, Ezzari M, et al. Global and regional burden of disease risk factors: systematic analysis of population health data. Lancet 2001;367:1747–57.
11. Greden JF, Riba MB, McInnis MG. Treatment resistant depression: a roadmap for effective care. Washington, DC: American Psychiatric Publishing, 2011.
12. Greden JF. The burden of disease for treatment-resistant depression. J Clin Psychiatry 2001;62(Suppl 16):26–31.

13. Dunner DL, Rush AJ, Russell JM, et al. Prospective, long-term, multicenter study of the naturalistic outcomes of patients with treatment-resistant depression. J Clin Psychiatry 2006;67(5):688–95.

14. Fekadu A, Wooderson SC, Markopoulo K, et al. What happens to patients with treatment-resistant depression? A systematic review of medium to long term outcome studies. J Affect Disord 2009;116(1–2):4–11.

15. Gaynes BN, Warden D, Trivedi MH, et al. What did STAR*D teach us? Results from a large-scale, practical, clinical trial for patients with depression. Psychiatr Serv 2009;60(11):1439–45.

16. Wooderson SC, Juruena MF, Fekadu A, et al. Prospective evaluation of specialist inpatient treatment for refractory affective disorders. J Affect Disord 2011;131(1–3): 92–103.

17. Fava GA, Offidani E. The mechanisms of tolerance in antidepressant action. Prog Neuropsychopharmacol Biol Psychiatry 2011;35(7):1593–602.

18. Whitaker R. Anatomy of an epidemic. New York: Crown, 2010.

19. Andrews PW, Kornstein SG, Halberstadt LJ, et al. Blue again: perturbational effects of antidepressants suggest monoaminergic homeostasis in major depression. Front Psychol 2011;2(Article 159):1–24.

20. Young AM, Goudie AJ. Adapative processes regulating tolerance to behavioral effects of drugs. In: Bloom FE, Kupfer DJ, editors. Psychopharmacology. New York: Raven Press, 1995;733–42.

21. Hyman SE, Nestler EJ. Initiation and adaptation: a paradigm for understanding psychotropic drug action. Am J Psychiatry 1996;153(2):151–62.

22. Souery D, Oswald P, Massat I, et al. Clinical factors associated with treatment resistance in major depressive disorder: results from a European multicenter study. J Clin Psychiatry 2007;68(7):1062–70.

23. Gorwood P, Rouillon F, Even C, et al. Treatment response in major depression: effects of personality dysfunction and prior depression. Br J Psychiatry 2010;196(2): 139–42.

24. Holzel L, Harter M, Reese C, et al. Risk factors for chronic depression—a systematic review. J Affect Disord 2011;129(1–3):1–13.

25. Rush AJ, Trivedi MH, Wisniewski SR, et al. Acute and longer-term outcomes in depressed outpatients requiring one or several treatment steps: a STAR*D report. Am J Pscyhiatry 2006;163(11):1905–17.

26. Kennedy N, Paykel ES. Residual symptoms at remission from depression: impact on long-term outcome. J Affect Disord 2004;80(2–3):135–44.

27. Stahl SM. Why settle for silver, when you can go for gold? Response vs. recovery as the goal of antidepressant therapy. J Clin Psychiatry 1999;60(4):213–4.

28. Ferrier IN. Treatment of major depression: is improvement enough? J Clin Psychiatry 1999;60(Suppl 6):10–4.

29. McIntyre RS, O'Donovan C. The human cost of not achieving full remission in depression. Can J Psychiatry 2004;49(3 Suppl 1):10S–16S.

30. Keitner GI, Ryan CE, Solomon DA. Realistic expectations and a disease management model for depressed patients with persistent symptoms. J Clin Psychiatry 2006;67:1412–21.

31. Fava GA. Can long-term treatment with antidepressant drugs worsen the course of depression? J Clin Psychiatry 2003;64(2):123–33.

32. Joyce PR, Mulder RT, Cloninger CR. Temperament predicts clomipramine and desipramine response in major depression. J Affect Disord 1994;30(1):35–46.

33. Joyce PR, Paykel ES. Predictors of drug response in depression. Arch Gen Psychiatry 1989;46(1):89–99.

34. Scott J, Williams JM, Brittlebank A, et al. The relationship between premorbid neuroticism, cognitive dysfunction and persistence of depression: a 1-year follow-up. J Affect Disord 1995;33(3):167–72.

35. Steunenberg B, Beekman ATF, Deeg DJH, et al. Personality predicts recurrence of late-life depression. J Affect Disord 2010;123:164–72.

36. Reynaert C, Janne P, Vause M, et al. Clinical trials of antidepressants: the hidden face: where locus of control appears to play a key role in depression outcome. Psychopharmacology [Berl] 1995;119(4):449–54.

37. Sullivan MD, Katon WJ, Russo JE, et al. Patient beliefs predict response to paroxetine among primary care patients with dysthymia and minor depression. J Am Board Fam Pract 2003;16(1):22–31.

38. Sirey JA, Bruce ML, Alexopoulos GS, et al. Stigma as a barrier to recovery: Perceived stigma and patient-rated severity of illness as predictors of antidepressant drug adherence. Psychiatr Serv 2001;52(12):1615–20.

39. Mintz DL, Belnap BA. What is psychodynamic psychopharmacology? An approach to pharmacological treatment resistance. In: Plakun EM, editor. Treatment resistance and patient authority: an Austen Riggs reader. New York: Norton, 2011. p. 42–65.

40. Bagby RM, Ryder AG, Cristi C. Psychosocial and clinical predictors of response to pharmacotherapy for depression. J Psychiatry Neurosci 2002;27(4):250–7.

41. Ezquiaga E, Garcia A, Bravo F, et al. Factors associated with outcome in major depression: a 6-month prospective study. Soc Psychiatry Psychiatr Epidemiol 1998;33(11):552–7.

42. Keitner GI, Heru AM, Glick ID. Clinical manual of couples and family therapy. Washington, DC: American Psychiatric Publishing; 2010.

43. Shelton RC, Osuntokun O, Heinloth AN, et al. Therapeutic options for treatment-resistant depression. CNS Drugs 2010;24(2):131–61.

44. Lam RW, Kennedy SH, Grigoriadis S, et al. Canadian Network for Mood and Anxiety Treatments (CANMAT) clinical guidelines for the management of major depressive disorder in adults. III. Pharmacotherapy. J Affect Disord 2009;117(Suppl 1):S26–43.

45. Thakur M, Grossman I, McCrory DC, et al. Review of evidence for genetic testing for CYP450 polymorphisms in management of patients with nonpsychotic depression with selective serotonin reuptake inhibitors. Genet Med 2007;9(12):826–35.

46. Souery D, Serretti A, Calati R, et al. Switching antidepressant class does not improve response or remission in treatment-resistant depression. J Clin Psychopharmacol 2011;31(4):512–6.

47. Crossley NA, Bauer M. Acceleration and augmentation of antidepressants with lithium for depressive disorders: two meta-analyses of randomized, placebo-controlled trials. J Clin Psychiatry 2007;68(6):935–40.

48. Nierenberg A, Fava M, Trivedi MH, et al. A comparison of lithium and T3 augmentation following two failed medication treatments for depression: a STAR*D Report. Am J Psychiatry 2006;163:1519–30.

49. Guzzetta F, Tondo L, Centorrino F, et al. Lithium treatment reduces suicide risk in recurrent major depressive disorder. J Clin Psychiatry 2007;68(3):380–3.

50. Nelson JC, Papakostas GI. Atypical antipsychotic augmentation in major depressive disorder: a meta-analysis of placebo-controlled randomized trials. Am J Psychiatry 2009;166(9):980–91.

51. Cooper-Kazaz R, Lerer B. Efficacy and safety of triiodothyronine supplementation in patients with major depressive disorder treated with specific serotonin reuptake inhibitors. Int J Neuropsychopharmacol 2008;11(5):685–99.

52. Folkerts HW, Michael N, Tolle R, et al. Electroconvulsive therapy vs. paroxetine in treatment-resistant depression—a randomized study. Acta Psychiatr Scand 1997; 96(5):334–42.

53. Devanand DP, Sackeim HA, Prudic J. Electroconvulsive therapy in the treatment-resistant patient. Psychiatr Clin North Am 1991;14(4):905–23.

54. Eschweiler GW, Vonthein R, Bode R, et al. Clinical efficacy and cognitive side effects of bifrontal versus right unilateral electroconvulsive therapy (ECT): a short-term randomised controlled trial in pharmaco-resistant major depression. J Affect Disord 2007;101(1–3):149–57.

55. Rush AJ, Marangell LB, Sackeim HA, et al. Vagus nerve stimulation for treatment-resistant depression: a randomized, controlled acute phase trial. Biol Psychiatry 2005;58(5):347–54.

56. Rush AJ, Sackeim HA, Marangell LB, et al. Effects of 12 months of vagus nerve stimulation in treatment-resistant depression: a naturalistic study. Biol Psychiatry 2005;58(5):355–63.

57. Kennedy SH, Giacobbe P. Treatment resistant depression—advances in somatic therapies. Ann Clin Psychiatry 2007;19(4):279–87.

58. Taylor SF, Goldman M, Maixner DF, et al. Device-related neuromodulation in treatment resistant depression. In: Greden JF, Riba MB, McInnis MG, editors. Treatment resistant depression: a roadmap for effective care. Washington, DC: American Psychiatric Publishing; 2011. p. 213–35.

59. Shuchman M. Approving the vagus-nerve stimulator for depression. N Engl J Med 2007;356(16):1604–7.

60. Sackeim HA, Rush AJ, George MS, et al. Vagus nerve stimulation (VNS) for treatment-resistant depression: efficacy, side effects, and predictors of outcome. Neuropsychopharmacology 2001;25(5):713–28.

61. George MS, Rush AJ, Marangell LB, et al. A one-year comparison of vagus nerve stimulation with treatment as usual for treatment-resistant depression. Biol Psychiatry 2005;58(5):364–73.

62. Grunhaus L, Schreiber S, Dolberg OT, et al. A randomized controlled comparison of electroconvulsive therapy and repetitive transcranial magnetic stimulation in severe and resistant nonpsychotic major depression. Biol Psychiatry 2003;53(4):324–31.

63. Avery DH, Holtzheimer PE 3rd, Fawaz W, et al. A controlled study of repetitive transcranial magnetic stimulation in medication-resistant major depression. Biol Psychiatry 2006;59(2):187–94.

64. Rossini D, Lucca A, Zanardi R, et al. Transcranial magnetic stimulation in treatment-resistant depressed patients: a double-blind, placebo-controlled trial. Psychiatry Res 2005;137(1–2):1–10.

65. Loo C, Mitchell P, Sachdev P, et al. Double-blind controlled investigation of transcranial magnetic stimulation for the treatment of resistant major depression. Am J Psychiatry 1999;156(6):946–8.

66. Boutros NN, Gueorguieva R, Hoffman RE, et al. Lack of a therapeutic effect of a 2-week sub-threshold transcranial magnetic stimulation course for treatment-resistant depression. Psychiatry Res 2002;113(3):245–54.

67. Poulet E, Brunelin J, Boeuve C, et al. Repetitive transcranial magnetic stimulation does not potentiate antidepressant treatment. Eur Psychiatry 2004;19(6):382–3.

68. Holtzheimer PE, Avery D, Schlaepfer TE. Antidepressant effects of repetitive transcranial magnetic stimulation. Br J Psychiatry 2004;184:541–2.

69. Fitzgerald PB, Benitez J, de Castella A, et al. A randomized, controlled trial of sequential bilateral repetitive transcranial magnetic stimulation for treatment-resistant depression. Am J Psychiatry 2006;163(1):88–94.

70. Wassermann EM. Risk and safety of repetitive transcranial magnetic stimulation: report and suggested guidelines from the International Workshop on the Safety of Repetitive Transcranial Magnetic Stimulation, June 5–7, 1996. Electroencephalogr Clin Neurophysiol 1998;108(1):1–16.

71. Sachdev PS, Sachdev J. Long-term outcome of neurosurgery for the treatment of resistant depression. J Neuropsychiatry Clin Neurosci 2005;17(4):478–85.

72. Mayberg HS, Lozano AM, Voon V, et al. Deep brain stimulation for treatment-resistant depression. Neuron 2005;45(5):651–60.

73. Trivedi RB, Nieuwsma JA, Williams JW Jr. Examination of the utility of psychotherapy for patients with treatment resistant depression: a systematic review. J Gen Intern Med 2010;26(6):643–50.

74. Thase ME, Friedman ES, Biggs MM, et al. Cognitive therapy versus medication in augmentation and switch strategies as second-step treatments: a STAR*D report. Am J Psychiatry 2007;164(5):739–52.

75. Scott J, Teasdale JD, Paykel ES, et al. Effects of cognitive therapy on psychological symptoms and social functioning in residual depression. Br J Psychiatry 2000;177: 440–6.

76. Harley R, Sprich S, Safren S, et al. Adaptation of dialectical behavior therapy skills training group for treatment-resistant depression. J Nerv Ment Dis 2008;196(2): 136–43.

77. Kennedy SH, Segal ZV, Cohen NL, et al. Lithium carbonate versus cognitive therapy as sequential combination treatment strategies in partial responders to antidepressant medication: an exploratory trial. J Clin Psychiatry 2003;64(4):439–44.

78. Blackburn IM, Moore RG. Controlled acute and follow-up trial of cognitive therapy and pharmacotherapy in out-patients with recurrent depression. Br J Psychiatry 1997;171:328–34.

79. Wiles NJ, Hollinghurst S, Mason V. A randomized controlled trial of cognitive behavioural therapy as an adjunct to pharmacotherapy in primary care based patients with treatment resistant depression: a pilot study. Behav Cogn Psychotherapy 2008;36:21–33.

80. Keitner GI, Miller IW, Epstein NB, et al. Family functioning and the course of major depression. Compr Psychiatry 1987;28(1):54–64.

81. Keitner GI, Miller IW. Family functioning and major depression: an overview. Am J Psychiatry 1990;147 (9):1128–37.

82. Keitner GI, Ryan CE, Miller IW, et al. Role of the family in recovery and major depression. Am J Psychiatry 1995;152 (7):1002–8.

83. Clarkin JF, Glick ID, Haas GL, et al. A randomized clinical trial of inpatient family intervention. J Affect Dis 1990;18:17–28.

84. Jacobson NS, Dobson K, Fruzzetti AE, et al. Martial therapy as a treatment for depression. J Consult Clin Psychol 1991;59(4):547–57.

85. Beach S, O'Leary D. The treatment of depression occurring in the context of marital discord. Behav Ther 1986;17:43–9.

86. Leff J, Vearnals S, Wolff G, et al. The London Depression Intervention Trial. Randomized controlled trial of antidepressants v. couple therapy in the treatment and maintenance of people with depression living with a partner: clinical outcome and costs. Br J Psychiatry 2000;177:95–100.

87. Keitner GI, Archambault R, Ryan CE, et al. Family therapy and chronic depression. J Clin Pract 2003;59(8):873–84.

88. Miller IW, Keitner GI, Ryan CE, et al. Treatment matching in the post hospital care of depressed patients. Am J Psychiatry 2005;162:2131–8.

89. Hartmann M, Bazner E, Wild B, et al. Effects of interventions involving the family in the treatment of adult patients with chronic physical diseases: a meta-analysis. Psychother Psychosom 2010;79(3):136–48.

90. Andrews G. Should depression be managed as a chronic disease? BMJ 2001; 322(7283):419–21.

91. Katon W, Guico-Pabia C. Improving quality of depression care using organized systems of care: a review of the literature. Prim Care Comp CNS Disord 2011;13(1): pii: PCC 10x0109blu.

92. Ofman JJ, Badamgarav E, Henning JM, et al. Does disease management improve clinical and economic outcomes in patients with chronic diseases? A systematic review. Am J Med 2004;117(3):182–92.

93. Neumeyer-Gromen A, Lampert T, Stark K, et al. Disease management programs for depression: a systematic review and meta-analysis of randomized controlled trials. Med Care 2004;42(12):1211–21.

94. Gilbody S, Bower P, Fletcher J, et al. Collaborative care for depression: a cumulative meta-analysis and review of longer-term outcomes. Arch Intern Med 2006;166(21): 2314–21.

95. Williams JW Jr, Gerrity M, Holsinger T, et al. Systematic review of multifaceted interventions to improve depression care. Gen Hosp Psych 2007;29:91–116.

96. Ryan CE, Keitner GI, Bishop S. An adjunctive management of depression program for difficult-to-treat depressed patients and their families. Depress Anxiety 2009; 27(1):27–34.

97. Yeung A, Feldman G, Fava M. Self-management of depression: a manual for mental health and primary care professionals. New York: Cambridge University Press, 2010.

98. Lam RW, Fiteau M, Milev R. Clinical effectiveness: the importance of psychosocial functioning outcomes. J Affect Disord 2011;132:S9–S13.

99. Patten S, Grigoriadis S, Beaulieu S. Clinical effectiveness, construct and assessment. J Affect Disord 2011;132:S3–S8.

100. Zimmerman M, Galione JN, Attiullah N, et al. Depressed patients' perspectives of 2 measures of outcome: the Quick Inventory of Depressive Symptomatology (QIDS) and the Remission from Depression Questionnaire (RDQ). Ann Clin Psychiatry 2011;23(3):208–12.

101. Harris A, Cronkite R, Moos R. Physical activity, exercise coping, and depression in a 10-year cohort study of depressed patients. J Affect Disord 2006;93:79–85.

102. Trivedi MH, Greer TL, Church TS, et al. Exercise as an augmentation treatment for nonremitted major depressive disorder: a randomized, parallel dose comparison. J Clin Psychiatry 2011;72(5):677–84.

Index

Note: Page numbers of article titles are in **boldface** type.

Psychiatr Clin N Am 35 (2012) 267–277
doi:10.1016/S0193-953X(12)00012-3
0193-953X/12/$ – see front matter © 2012 Elsevier Inc. All rights reserved.

psych.theclinics.com

Printed and bound by CPI Group (UK) Ltd, Croydon, CR0 4YY

22/10/2024

01777341-0001